Essential Epidemi
An Introduction for Students and Health Profess
Second Edition

Penny Webb, MA (Cambridge), DPhil (Oxford), is a Senior Research Fellow at the Queensland Institute of Medical Research and Associate Professor in the School of Population Health, University of Queensland. She has worked as a visiting scientist at the International Agency for Research on Cancer, France, and Harvard University, USA and has published more than 120 original research papers in the field of cancer epidemiology.

Chris Bain, MB BS (UQ), MPH, MSc (Harvard) is Reader in Epidemiology in the School of Population Health, University of Queensland. He has been teaching epidemiology to public health and medical students for over 3 decades and has co-authored a book on how to conduct a systematic review as well as more than 100 original epidemiology research papers. He has worked at Harvard in the USA and as a visiting researcher at the London School of Hygiene and Tropical Medicine and at the Universities of Cambridge, Oxford and Bristol in the UK.

Essential Epidemiology

An Introduction for Students and Health Professionals

Second Edition

Penny Webb

Senior Research Fellow and Head,
Gynaecological Cancers Group,
Queensland Institute of Medical Research,
Brisbane, Australia

and

Chris Bain

Reader in Epidemiology,
School of Population Health,
University of Queensland,
Brisbane, Australia

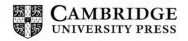

CAMBRIDGE
UNIVERSITY PRESS

CAMBRIDGE
UNIVERSITY PRESS

University Printing House, Cambridge CB2 8BS, United Kingdom

Published in the United States of America by Cambridge University Press, New York

Cambridge University Press is part of the University of Cambridge.

It furthers the University's mission by disseminating knowledge in the pursuit of education, learning and research at the highest international levels of excellence.

www.cambridge.org
Information on this title: www.cambridge.org/9780521177313

First published 2011
3rd printing 2013

Printed in Spain by Grafos S.A. Arta Sobre Papel, Barcelona

A catalogue record for this publication is available from the British Library

Library of Congress Cataloguing in Publication data
Webb, Penny, 1963–
Essential epidemiology : an introduction for students and health professionals /
Penny Webb and Chris Bain. – 2nd ed.
     p. ; cm.
Includes bibliographical references and index.
ISBN 978-0-521-17731-3 (pbk.)
1. Epidemiology.   I. Bain, Chris, 1947–   II. Title.
[DNLM: 1. Epidemiologic Methods.   2. Epidemiology.   WA 105]
RA651.W385   2011
614.4 – dc22   2010040293

ISBN 978-0-521-17731-3 Paperback

Additional resources for this publication at www.cambridge.org/webb

---

Every effort has been made in preparing this book to provide accurate and up-to-date information which is in accord with accepted standards and practice at the time of publication. Although case histories are drawn from actual cases, every effort has been made to disguise the identities of the individuals involved. Nevertheless, the authors, editors and publishers can make no warranties that the information contained herein is totally free from error, not least because clinical standards are constantly changing through research and regulation. The authors, editors and publishers therefore disclaim all liability for direct or consequential damages resulting from the use of material contained in this book. Readers are strongly advised to pay careful attention to information provided by the manufacturer of any drugs or equipment that they plan to use.

Contents

Foreword

As a core discipline of public health, epidemiology provides a perspective and methodological approach relevant to all settings requiring rigorous evidence for health and wellbeing. Excellent introductory texts such as this are therefore invaluable to a range of audiences, including students and teachers, practitioners and researchers. The text leads the reader through the history, perspective, concepts and methods of epidemiology and some key public health applications, in a steady, clear fashion. It is nicely paced with worked examples, illustrative questions and tables and frequent practical asides. The style is easy, accessible and not at all dry, which will be particularly valuable for those whose first language is not English. Underlying this approachability, however, is a strong methodological rigour, reflecting the wide international research experience of the authors that informs their writing and teaching.

The second edition of this highly successful book is fully updated and includes expanded sections dealing with new terminology, current themes such as genetic epidemiology, life expectancy and global burden, and the importance of systematic reviews as a key public health tool for assessing causality and setting policy. It will be an excellent reader or background text for undergraduate and graduate students in epidemiology and public health.

Carol Brayne
Professor of Public Health Medicine
University of Cambridge

Preface

Preface to the first edition

This book has grown out of our collective experience of teaching introductory epidemiology both in the classroom and to distance students enrolled in public health and health studies programmes in the School of Population Health (formerly the Department of Social and Preventive Medicine), University of Queensland. It began life as a detailed set of course notes that we wrote because we could not find a single epidemiology text that covered all of the areas we felt were important in sufficient detail. As the notes were to be used primarily by distance students, we tried hard to make them accessible with lots of examples, minimal jargon and equations, and by engaging readers in 'doing' epidemiology along the way. Feedback from students and colleagues convinced us that the notes were both approachable and practical. We have built on this, and offer this text as a practical introduction to epidemiology for those who need an understanding of health data they meet in their everyday working lives, as well as for those who wish to pursue a career in epidemiology.

Acknowledgements

If we were to name everyone who had contributed in some way to this book the list would be endless. We would, however, like to acknowledge some of the great teachers (and their books) from whom we have learned most of what we know, and the books we have relied heavily on for our teaching. These include Brian MacMahon (*Epidemiology: Principles and Methods*, MacMahon and Pugh, 1970), Olli Miettinen, Charlie Hennekens (*Epidemiology in Medicine*, Hennekens and Buring, 1987), Ken Rothman (*Modern Epidemiology*, 1986), *Foundations of Epidemiology* (Lilienfeld and Lilienfeld, 1980), and *Epidemiology* (Gordis, 1996). We would also like to thank our colleagues and friends, especially the Fellows from the NHMRC Capacity Grant in Longitudinal Study Methods in the School of Population Health, University of Queensland, and the staff and students from the Cancer and Population Studies Group at the Queensland Institute of Medical

Research who willingly read drafts of the text and whose constructive feedback helped shape the final version. Particular thanks go to Adrian Sleigh (Australian National University) who authored Chapters 4 [Chapter 13 in the second edition] and 12 and also contributed to Chapter 15 [Chapter 16 in the second edition], Susan Jordan (QIMR) who helped with pulling everything together and Christine Howes (Bristol, UK) who drew all otherwise non-attributed illustrations. Finally, we would like to acknowledge the School of Population Health, University of Queensland, which provided the intellectual environment that led to this book as well as financial support to cover the costs of preparing the final draft.

Preface to the second edition

This first revision of our text reflects evolution, not revolution. We have listened to the feedback we have received from instructors and students and have tried to simplify and clarify some of the trickier bits of the original text while maintaining a very 'hands-on' approach. We have added new material to reflect contemporary epidemiological practice in public health and have re-ordered some of the existing elements to improve the flow and enhance the continuity between chapters. New and expanded topics include a look at how we measure the burden of disease, greater discussion of issues relevant to ethics and privacy, and appendices covering life tables and calculation of confidence intervals for common epidemiological measures. We have also added a glossary and developed an accompanying website with useful materials including additional test questions and answers, resources for teachers and useful links to a variety of web-based data sources and other epidemiological sites. The website can be accessed at www.cambridge.org/webb.

Our overall aims are, however, unchanged – to show the role of epidemiology across a broad range of health monitoring and research activities and to give students a good understanding of the fundamental principles common to all areas of epidemiology including the study of both infectious and chronic diseases as well as public health and clinical epidemiology. To this end, we have maintained the general structure of the original text. As previously, Chapter 1 is a general introduction that both answers the question 'what is epidemiology and what can it do?' and presents the main concepts that are the focus of the rest of the book.

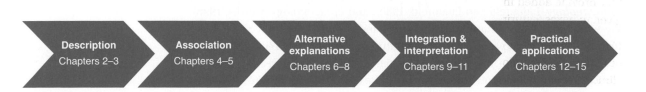

Description	Association	Alternative explanations	Integration & interpretation	Practical applications
Chapters 2–3	Chapters 4–5	Chapters 6–8	Chapters 9–11	Chapters 12–15

The first sections cover the basic principles and underlying theory of epidemiology in a very 'hands-on' way.

We start by looking at how we can measure disease and, new to this edition, the overall burden of disease in a population (Chapter 2), followed by a look at the role of descriptive epidemiology in describing health patterns (Chapter 3). We move on to look at the types of study that we use to identify potential causes of disease including an expanded discussion of the potential of record linkage (Chapter 4) and how we quantify the associations between cause and outcome (Chapter 5). In response to feedback from the first edition, we then present a separate look at the role of chance in epidemiology (Chapter 6), a simplified discussion of the thorny issue of error and bias (Chapter 7) and a practical overview of the problem of confounding (Chapter 8). This leads to the next section where we integrate this information in a practical look at how we read and interpret epidemiological reports (Chapter 9), think about assessing causality (Chapter 10) and finally synthesise a mass of information in a single review (Chapter 11). In the final section we look at some specific applications of epidemiology including the study of outbreaks (Chapter 12), surveillance (Chapter 13), prevention – including an expanded discussion of how we can assess the impact of different preventive interventions on the health of a population (Chapter 14), and screening (Chapter 15), while Chapter 16 concludes with a fresh look at what epidemiology is and what it can do to help address the health concerns facing the world today.

Symbols

Throughout the book we have used **bold** typeface to indicate terms included in the glossary and the following symbols are used to define key elements within the text.

We strongly believe that the best way to learn anything is by actually doing it and so have included questions within the text for those who like to test their understanding as they go. Because we also know how frustrating it is to have to search for answers, we have provided these immediately following the questions for those in a hurry to proceed.

We have used numerous real-life examples from all around the world to illustrate the key points and to provide additional insights in some areas. Extra examples that provide added interest and complement the main message in the text are given in boxes featuring this symbol.

Many books present clinical epidemiology as a separate discipline from public health epidemiology – a distinction that is strengthened by the fact that clinical epidemiologists have developed their own names for many standard epidemiological terms. In practice all epidemiology is based on the same under-lying principles, so we have integrated the two approaches throughout the book but have also highlighted specific examples more relevant to the clinical situa-tion. (Please note that this book does not offer a comprehensive coverage of clin-ical epidemiology; rather we aim to show the similarity of the two areas where they overlap.)

We have deliberately tried to keep the main text free of unnecessary detail and equations but have included some epidemiological 'extras'. This material is not essential to the continuity of the core text but provides some additional infor-mation for those who like to see where things have come from or want a more detailed perspective.

Acknowledgements for the second edition

We are again indebted to the many people who have provided input at all stages of the development of this book. In addition to those named previously, a few deserve a special mention. Our former colleague and co-author of the first edi-tion, Sandi Pirozzo, has moved on to a rewarding new career post-epidemiology; we remain grateful for her prior contributions and for her continuing friendship and interest. Adrian Sleigh has kindly updated the chapter on Outbreaks that he wrote for the first edition and has also contributed valuable insights to the chapter on Surveillance and the final chapter. Discernible improvements in the cohesion and internal 'sign-posting' of the book reflect excellent critiques and suggestions we received from Michael O'Brien and Kate Van Dooren, the for-mer an educator and the latter a doctoral student within the School of Popula-tion Health. Kate also provided much practical support which enabled this revi-sion. Finally, our expanded consideration of the 'Burden of Disease' approach has benefited from interactions with, and teaching materials developed by mem-bers of the Burden of Disease group at the School of Population Health, espe-cially Theo Voss, Steven Begg and Alan Lopez. Finally we thank the many users of the first edition, particularly the team from Otago University in New Zealand, who provided the critical feedback that has directly led to this new and hopefully improved edition.

Epidemiology is . . .

Box 1.1 Epidemiology is . . .

'The science of epidemics' (*Concise Oxford Dictionary*, 1964)

'The science of the occurrence of illness' (Miettinen, 1978)

'The study of the **distribution** and **determinants** of disease in humans' (MacMahon and Pugh, 1970)

'The study of the distribution and determinants of **health-related states or events** in specified populations, and the **application of this study to control of health problems**' (Porta, 2008)

So what is epidemiology anyway? As shown in Box 1.1, the *Concise Oxford Dictionary* (1964) defined it accurately, but not very helpfully, as 'the science of epidemics'. In 1970, MacMahon and Pugh came up with something a bit more concrete: 'the study of the *distribution* and *determinants* of disease'. Their definition succinctly identifies the two core strands of traditional epidemiology: *who* is developing disease (and *where* and *when*), and *why* are they developing it? The final definition, from the *Dictionary of Epidemiology* (Porta, 2008) takes it two steps further by broadening the scope to include health in general, not just disease, as well as highlighting the direct role of epidemiology in disease control.

Epidemiology, therefore, is about measuring health, identifying the causes of ill-health and intervening to improve health; but what do we mean by 'health'? Back in 1948, the World Health Organization (WHO, 1948) defined it as ' . . . a state of physical, mental and social well-being'. Now, while this view is clearly what we hope for as individuals, the inclusion of 'mental and social well-being' would until recently have induced despair in epidemiologists. In practice what we usually measure is *ill-health* or disease: more disease equals poorer physical health, and this focus is reflected in the content of most routine reports of health data and in many of the health measures that we will consider here. However, methods that do attempt to capture the more elusive components of mental and social wellbeing are now emerging. Instead of simply measuring 'life expectancy', the WHO introduced the concepts of 'health-adjusted life expectancy' (HALE) and subsequently 'disability-adjusted life years' (DALYs) to allow better international comparisons of the effectiveness of health systems. In doing so they recognised that it is not longevity per se that we seek, but a long and healthy life. We will discuss these and other measures in more detail in Chapter 2.

Perhaps epidemiology's most fundamental role is to provide a logic and structure for the analysis of health problems both great and small. It also emphasises the sound use of numbers – we have to count and we have to think. We have to think about what is worth counting and how best to count it, about what is practical and, importantly, about how well we (or others) finally measured whatever it was we set out to measure, and what it all means. Accurate measurement of health is clearly the cornerstone of the discipline, but we believe the special value of epidemiology flows from a way of thought that is open, alert to the potential for error, willing to consider alternative explanations and, finally, constructively critical and pragmatic.

We offer this book as an aid to such thought. It does not aim to turn you into a practising epidemiologist overnight but will give clear directions if that is where you decide to go. Its primary goal is to help you interpret the mass of epidemiological literature and the various types of health data that you may come across. We hope that you will see, by reading and by doing, that the fundamental

Table 1.1 Numbers of people who became ill after eating various foods at a youth camp.

Food	People who ate the food		People who didn't eat the food	
	Total	Number ill	Total	Number ill
Friday dinner:				
Hot chicken	343	156	231	74
Peas	390	175	184	55
Potato fries	422	184	152	46
Saturday lunch:				
Cold chicken	202	155	372	75
Salad	385	171	189	59
Saturday dinner:				
Fruit salad	324	146	250	84

(Adapted from Hook *et al.*, 1996, with permission from John Wiley and Sons.)

concepts and tools of epidemiology are relatively simple, although the tasks of integrating, synthesising and interpreting health information are more challenging. But before we go any further, let us do some public health epidemiology.

A case of food poisoning

Epidemiology is a bit like detective work in that we try to find out why and how disease occurs. Our first example illustrates this. After an outbreak of food poisoning at a youth camp, the local public health unit was called in to identify the cause (Hook *et al.*, 1996). They first asked everyone at the camp what they had eaten prior to the outbreak and some results of this investigation are shown in Table 1.1.

Looking at the numbers in Table 1.1, it is difficult to see which of the foods might have been responsible for the outbreak. (Note that everyone is recorded as either having eaten or not eaten each food; and that most people will have eaten more than one of the foods.) More people became ill after eating potato fries than after eating cold chicken (184 versus 155) – but then more people ate the fries (422 versus 202). How then can we best compare the two foods? One simple way to do this is to calculate the *percentage* of people who became ill among those who ate (or did not eat) each type of food. For example, 156 out of 343 people who ate hot chicken became ill and

$$156 \div 343 = 0.45 = 45\%$$

So 45% of people who ate hot chicken became sick. This is known as the **attack rate** for hot chicken, i.e. 45% of hot-chicken eaters were 'attacked' by food poisoning.

Calculate the attack rates for the other foods. Which food has the highest attack rate?

Although cold chicken has the highest attack rate (77%), not everyone who ate it (or, more precisely, who *reported* eating it) became ill and 20% or one in five people who did *not* eat cold chicken still became ill. This is to be expected; no matter what the cause of concern, it is rare that everyone who is exposed to it will show the effects (in this case, become ill). What can help here is to work out how much *more likely* people who ate a particular food were to become ill than those who did not eat it. For example, 45% of people who ate hot chicken became ill, compared with 32% of people who did not eat hot chicken. Hot-chicken eaters were therefore 1.4 times (45% ÷ 32% = 1.4) more likely to become ill than people who did not eat hot chicken. This measure gives us the risk of sickness in hot-chicken eaters *relative* to non-eaters, hence its name – **relative risk**.

Calculate the relative risk of developing food poisoning associated with each of the other food items. Which food is associated with the highest relative risk of sickness?

We can now conclude that the food item most likely to have been responsible for the outbreak was the cold chicken – people who ate this were almost four times more likely to become ill than those who did not. This is quite a strong relative risk; in comparison, eating any of the other foods was associated with no more than one and a half times the risk of disease. The relevant data, including the attack rates and relative risks, are summarised in Table 1.2, which is much more informative than the raw numbers of Table 1.1.

In identifying the cause of the outbreak you have just solved an epidemiological problem. The 'attack rates' and 'relative risks' that you used are fairly simple to calculate and are two very useful epidemiological measures. We will discuss them further in Chapters 2 and 5 and they will appear throughout the book.

Subdisciplines of epidemiology

The outbreak investigation above is an example of what might be called *public health epidemiology*, or *infectious disease epidemiology*, with the first name reflecting the broad field of application and the second the nature of both the aetiological (causal) agent and the disease. It is quite common now to specify such sub-fields of epidemiology, which range on the one hand from *nutritional* through *social* to *environmental epidemiology*, and on the other from *cancer* to

Table 1.2 Numbers of people who became ill after eating various foods at a youth camp and attack rates and relative risks for each food.

	People who ate the food			People who didn't eat the food			
Food	Total	Number ill	Attack rate	Total	Number ill	Attack rate	Relative risk[a]
Friday dinner:							
Hot chicken	343	156	45%	231	74	32%	1.4
Peas	390	175	45%	184	55	30%	1.5
Potato fries	422	184	44%	152	46	30%	1.4
Saturday lunch:							
Cold chicken	202	155	77%	372	75	20%	3.8
Salad	385	171	44%	189	59	31%	1.4
Saturday dinner:							
Fruit salad	324	146	45%	250	84	34%	1.3

[a] Note, RR are calculated using the exact percentages and not the rounded values shown.
(Adapted from Hook *et al.*, 1996, with permission from John Wiley and Sons.)

injury or *perinatal epidemiology*: the former grouping being exposure-oriented and the latter focused on the particular disease or outcome. Nonetheless, the core methods and techniques of epidemiology remain common to all subdisciplines, so the contents of this book are relevant to all. Setting sub-speciality boundaries largely reflects the explosion of knowledge in these areas, although some areas do present special challenges. For example, capturing a person's usual diet is remarkably challenging and the subsequent data analysis equally so; epidemiologists coming fresh to the field of nutritional epidemiology will need to develop experience and expertise in that specific area. As you read on you will meet examples from a wide cross-section of health research and the common threads of logic, study design and interpretation will, we trust, become apparent.

It is of some interest to know a bit more about a few of the special epidemiologies. *Occupational epidemiology* has the longest history of all, with influential early observations of diseases linked to occupations such as mining appearing in the sixteenth century, and a systematic treatise on occupational diseases was published by Ramazzini back in 1700 (Rosen, 1958). Occupational health research in general, and epidemiology in particular, continue to contribute to enhancing workplace health today. Seminal contributions in the field include identification of the pulmonary (lung) hazards of asbestos for miners and construction workers (Selikoff *et al.*, 1965) and the work practices that led to an epidemic of a rare fatal cancer in workers in the polyvinyl chloride industry (Makk *et al.*, 1974). Company records of job tasks can provide measures of past exposure among employees, allowing researchers to look back in time and link, for example, past asbestos exposure to subsequent deaths in the workforce. (This type of study is a *historical cohort design* – see Chapter 4. It is only possible when there are good records of both exposure and outcome, usually death, and for this reason has proved particularly useful in occupational studies where such records often do exist.)

Far more modern are the subdisciplines of *molecular epidemiology* and *clinical epidemiology*. The former aims to weld the population perspective of epidemiology with our rapidly increasing understanding of how variations in genes and their products affect the growth, form and function of cells and tissues. It thus has the potential for defining genetic contributions to disease risk and can also provide biological markers of some exposures (e.g. changes to DNA following exposure to tobacco smoke). In contrast, clinical epidemiology does not rely on advanced technology but differs from other branches of epidemiology in its focus on enhancing clinical decisions to benefit *individual patients*, rather than improving the health of *populations*. For this reason, clinical epidemiology is sometimes regarded as a completely separate discipline, a view which is encouraged by the fact that it has developed its own names for many standard epidemiological measures. The foundations are, however, identical to those of public health epidemiology and when appropriate we will discuss the two in parallel, highlighting any differences in language or approach along the way.

On epidemics

If we take the word 'epidemiology' itself, its origins from '*epidemic*' are clear. If we talk about an epidemic we immediately conjure up pictures of an acute outbreak of infectious disease but, both for practical and for etymological reasons, it seems reasonable to use the term to describe a notable excess of any disease over time. Many developed countries could, for example, be described as undergoing an epidemic of lung cancer over the last few decades (Figure 1.1). Notably the pattern of lung cancer over time differs for men and women; rates in men rose sharply between 1950 and 1980 but have been falling for some years now, while those in women rose later and are only just starting to fall – a consequence of the fact, that as a group, women took up smoking more recently than men. To describe this excessive occurrence of disease (or death) as an 'epidemic' captures some of the urgency the numbers demand.

The derivation of the word 'epidemiology' itself is from the Greek *epi*, upon, *demos*, the people, and *logia*, study. Literally, therefore, it means the 'study (of what is) upon the people'. Such study suggests a simple set of questions that have long lain at the heart of epidemiology.

- **What** disease/condition is present in excess?
- **Who** is ill?

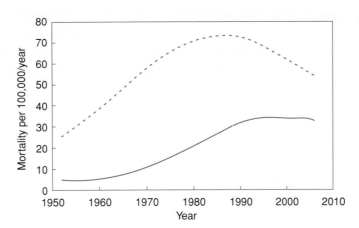

Figure 1.1 Time trends in lung cancer mortality rates (age-standardised to the 1970 US population) for white males (- - - - -) and females (———). (Drawn from: Devesa *et al.*, 1999 and CDC Wonder Database (CDC), accessed 8 January 2010.)

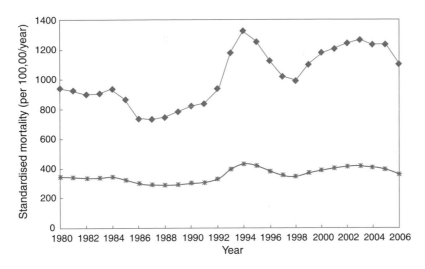

Figure 1.2 Changes in all-cause mortality at ages 0–64 years in the Russian Federation from 1980–2006 (♦, men; *, women). (Data from the European Health for All Database. WHO Regional Office for Europe, Copenhagen, Denmark, accessed via http://data.euro.who.int/ hfadb/, 30 December 2009.)

- **Where** do they live?
- **When** did they become ill?
- **Why** did they become ill?

The first question reflects the need for a sound, common definition of a disease so that like is compared with like. Epidemiology is all about comparison – without some reference to what is usual, how can we identify excess? The next three questions form the mantra of **descriptive epidemiology**: '*person, place and time*'. As Figure 1.2 shows, an 'epidemic of premature mortality' occurred in the mid-1990s among young and middle-aged men in Russia and again in the early 2000s. This description captures the essence of the problem and prompts the next question: what caused these epidemics? What changed in the circumstances of younger Russian men to reverse the pattern of falling mortality in the

Table 1.3 An historical event.

SES[a]	Adult males		Adult females		Children (both sexes)		Total population	
	Total	% Dead	Total	% Dead	Total	% Dead	Total	% Dead
High	175	67.4	144	2.8	6	–	325	37.5
Medium	168	91.7	93	14.0	24	–	285	58.6
Low	462	83.8	165	53.9	79	65.8	706	74.8
Other	885	78.3	23	13.0	0	–	908	76.7
Total	1690	80.0	425	25.6	109	47.7	2224	68.0

[a] SES, socioeconomic status.

(*Source:* http://www.anesi.com; for full details see reference list.)

early 1980s and then cause it to almost double in less than 10 years? And why did this happen again in the late 1990s? Other data show that there were no such mortality changes in Western Europe, nor among older Russian men or infants, nor (to the same extent) in Russian women. This simple graph captures a public health disaster for Russia and prompts urgent causal speculation: *why did this happen?* Solving and responding to this final question is critical for public health progress, but there is clearly no simple solution. In this case, a high proportion of the deaths were linked to excess consumption of alcohol: increases in mortality coincided with periods of economic and societal crisis, and rates fell when the economic situation improved (Zaridze *et al.*, 2009). This example highlights the central importance of paying close attention to descriptive data that provide a 'community diagnosis' or take the public health 'pulse' of a nation. Much can be gleaned from apparently simple data to give a quite precise description of the health event or state of interest, as the following exercise shows.

An historical epidemic

Table 1.3 shows some data that relate to an actual human experience. It tells you how many people there were in various age, sex and socioeconomic groups and what percentage of these people died during the 'epidemic'. The challenge is to use these data to describe the event systematically in terms of **whom** this happened to (we have no data on place or time) and then to think about the sort of event that might have induced such a pattern.

The following questions are designed to help you identify key features of the data.

1. What is distinctive about this isolated population with regard to
   • the numbers of men and women (sex distribution),
   • the numbers of adults and children (age distribution) and
   • the numbers in each socioeconomic group (socioeconomic distribution)?

2. What strikes you about the percentage of people who died (the 'death rate')? Is this different for (a) adults and children, (b) men and women, (c) high and low socioeconomic status (SES) and (d) any particular combinations of the above?

3. How many times more likely were
   • men to die than women and
   • those of low SES to die than those of high SES?

4. To what historical event might these data refer?

Table 1.3 displays more complicated data than Table 1.2, since you had to consider the joint effects of three factors (sex, socioeconomic status and age) on mortality. The sequence of questions aims to underline a general principle in describing such tables, i.e. to look at overall patterns first, then move on to more detail (see Box 1.2 on the next page). We all see things in different ways, but until you develop your own style this approach is one that can help you avoid becoming lost in the array of possible relationships. You need first to grasp the size of the *whole group* under study and how many died; then check the overall patterns (numbers and mortality rates) across each 'exposure' separately (sex, SES, age). These are sometimes called the 'marginal' rates based on row and column totals; e.g. first look at the rates for all adult males, ignoring their SES, or for all people of high SES, ignoring their age and sex. Only then consider the more complex 'inner' set of joint effects such as the influence of SES on mortality among women.

In tackling this and the previous problem you have already done some serious epidemiology: you have *described* data, *interpreted* the patterns you observed and used *epidemiological measures* to help do this. We will build on this throughout the book, but first let's step back a little and see what other lessons we can learn from the past.

The beginnings[1]

The 'great man' approach has fallen out of favour in modern historical practice; however, linking historical events to people adds character so we will focus on some of the main players in this brief overview of the development of population health and epidemiology.

---

[1] The material in this section is drawn from a mix of primary and secondary sources, with the latter including a number of texts, most helpful being those of Stolley and Lasky (1995) and Lilienfeld and Lilienfeld (1980).

Box 1.2 An historical event

Things to note about the population include
- the predominance of adult males $(1{,}690 \div 2{,}224 = 76\%)$, the much smaller proportion of adult females (19%) and the very few children;
- the substantial excess of persons of low SES (men and children in particular); and
- the total population (2,224) is quite large – a village, small town, an army barracks . . . ?

Things to note about the 'death rates' include the following.
- The overall death rate is very high – more than two-thirds died. (Note: these death rates are essentially identical in form to the attack rates in Table 1.2.)
- Overall, death rates increased with decreasing SES.
- The death rate in men (80.0%) was much higher than that in women (25.6%); the death rate in children was between these two.
- In men, the death rate was high in all socioeconomic classes, although those of high SES fared better than the rest; in women, the death rate was always less than that for males of equivalent SES, but it increased strikingly from high to medium to low SES.
- The only children to die were of low SES.

Overall, the relative risk (RR) for men versus women is	$80.0 \div 25.6 = 3.1$
The RR for low versus high SES is	$74.8 \div 37.5 = 2.0$
The RR for women of low SES versus women of high SES is	$53.9 \div 2.8 = 19.3$
The RR for men of low SES versus women of high SES is	$83.8 \div 2.8 = 29.9$

A disaster has occurred, causing a high death rate that predominantly affected men (of all social classes) and, to a lesser extent, women and children of low social class. Overall there is a modest benefit of belonging to a higher social stratum, and among women this protection was exceptionally strong (a 19-fold higher risk of dying for low versus high SES).

Such substantial differences in risk reflect powerful preventive effects and in this instance it was a mix of social custom and the physical consequences of social stratification. The event was the sinking of the Titanic, where those of higher SES (the first class passengers) were situated on the upper decks and were therefore closer to the lifeboats than those of medium and low SES (those travelling second and third class, respectively). The males gallantly helped the females and children into the lifeboats first. Those of 'other' SES were the crew.

Box 1.3 On airs, waters and places

Whoever wishes to investigate medicine properly, should proceed thus: in the first place to consider the seasons of the year, and what effects each of them produces ... Then the winds, the hot and the cold, especially such as are common to all countries, and then such as are peculiar to each locality. We must also consider the qualities of the waters ... In the same manner, when one comes into a city to which he is a stranger, he ought to consider its situation, how it lies as to the winds and the rising of the sun; for its influence is not the same whether it lies to the north or the south, to the rising or to the setting sun. These things one ought to consider most attentively, and concerning the waters which the inhabitants use, whether they be marshy and soft, or hard, and running from elevated and rocky situations, and then if saltish and unfit for cooking; and the ground, whether it be naked and deficient in water, or wooded and well watered, and whether it lies in a hollow, confined situation, or is elevated and cold; and the mode in which the inhabitants live, and what are their pursuits, whether they are fond of drinking and eating to excess, and given to indolence, or are fond of exercise and labour ...

(Extracted from Hippocrates of Cos, 400 BC.)

Good epidemiological practice and reasoning started long ago. Perhaps the first proto-epidemiologist (*proto* because he did not actually count anything) was Hippocrates of Cos (460–375 BC), who recognised that both environmental and behavioural factors could affect health (see Box 1.3).

The Dark Ages and Middle Ages (AD 500–1500) have little to say to us, other than in the development of causal reasoning, which we will set aside until later in the book (Chapter 10). The introduction of more quantitative methods into epidemiology, and, in fact, into biology and medicine in general, has been attributed to John Graunt (1620–1674), a haberdasher and early Fellow of the Royal Society in London, although his friend William Petty may well have been a seminal influence too. In 1662 Graunt published his *Natural and Political Observations Mentioned in a Following Index and Made Upon the Bills of Mortality*. He studied parish christening registers and the 'Bills of Mortality', and noted many features of birth and death data, including the higher numbers of both male births and deaths in comparison with females, the high rates of infant mortality and seasonal variations in mortality. He also provided a numerical account of the impact of the plague in London and made the first attempts to estimate the size of the population. In an attempt to define a 'law of mortality' he constructed the first life-table (Table 1.4). This summarised the health of a population in terms of the chance of an individual surviving to a particular age. Notice that at this time only

Table 1.4 An historical example of a life-table.

Exact age (years)	Deaths	Survivors	Chance of living to that age (%)
0	–	100	
6	36	64	64
16	24	40	40
26	15	25	25
36	9	16	16
46	6	10	10
56	4	6	6
66	3	3	3
76	2	1	1
86	1	0	

(Adapted from Graunt, 1662.)

three out of every hundred people reached the age of 66, and the majority of deaths occurred in early life. This technique was a forerunner of that used by life insurance companies for calculating insurance premiums today, as well as a fundamental approach to measuring a population's health. As you will see when we come back to consider life-tables in more detail in Chapter 2 (see also Appendix 5 for details of how to construct a life-table), things have improved considerably since Graunt's time, with about 85 of every 100 men and 90 of every 100 women now making it to the age of 66 in developed countries such as Australia.

During the nineteenth century, the collection and use of health statistics for what we now call 'descriptive epidemiology' continued to develop in England and also, briefly, in France. Of particular influence as a teacher was Pierre Charles-Alexandre Louis (1787–1872), who conducted some of the earliest epidemiological studies of treatment effectiveness when he demonstrated that bloodletting did not aid recovery from disease. Among his students was William Farr (1807–1883), physician, statistician and director of the Office of the Registrar General for England and Wales from 1837, its second year of operation. Farr studied levels of mortality in different occupations and institutions and in married and single persons, as well as other facets of the distribution of disease. He published these and other findings in the *Annual Reports of the Registrar General*, and the present UK system of vital statistics stems directly from his work.

John Snow (1813–1858), a physician and contemporary of Farr, was better known at the time for giving chloroform to Queen Victoria during childbirth, but is now remembered for his pioneering work in elucidating the mode of transmission of cholera (Snow, 1855). This remains a classic and exciting example of epidemiological detection and some of Snow's personal account of it is given below and again later in the chapter. His initial observations were based on a series of reports of individual cases of cholera and, in every instance, he was able to link the case to contact with another infected person (or their goods), thereby demonstrating that the disease could spread from person to person. He then surmised, contrary to popular belief at the time, that cholera could be transmitted through polluted water, a view that was strengthened by his observations linking a terrible outbreak of cholera around Broad Street, London, in 1854, to the local water pump (Box 1.4).

Box 1.4 John Snow and the Broad Street Pump (1854)

Within two hundred and fifty yards of the spot where Cambridge Street joins Broad Street, there were upwards of five hundred fatal attacks of cholera in ten days … The mortality would undoubtedly have been much greater had it not been for the flight of the population … so that in less than six days from the commencement of the outbreak, the most afflicted streets were deserted by more than three-quarters of their inhabitants.

There were a few cases of cholera in the neighbourhood of Broad Street, Golden Square, in the latter part of August; and the so-called outbreak, which commenced in the night between the 31st of August and the 1st of September, was, as in all similar instances, only a violent increase of the malady. As soon as I became acquainted with the situation and extent of this eruption of cholera, I suspected some contamination of the water of the much-frequented street-pump in Broad Street … but on examining the water … I found so little impurity in it of an organic nature, that I hesitated to come to a conclusion. Further inquiry, however, showed me that there was no other circumstance or agent common to the circumscribed locality in which this sudden increase of cholera occurred, and not extending beyond it, except the water of the above mentioned pump.

On proceeding to the spot, I found that nearly all the deaths had taken place within a short distance of the pump. There were only ten deaths in houses situated decidedly nearer to another street pump. In five of these cases the families of the deceased persons informed me that they always sent to the pump in Broad Street, as they preferred the water to that of the pump which was nearer. In three other cases, the deceased were children who went to school near the pump in Broad Street. Two of them were known to drink the water; and the parents of third think it probable that it did so. The other two deaths, beyond the district which this pump supplies, represent only the amount of mortality from cholera that was occurring before the irruption

(continued)

Box 1.4 *(continued)*

took place . . . (*Snow used a spot map to show the spread of cases in relation to this and other pumps.*) I had an interview with the Board of Guardians of St James's parish, on the evening of Thursday, 7th September, and represented the above circumstances to them. In consequence of what I said, the handle of the pump was removed on the following day.

Snow was also able to explain why some groups of people within the area did not develop cholera:

The Workhouse in Poland Street is more than three-fourths surrounded by houses in which deaths from cholera occurred, yet out of five hundred and thirty-five inmates, only five died of cholera, . . . The workhouse has a pump well on the premises, . . . and the inmates never sent to Broad Street for water. If the mortality in the workhouse had been equal to that in the streets immediately surrounding it on three sides, upwards of one hundred persons would have died. (*Note Snow's comparison of the 'observed' number of cases with the number 'expected'.*)

There is a Brewery in Broad Street, near to the pump, and on perceiving that no brewery men were registered as having died of cholera, I called on Mr Huggins, the proprietor. He informed me that there were above seventy workmen employed in the brewery, and that none of them had suffered from cholera . . . The men are allowed a certain quantity of malt liquor, and Mr Huggins believes they do not drink water at all . . .

The limited district in which this outbreak of cholera occurred, contains a great variety in the quality of the streets and houses; Poland Street and Great Pulteney Street consisting in a great measure of private houses occupied by one family, whilst Husband Street and Peter Street are occupied by the poor Irish. The remaining streets are intermediate in point of respectability. The mortality appears to have fallen pretty equally amongst all classes, in proportion to their number.

(Extracted from Snow, 1855.)

Snow went to a lot of trouble to explain why some people developed cholera when they were believed *not* to have drunk the water from the Broad Street pump. He attributed these cases to the use of water from the pump in the local public houses, dining rooms and coffee shops. He was also able to explain why some groups of people within the area did not develop cholera when they lived in the affected area. If these low-risk groups (brewery workers, workhouse dwellers) had been users of the nearby Broad Street pump, Snow's hypothesis would have been in tatters. His findings among the 'exceptions' of both sorts thus bolster his arguments considerably: for the most part he found convincing explanations

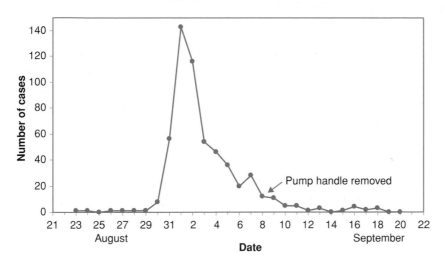

Figure 1.3 The Broad Street cholera epidemic, 1854. (Drawn from: Snow, 1855.)

for why some people apparently at risk did not fall ill, and so too for the small group not living near the pump who did contract cholera. His openness to collecting all the facts, not just those that obviously supported his contention, is a salutary reminder of what constitutes good science – and that effective public health action requires realistic information about the problem at hand.

In addition to mapping the distribution of cases by place, Snow tabulated the numbers of cases and deaths over time. His time data are displayed graphically, showing what is called an 'epidemic curve', in Figure 1.3.

When did the epidemic start? When did it end? What role did Snow's dramatic removal of the pump handle on 8 September play in interrupting its course?

The epidemic curve shows that the rise above the preceding baseline began on 30 August, with a dramatic increase over the next two days. And although the fall from the peak starts shortly thereafter, case numbers are high for quite some days later, not getting close to the preceding baseline until two weeks from the commencement. The epidemic had waned substantially before Snow's intervention on 8 September, probably largely due to the flight of much of the populace. However, since the graph shows the total *number* of cases occurring and does not take into account the size of the population, the *rate* of disease (the number of new cases occurring among the smaller number of people remaining in the area) could still have been fairly high. Snow's action may therefore truly have contributed to containment of the outbreak.

The second half of the nineteenth century saw the expansion of epidemiology in the direct service of public health in the UK, with a similar trend in the USA starting early the next century. Infectious diseases remained the core

Figure 1.4 Age-standardised death rates from lung cancer in relation to the number of cigarettes smoked per day, British Doctors Study, 1951–1961. (Reproduced from: Doll and Hill, *BMJ*, 1964;1: 1399–1410, with permission from BMJ Publishing Group Ltd.)

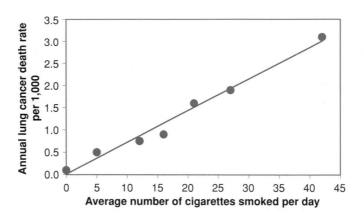

interest until the early 1900s when Joseph Goldberger, a Hungarian physician working in the US Public Health Service, showed that pellagra[2] was not infectious but of dietary origin and Wade Hampton Frost, another pioneer in the field, articulated the value of non-experimental epidemiology in discovering disease origins. Then in 1950, the publication of two case–control studies of lung cancer, by Richard Doll (epidemiologist) and Austin Bradford Hill (statistician) in the UK and Ernest Wynder (medical student) and Evart Graham (surgeon) in the USA, publicly marked the start of modern epidemiology.

Both papers (Doll and Hill, 1950; Wynder and Graham, 1950) showed that patients with lung cancer (*cases*) tended to smoke much more than people without lung cancer (*controls*). Doll and Hill then set out to confirm their findings using a different, prospective design (a *cohort study*). They wrote to a large number of British doctors to find out how much they smoked and then 'followed' them (by mail and death records) over subsequent years to see what they died from. They again showed quite clearly that those who smoked cigarettes were much more likely to die of lung cancer than those who did not smoke, and the more they smoked the higher their risk (Figure 1.4). What is now known as the 'British Doctors Study' ran for more than 50 years (Doll *et al.*, 2004). Unfortunately, in spite of this and other clear evidence of the harmful effects of smoking, it was many years before attempts to discourage people from smoking were made, and it is only recently that tobacco companies have begun to admit that their products cause disease.

Twenty years after those key case–control studies came the publication of the first comprehensive and widely influential disciplinary text: *Epidemiology: Principles and Methods* by Brian MacMahon and Thomas Pugh (1970). Highly readable and erudite, it remains a benchmark for successors.

---

[2] A disease common in poorer areas, characterised by diarrhoea, dermatitis, dementia and ultimately death.

What does epidemiology offer?

You will have discerned parts of the answer to this question from what you have already read and done in reaching this point. Here we recap and expand to bring the elements together more directly and fully, and thereby effectively map the content of the rest of the book. This section sketches the broad purposes of epidemiology and the next aims to illuminate these through some concrete examples.

A large part of public health is about identifying health problems within a community (who is becoming ill, where and when?), identifying what is causing the problems and then testing possible solutions to try to resolve or reduce the problem. Epidemiology is fundamental in providing the data needed to make public health judgements in each of these areas and the data come from studies of 'populations' (groups of people) of all sorts and sizes. Epidemiology largely deals with descriptions and comparisons of groups of people who vary widely in their genetic make-up, behaviour and environments. The great challenge for epidemiologists is to deal with such multiple influential health-modifiers in a systematic and logical way that produces information of practical value (to improving a community's health). How this challenge is met is what this book is all about.

Description of health status of populations

The observation and recording of health status makes it possible to identify sudden (and not-so-sudden) changes in the level of disease over time that might point to a need for action or further investigation. Similarly, differences between groups of people in one area, or between different geographical areas, can also give clues regarding the causes of disease (or health) in those groups. Such *descriptive statistics* are also important for health authorities and planners who need to know the nature and size of the health challenges faced by their communities.

Causation

Once a problem has been identified, we need to know what causes it, and probably the best-recognised use of epidemiology is in the search for the causes of disease. In some cases strong genetic factors have been identified, as for example with cystic fibrosis, a lung disease that occurs because of specific genetic defects. In other instances major environmental factors are crucial, such as asbestos in the development of lung mesothelioma (a rare form of lung cancer). In general, though, there is almost always some interaction between genetic and environmental factors in the causation of disease. Epidemiological tools are central to the identification of modifiable factors that will allow preventive interventions. (Note that in epidemiology and public health there remains some confusion over what is meant by *environmental factors*. We, and most others, take this to mean the sum of all non-genetic factors, including psychological, behavioural, social and cultural traits.)

Evaluation of interventions

Once we have identified a factor that causes disease, we then want to know whether we can reduce a population's exposure to this factor and so prevent the occurrence of disease – a 'primary' prevention programme (we will discuss prevention further in Chapter 14). Epidemiology has a core role to play in this process and is also key to the evaluation of different treatments for a particular disease (an aspect of both mainstream and clinical epidemiology) and assessments of the effectiveness of health services.

Natural history and prognosis

Epidemiologists are also concerned with the *natural history*, or the course and outcome, of disease, both in individuals and in groups. *Prognosis* often implies the course of disease after treatment, but the terms tend to be used rather interchangeably. Such knowledge has obvious value for discussing treatment options with individual patients, as well as for planning and evaluating interventions. Of particular interest is whether early disease is present for long before symptoms drive someone to seek medical attention. If this 'sub-clinical' disease can be detected and if, as a result, treatment is more effective, this opens the way for screening programmes that aim to improve treatment outcomes. (We will discuss screening further in Chapter 15.)

What do epidemiologists do?

How then are these objectives of epidemiological research attained? Let us look briefly at some more examples of what the practice of epidemiology can yield across some of its main dimensions.

Descriptive studies: person, place and time

By 'person'

In some countries there is concern over health differences between indigenous people and the rest of the population. Figure 1.5 shows Australian mortality data comparing Indigenous with non-Indigenous people. The bars show how many times higher mortality from circulatory, respiratory and infectious

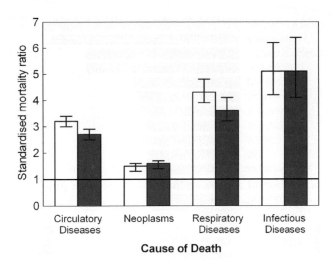

Figure 1.5 Age-standardised mortality ratios for selected diseases in the Indigenous compared to the non-Indigenous population in Australia, 2001 to 2005. (Drawn from: Pink and Allbon, 2008.) The bars indicate how much higher mortality was among Indigenous men (open bars) and women (solid bars) compared to non-Indigenous people. The vertical lines indicate 95% confidence intervals for these estimates (a measure of how certain the figures are).

diseases and cancer is in Indigenous men and women in Australia compared to non-Indigenous Australians (the horizontal line at the level '1' indicates the point where mortality rates in Indigenous and non-Indigenous people would be equal).

How many times higher is mortality from circulatory diseases in Indigenous males than in non-Indigenous males?

What is the obvious striking fact about relative mortality in Indigenous people in general?

Mortality for circulatory diseases in Indigenous men is just over three times that in non-Indigenous men and the difference for women is almost as great. The data presented indicate a much worse health situation for Indigenous Australians than for the non-Indigenous population. (Note: these **standardised mortality ratios** are similar to the relative risk in the food poisoning example earlier. They show how many times more likely it was for an Indigenous Australian to die compared with a non-Indigenous Australian in 2001–2005. The process of standardisation also takes account of the fact that Indigenous Australians are, on average, younger than non-Indigenous people. We will discuss these measures further in Chapter 2.)

By 'place'

How 'healthy' is any given country in relation to the rest of the world – are things better or worse there compared with other countries? Figure 1.6 shows cardiovascular disease mortality rates in males in different countries. You can see that men in the Netherlands, for example, are considerably better off than those in the UK, New Zealand and particularly Poland and Hungary; but things could be

Figure 1.6 Circulatory disease mortality for males, about 2001. (Drawn from: AIHW, 2008.)

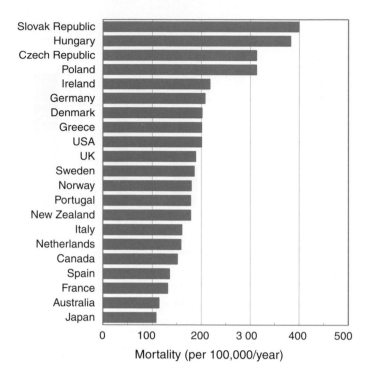

Mortality (per 100,000/year)

better – as shown by the lower rates in Spain, France, Australia and Japan. What is it about Japanese men that makes them less likely to die of cardiovascular disease than Dutch men? If we can work this out then perhaps we could reduce cardio-vascular mortality in the Netherlands to the level seen in Japan (provided that the differences are not purely genetic). By studying patterns of disease and relating them to variations in risk factors for the disease we can come up with possible reasons why some people or places have higher rates of disease than others or why disease rates have changed over time.

By 'time'

What emerges if we look at the changing patterns of mortality in a country over time? The graph in Figure 1.7 shows mortality trends for selected conditions and groups over almost three decades (1979–2006) in the USA.

What are the most notable features of Figure 1.7?

The picture we see is mixed, some good news, some concerning. The most obvious health success story is the consistent downward trend in deaths from heart attacks, with more than 100 fewer people in every 100,000 (half as many) dying from them at the end of the period. A less dramatic decline is seen for motor vehicle accidents. Deaths from AIDS rose until 1995 and have fallen since

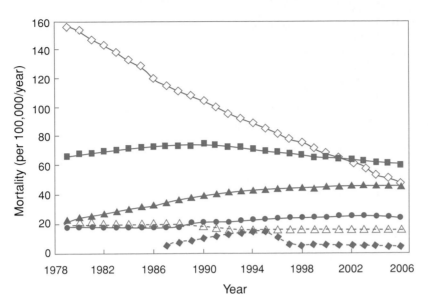

Figure 1.7 US mortality rates, 1979–2006, for heart attack (◇), lung cancer in males (■), lung cancer in females (▲), motor vehicle accidents (△), diabetes (•) and AIDS (◆). (Drawn from CDC Wonder (CDC), accessed 8 January 2010.)

(an epidemic where perhaps the worst is past, at least for the USA). The same is true for lung cancer in men, although on this scale it is not striking. Most worrying is the steady rise in lung cancer deaths among women.

However, these details don't give us the big picture. Some up, some down, some changing direction: what was happening to overall mortality in the USA during the period? Total mortality rates fell from about 1,000 to 810 per 100,000 per year, but we would not be able to fit this information onto the same graph without losing almost all the details we noted above. We could, of course, draw a separate graph showing the total death rate, but we can do both by changing the scale of the vertical axis, as in Figure 1.8.

Instead of a linear scale (1, 2, 3, 4, ...), we have now used a 'log' (logarithmic) scale (1, 10, 100, 1,000, ...) where the distance between 1 and 10 (a 10-fold difference) is the same as the distance between 10 and 100 (also a 10-fold difference) and so on. Now we can fit mortality rates as different as 4.0/100,000 (AIDS mortality in 2006) and 1,000/100,000 (all-cause mortality in 1979) on the same page. It also allows us to compare *relative* changes in mortality rates directly, with parallel slopes reflecting equal rates of change. The fall in heart attacks looks much less dramatic now: the drop is only about 2%–3% per year but, as Figure 1.7 showed, this led to a large absolute benefit, because the death rate was so high to start with. The rate of change for AIDS looks much steeper on a log scale because the percentage change is greater, but the absolute benefits are clearly much less. In public health we need to think on both relative and absolute scales: they tell us different things that are useful for different purposes. We will take this further later in the book.

Figure 1.8 US mortality rates (log scale), 1979–2006 for all causes (○), heart attack (◇), lung cancer in males (■), lung cancer in females (▲), motor vehicle accidents (△), diabetes (●) and AIDS (◆) (Drawn from: CDC Wonder (CDC), accessed 8 January 2010.)

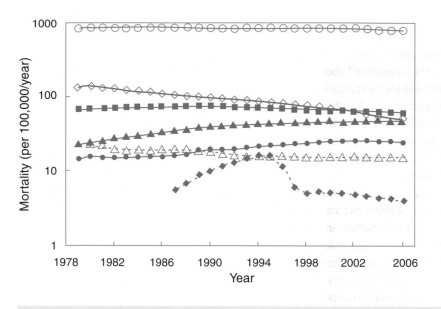

Box 1.5 Smallpox

The elimination of smallpox had a major impact on the health of millions of people, especially in many of the poorest countries. Descriptive epidemiology played a major role by providing information about the distribution of cases (*jointly by person, place and time*) and levels of transmission, by mapping outbreaks and by evaluating control measures. In 1967, there were 10–15 million new cases and 2 million deaths from smallpox in 31 countries. By 1976, smallpox was being reported in only two countries and the last naturally occurring case was recorded in 1977. Elimination of this scourge was helped by simple but painstaking case-finding and counting.

See Box 1.5 for a practical example of how simple descriptive epidemiology can help to solve a major global health problem.

Analytic studies

Ideas generated by such *descriptive* work can then be tested further in *analytic* studies, looking for associations between potential causal agents and diseases. This research is based on facts collected from groups of individuals, not large-scale population statistics. Are people with higher blood pressure more likely to develop coronary heart disease than those with normal blood pressure? Are people who smoke more likely to develop lung cancer than those who do not? Even

Box 1.6 The Nurses' Health Study

This cohort study of 120,000 US nurses was started in 1976 by Frank Speizer of the Channing Laboratory, Harvard Medical School. The study was initially funded for five years to study whether the oral contraceptive pill caused breast cancer, but the nurses are still being followed over 30 years later. Hundreds of scientific papers have been published, covering scores of diseases and exposures and investigating their inter-relationships. The study has been particularly influential in the field of diet and disease (nutritional epidemiology), owing to diet questionnaires that the nurses have been completing since 1980. As with other long-term follow-ups of cohorts, such as the British Doctors Study of Doll and Hill, its success is jointly dependent on the enthusiasm and commitment of researchers and participants. For the latter this has extended to providing blood, toenail clippings (for measurement of trace metals) and samples of tapwater over the years! This human side to epidemiology does not feature much in textbooks but is fundamental to successful fieldwork.

more usefully, how *much* more likely is a smoker to develop lung cancer than a non-smoker? Does risk depend on the number of cigarettes smoked? That is, how *strong* is the effect of the exposure; and does it increase with higher levels of exposure? In the British Doctors Study mentioned earlier, Doll and Hill found that the risk of lung cancer increased steadily as people smoked more cigarettes (Figure 1.4). This adds weight to the idea that smoking cigarettes really does affect the chance that an individual will develop lung cancer. In Box 1.6 you will find a brief account of another cohort study which has studied many exposures and diseases over the past three decades.

Once we have found an association, the challenge is then to evaluate this in order to determine whether something really *causes* disease or is linked to it only secondarily. If we find that people with a peptic ulcer drink a lot of milk, does this mean that drinking milk causes ulcers or simply that people with an ulcer drink milk to ease their pain? In Chapter 10 we will look more deeply at this challenge.

Intervention studies

Finally, epidemiologists evaluate new preventive measures, programmes or treatments that are designed to reduce ill health or promote good health. They also monitor the effectiveness of these 'intervention' programmes after they have been implemented: do they actually achieve the good they set out to do? These programmes can include evaluations of different health promotion strategies targeted at individuals or whole communities, or clinical trials of new drugs designed to cure disease. Does taking aspirin reduce your chance of having a heart attack? Which of several strategies is better at helping people give up smoking? Is one drug better than another for treating a heart attack?

A natural experiment

We will end this chapter with another example from John Snow's *On the Mode of Communication of Cholera* (1855) because, although this text is more than 150 years old, the methods he used and his combination of flair, skill, logic and dogged persistence remain the cornerstones of modern epidemiology. His work also exemplifies, in more detail than modern papers, the logical dissection of evidence about disease patterns to identify practical preventive strategies – which is still the key function of epidemiology – and it gives an excellent sense of the role and utility of epidemiology in practical public health.

In the early 1850s, London was cholera-free for a number of years and during that period one of the major water supply companies (the Lambeth Company) moved their waterworks out of London, thereby obtaining water free of the sewage of the city. During the next major cholera outbreak in 1853–1854 Snow was able to obtain information about the number of deaths occurring in the different sub-districts of London and he found that cholera mortality was lower in areas supplied by water from the Lambeth Company than in those supplied by the Southwark and Vauxhall water company which continued to take water from Battersea in the city. He did not stop there, but went on to conduct his 'Grand Experiment' (see Box 1.7).

Conclusions

Again we have a vivid picture of a master epidemiologist at work. Not satisfied that his hypothesis had been adequately tested, Snow identified the opportunity to conduct an even more rigorous test – his '*Grand Experiment*' – and in doing so he addressed the major epidemiological issues that still concern us today.

- He identified a situation in which people were unknowingly divided into two groups differing only in the source of their water, thereby creating what was effectively a **randomised trial** (we will look at the different types of epidemiological study in Chapter 4).
- In doing so, he realised the importance of ruling out other differences between the groups (e.g. sex, age, occupation, socioeconomic status) that could explain any mortality differences (a problem known as **confounding** that we will come back to in Chapter 8).
- He worked long and hard to acquire *accurate information* about both the water supply and the number of cholera deaths in each house – we will

Box 1.7 A grand experiment

Although the facts … afford very strong evidence of the powerful influence which the drinking water containing the sewage of a town exerts over the spread of cholera, when that disease is present, yet the question does not end here; for the intermixing of the water supply of the Southwark and Vauxhall Company with that of the Lambeth Company, over an extensive part of London, admitted of the subject being sifted in such a way as to yield the most incontrovertible proof on one side or the other … A few houses are supplied by one Company and a few by the other, according to the decision of the owner or occupier at that time when the Water Companies were in active competition … Each Company supplies both rich and poor, both large houses and small; there is no difference either in the condition or occupation of the persons receiving the water of the different Companies. Now it must be evident that, if the diminution of cholera, in the districts partly supplied with the improved water, depended on this supply, the houses receiving it would be the houses enjoying the whole benefit of the diminution of the malady, whilst the houses supplied with the water from Battersea Fields would suffer the same mortality as they would if the improved supply did not exist at all. As there is no difference whatever, either in the houses or the people receiving the supply of the two water Companies, or in any of the physical conditions with which they are surrounded, it is obvious that no experiment could have been devised which would more thoroughly test the effect of water supply on the progress of cholera than this which circumstances placed ready made before the observer.

The experiment, too, was on the grandest scale. No fewer than three hundred thousand people of both sexes, of every age and occupation, and of every rank and station, from gentlefolk down to the very poor, were divided into two groups without their choice, and, in most cases, without their knowledge; one group being supplied with water containing the sewage of London, and amongst it, whatever might have come from the cholera patients, the other group having water quite free from such impurity.

To turn this grand experiment to account, all that was required was to learn the supply of water to each individual house where a fatal attack of cholera might occur …

The epidemic of 1854

When the cholera returned to London in July of the present year … I resolved to spare no exertion … to ascertain the exact effect of the water supply on the progress of the epidemic, in the places where all the circumstances were so happily adapted for the inquiry … I accordingly asked permission at the

(*continued*)

Box 1.7 *(continued)*

General Register Office to be supplied with the addresses of persons dying of cholera, in those districts where the supply of the two Companies is intermingled in the manner I have stated above...I commenced my inquiry about the middle of August with two sub-districts of Lambeth...There were forty-four deaths in these sub-districts down to 12th August, and I found that thirty-eight of the houses in which these deaths occurred were supplied with water by the Southwark and Vauxhall Company, four houses were supplied by the Lambeth Company, and two had pump-wells on the premises and no supply from either of the Companies.

As soon as I had ascertained these particulars, I communicated them to Dr Farr, who was much struck with the result, and at his suggestion the Registrars of all the south districts of London were requested to make a return of the water supply of the house in which the attack took place, in all cases of death from cholera. This order was to take place after the 26th of August, and I resolved to carry my inquiry down to that date, so that the facts might be ascertained for the whole course of the epidemic.

The inquiry was necessarily attended with a good deal of trouble. There were very few instances in which I could at once get the information I required. Even when the water rates were paid by the residents, they can seldom remember the name of the Water Company till they have looked for the receipt. In the case of working people who pay weekly rents, the rates are invariably paid by the landlord or his agent, who often lives at a distance, and the residents know nothing about the matter. It would, indeed, have been almost impossible for me to complete the inquiry, if I had not found that I could distinguish the water of the two companies with perfect certainty by a chemical test. The test I employed was founded on the great difference in the quantity of chloride sodium [salt] contained in the two kinds of water, at the time I made the inquiry...

According to a return which was made to Parliament, the Southwark and Vauxhall Company supplied 40,046 houses from January 1st to December 31st, 1853, and the Lambeth Company supplied 26,107 houses during the same period; consequently, as 286 fatal attacks of cholera took place, in the first four weeks of the epidemic, in houses supplied by the former Company, and only 14 in houses supplied by the latter, the proportion of fatal attacks to each 10,000 houses was as follows. Southwark and Vauxhall 71, Lambeth 5. **The cholera was therefore fourteen times as fatal at this period amongst persons having the impure water of the Southwark and Vauxhall Company as amongst those having the purer water from Thames Ditton.**

(Excerpted from Snow, 1855.)

consider sources of data in Chapter 3 and will discuss the problem of error in Chapter 7.

- He *measured the occurrence of cholera* in the two groups of houses served by the different water companies – we will look further at measures such as these in Chapter 2.
- He calculated *how many times more common* cholera deaths were in those houses receiving the contaminated water – we will come back to this measure (again a **relative risk**) in Chapter 5.
- He then integrated all of his information to reach the conclusion that cholera was indeed *caused* by contaminated water – Chapter 10.

He did not stop there, but went on to make a series of clear practical recommendations to prevent transmission of cholera in future – sensible measures including the need for cleanliness and sterilisation that are still practised today.

Snow's work therefore sets the scene for the chapters to come. Chapters 2–8 cover the basic principles and underlying theory of epidemiology in a very 'hands-on' way, leading to Chapters 9–11, which integrate this information in a practical look at how we read and interpret epidemiological reports, think about assessing causality and finally synthesise a mass of information in a single review. Chapters 12–15 then look at some specific applications of epidemiology and Chapter 16 concludes with a fresh look at what epidemiology is and what it can do to help address the health concerns facing the world today.

But, before you move on, take a minute to stop and think. Imagine that someone asked you what epidemiology was and why it was useful. Could you now give them a satisfactory explanation in a few sentences?

REFERENCES

AIHW (Australian Institute of Health and Welfare). (2008). *Australia's Health 2008*. Cat. *no. AUS 99*. Canberra: AIHW.

CDC (Centers for Disease Control and Prevention), National Center for Health Statistics. Compressed Mortality File 1979–1998. CDC WONDER On-line Database, compiled from Compressed Mortality File CMF 1968–1988, Series 20, No. 2A, 2000 and CMF 1989–1998, Series 20, No. 2E, 2003. Accessed at http://wonder.cdc.gov/cmf-icd9.html on 8 January 2010 7:24:23 p.m. and Compressed Mortality File 1999–2006. CDC WONDER On-line Database, compiled from Compressed Mortality File 1999–2006 Series 20 No. 2L, 2009. Accessed at http://wonder.cdc.gov/cmf-icd10.html on 29 December 2009 10:50:10 p.m..

Concise Oxford Dictionary, 5th edn. (1964). Oxford: Oxford University Press.

Devesa, S. S., Grauman, D. J., Blot, W. J. *et al.* (1999). *Atlas of Cancer Mortality in the United States: 1950–1994*. Washington DC: US Government Print Office.

Doll, R. and Hill, A. B. (1950). Smoking and carcinoma of the lung. *British Medical Journal*, **2**: 739–748.

Doll, R. and Hill, A. B. (1964). Mortality in relation to smoking: ten years' observations of British doctors. *British Medical Journal*, **1**: 1399–1410, 1460–1467.

Doll, R., Peto, R., Boreham, J. and Sutherland, I. (2004). Mortality in relation to smoking: 50 years' observations on male British doctors. *British Medical Journal*, doi: 10.1136/bmj.38142.554479.AE (published 22 June 2004).

Graunt, J. (1662). *Natural and Political Observations Mentioned in a Following Index and Made Upon the Bills of Mortality.* London. (http://www.books-on-line.com)

Hippocrates of Cos. (400 BC). *On Airs, Waters, and Places.* Translated by Francis Adams. (http://classics.mit.edu)

Hook, D., Jalaludin, B. and Fitzsimmons, G. (1996). *Clostridium perfringens* food-borne outbreak: an epidemiological investigation. *Australian and New Zealand Journal of Public Health*, **20**: 119–122.

Lilienfeld, A. M. and Lilienfeld, D. E. (1980). *Foundations of Epidemiology*, 2nd edn. New York: Oxford University Press.

MacMahon, B. and Pugh, T. F. (1970). *Epidemiology – Principles and Methods.* Boston: Little Brown.

Makk, L., Creech, J. L., Whelan, J. G. and Johnson, M. D. (1974). Liver damage and angiosarcoma in vinyl chloride workers – a systematic detection program. *Journal of the American Medical Association*, **230**: 64–68.

Miettinen, O. S. (1978). *Course Notes – Principles of Epidemiologic Research.* Harvard School of Public Health.

Pink, B. and Allbon, P. (2008). *The Health and Welfare of Australia's Aboriginal and Torres Strait Islander Peoples.* Canberra: Australian Bureau of Statistics and Australian Institute of Health and Welfare.

Porta, M. (Ed.) (2008). *A Dictionary of Epidemiology*, 5th edn. New York: Oxford University Press.

Rosen, G. (1958). *A History of Public Health.* New York: MD Publications.

Selikoff, I. J., Churg, J. and Hammond, E. C. (1965). Relation between exposure to asbestos and mesothelioma. *New England Journal of Medicine*, **272**: 560–565.

Snow, J. (1855). *On the Mode of Communication of Cholera*, 2nd edn. London: Churchill. (http://www.ph.ucla.edu/epi/snow/snowbook.html)

Stolley, P. D. and Lasky, T. (1995). *Investigating Disease Patterns: the Science of Epidemiology.* New York: Scientific American Library.

WHO (World Health Organization). (1948). Text of the constitution of the World Health Organization. *Official Record World Health Organization*, **2**: 100.

www.anesi.com/titanic.htm, The Titanic casualty figures (and what they mean). Accessed 30 December 2009.

Wynder, E. L. and Graham, E. A. (1950). Tobacco smoking as a possible etiologic factor in bronchiogenic carcinoma. A study of six hundred and eighty-four proved cases. *Journal of the American Medical Association*, **143**: 329–336.

Zaridze, D., Maximovitch, D., Lazarev, A. *et al.* (2009). Alcohol poisoning is a main determinant of recent mortality trends in Russia: evidence from a detailed analysis of mortality statistics and autopsies. *International Journal of Epidemiology*, **38**: 143–153.

2

How long is a piece of string?
Measuring disease frequency

Description	Association	Alternative explanations	Integration & interpretation	Practical applications
Chapter 2: Measuring health	Chapters 4–5	Chapters 6–8	Chapters 9–11	Chapters 12–15

Box 2.1 Who drinks the most beer?

According to the Brewers Association of Japan, the Chinese now drink the most beer in the world (28,640 million litres in 2004) followed by the Americans (23,974 million litres). In contrast the Czech Republic ranked a lowly 15th in terms of total consumption (1,878 million litres) and Ireland didn't even make the top 25. This information may be useful for planning production, but do the Chinese and Americans really drink more beer than the rest of us? An alternative and possibly more informative way to look at these data is in terms of consumption *per capita*. When we do this, the USA falls to 13th position in the 'beer drinking league table' (82 litres per capita in 2004) and China falls way off the screen (a mere 22 litres per capita). The Czechs are now the champions (157 litres per capita), followed by the Irish (131 litres per capita) with Germany and Australia, two nations who tend to pride themselves on their beer drinking, ranked in 3rd (116 litres) and 4th (110 litres) place, respectively.

(*Source*: www.brewers.or.jp, accessed 10 October 2009.)

Many different measures are used by researchers and policy makers to describe the health of populations. You have already met some of these, for example the attack rate which was used to investigate the source of the outbreak investigation in the previous chapter. In this chapter we will introduce you to some more of the most commonly used measures so that you can use and interpret them correctly. We will first discuss the three fundamental measures that underlie both the attack rate and most of the other health statistics that you will come across in health-related reports and will then look at how they are calculated and used in practice. We will finish by considering some other more elaborate measures that attempt to get closer to describing the overall health of a population. As you will see, all of this is not always as straightforward as it might seem.

What are we measuring?

Although, as discussed in the previous chapter, we are primarily interested in 'health', this is a somewhat abstract concept. In practice, it is much easier to define ill-health or disease and this is what we usually measure. Lack of a particular disease does not necessarily imply 'health' but simply a lack of the disease of interest.

Before we can start to measure disease, we have to have a very clear idea of what it is that we are trying to determine. In general, the diagnosis of disease is based on a combination of *symptoms*, subjective indications of disease reported by the person themselves; *signs*, objective indications of disease apparent to

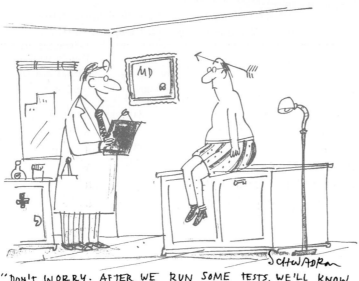

"DON'T WORRY. AFTER WE RUN SOME TESTS, WE'LL KNOW FOR SURE WHAT'S CAUSING YOUR HEADACHES."

the physician; and additional *tests*. Criteria for making a diagnosis can be very simple: the presence of antibodies against an infectious agent can indicate infection, and diagnosis of most cancers is fairly straightforward on the basis of tissue histology (examination with a light microscope); but for some diseases the diagnostic criteria are much more complex, involving combinations of signs and symptoms.

For health data to be meaningful, diagnostic criteria leading to a case definition have to be clear, unambiguous and easy to use under a wide range of circumstances. It is important to remember that different case definitions can lead to very different pictures. As shown in Figure 2.1, a study in the United Arab Emirates showed that the prevalence of gestational diabetes (diabetes during pregnancy) in a group of 3,500 women was much higher using one set of criteria to

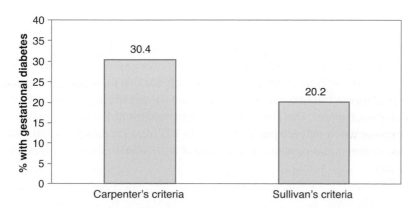

Figure 2.1 Percent of population with gestational diabetes according to two sets of diagnostic criteria. (Drawn from: Agarwal and Punnose, 2002.)

Table 2.1 Estimates of the number of people living with HIV/AIDS and the number of new HIV infections around the world in 2007.

Region	Population (×1000)	People living with HIV/AIDS (end of 2007)	New HIV infections (2007)
Sub-Saharan Africa	788,000	22,500,000	1,700,000
East Asia	1,550,000	800,000	92,000
Oceania	35,000	75,000	14,000
South and Southeast Asia	2,176,000	4,000,000	340,000
Eastern Europe & Central Asia	322,000	1,600,000	150,000
Western and Central Europe	486,000	760,000	31,000
North Africa & Middle East	395,000	380,000	35,000
North America	335,000	1,300,000	46,000
Caribbean	40,000	230,000	17,000
Latin America	529,000	1,600,000	100,000
Total	6,656,000	33,245,000	2,525,000

(*Data source:* UNAIDS, 2007 and Population Reference Bureau, 2007.)

diagnose diabetes (Carpenter's criteria, 30.4%) than another (O'Sullivan's criteria, 20.2%) (Agarwal and Punnose, 2002). If you want to compare information from different reports the first thing to check is that you are comparing apples with apples – have they all measured the same thing using the same criteria? This can be a particular problem when trying to compare patterns of disease over time because changes in diagnostic criteria can lead to sudden increases or decreases in the number of cases recorded.

The concepts: prevalence and incidence

Once we have defined what we mean by disease, we can then go on to measure how often it occurs.

In Table 2.1 we see the estimated number of people living with HIV/AIDS in the various regions of the world at the end of 2007, and the number of new cases of HIV infection that occurred during 2007. These data clearly show the huge burden borne by sub-Saharan Africa, which has five times more cases than any other region, but what can they tell us about the relative importance of HIV/AIDS in other regions? The East Asia and Western/Central Europe regions both had approximately 800,000 people living with HIV/AIDS at the end of 2007. How can we describe and compare the burden of HIV/AIDS in these populations more fully?

Table 2.2 The prevalence of HIV/AIDS and incidence of HIV infection around the world in 2007.

Region	Population (×1000)	People living with HIV/AIDS (end of 2007)	Prevalence (%)	New HIV infections (2007)	Incidence (per 100,000/yr)
Sub-Saharan Africa	788,000	22,500,000	2.86%	1,700,000	215.7
East Asia	1,550,000	800,000	0.05%	92,000	5.9
Oceania	35,000	75,000	0.21%	14,000	40.0
South and Southeast Asia	2,176,000	4,000,000	0.18%	340,000	15.6
Eastern Europe & Central Asia	322,000	1,600,000	0.50%	150,000	46.6
Western and Central Europe	486,000	760,000	0.16%	31,000	6.4
North Africa & Middle East	395,000	380,000	0.10%	35,000	8.9
North America	335,000	1,300,000	0.39%	46,000	13.7
Caribbean	40,000	230,000	0.58%	17,000	42.5
Latin America	529,000	1,600,000	0.30%	100,000	18.9
Total	6,656,000	33,245,000	0.50%	2,525,000	37.9

(*Data source:* UNAIDS, 2007 and Population Reference Bureau, 2007.)

What percentage of people in Western and Central Europe had HIV/AIDS at the end of 2007?

What percentage of people in Western and Central Europe became HIV-positive during 2007?

At the end of 2007, 760,000 of the 486,000,000 people in Western and Central Europe or 0.16% of the population were living with HIV/AIDS. During 2007, another 31,000 people or 0.0064% of the population became infected with HIV. Now 0.0064% is a very small number. It simply tells us that there were 0.0064 new HIV infections for every 100 people during 2007, so an alternative way to present the same information would be to multiply the numbers by 1,000 and say that there were 6.4 new infections in every 100,000 people ($6.4/100,000$ or $6.4/10^5$).[1]

What you calculated above were, first, the **prevalence** of *existing* HIV/AIDS in Western and Central Europe at the end of 2007 and, secondly, the **incidence** of *new* HIV infections in the same region during 2007. These measures give us two different ways of quantifying the amount of disease in a population. Table 2.2 shows the same information for each of the regions. These data confirm the high levels of HIV/AIDS in sub-Saharan Africa and show us that, despite the relatively low numbers of new cases in Oceania and the Caribbean, the small size of these populations means that the incidence there is also high (note that 70% of cases

---

[1] If you are not familiar with this nomenclature, the superscript number is simply a shorthand way to say how many zeros the number has. So, 10^2 would be 100, 10^5 is 100,000 and 10^6 is one million (1,000,000).

in Oceania occur in Papua New Guinea, which, with a population of only about 6.4 million, has an incidence of about 153 per 100,000/year). The data also show us that, although the actual *numbers* of cases in East Asia and Western/Central Europe are similar, the *prevalence* per 100 people (%) is much lower in East Asia (0.05%) than in Western and Central Europe. Like the example in Box 2.1, these data emphasise the need to take the size of a population into account when making comparisons between populations.

Prevalence

The **prevalence** of a disease tells us what proportion of a population actually has the disease at a specific point in time: an estimated 0.16% or 160 of every 100,000 people in Western and Central Europe had HIV/AIDS at the end of 2007. This is a snapshot of the situation at a single point in time and, for this reason, it is sometimes called the 'point' prevalence. Note that you may also see references to 'period prevalence', which measures the proportion of the population that had the disease *at any time during a specified period*. This is a complex measure that combines the prevalence (everybody who had the disease at the start of the period) and incidence (all of the new cases of disease during the period).

> *Prevalence* measures the amount of a disease in a population at a given point in time:
>
> $$\text{Prevalence} = \frac{\text{Number of people with disease at a given point in time}}{\text{Total number of people in the population}} \quad (2.1)$$

Prevalence measures are just one number (the number of people with disease) divided by another number (the total number of people in the population). They have no units, and are mostly reported simply as a proportion or a percentage (2.9% of Sub-Saharan Africans had HIV/AIDS at the end of 2007), but may also be shown as cases/population (390/100,000 North Americans had HIV/AIDS at the end of 2007). Note that the precise answer for the proportion of Sub-Saharan Africans with HIV/AIDS is 0.028553299... or 2.853299% but, for simplicity, we have *rounded* this to one decimal place, giving 2.9%.[2] (In our experience, people are sometimes confused by percentages because there is often more than one way in which they can be calculated and this can lead to problems with interpretation – see Box 2.2 for some additional guidance.) Although you will often see the

---

[2] If the first number that is cut off is between 0 and 4 you round *down* and if it is between 5 and 9 you round *up*. In this case the first number to go was a 5 so we rounded 2.8553299 *up* to 2.9. If, however, it had been 2.8453299 then we would have rounded down to 2.8. In practice it is rarely necessary to show results to more than two or three significant figures, i.e. numbers other than zero.

Box 2.2 A note about percentages

Imagine a study that gave the following results:

	Asthma	No asthma	Total
Non-smokers	40	360	400
Smokers	30	170	200
Total	70	530	600

There are two ways that we can look at these data. One way would be to calculate the percentages of (a) non-smokers and (b) smokers who have asthma – these are row percentages because we use the total of each row, the number of non-smokers or smokers, as the denominator (note: the *denominator* is the bottom half of a fraction and the *numerator* the top half):

	Asthma	No asthma	Total
Non-smokers	$40 \div 400 = 10\%$	$360 \div 400 = 90\%$	$400 = 100\%$
Smokers	$30 \div 200 = 15\%$	$170 \div 200 = 85\%$	$200 = 100\%$

This tells us that 10% of non-smokers and 15% of smokers have asthma.

Alternatively, we could use the same data to calculate the percentage of people with and without asthma who smoke – these are column percentages because now we use the total of each column, the number of people with or without asthma, as the denominator:

	Asthma	No asthma
Non-smokers	$40 \div 70 = 57\%$	$360 \div 530 = 68\%$
Smokers	$30 \div 70 = 43\%$	$170 \div 530 = 32\%$
Total	$70 = 100\%$	$530 = 100\%$

This tells us that 43% of people with asthma and only 32% of people without asthma are smokers.

It is very important to decide first which percentages are most relevant for a particular situation and then to calculate and interpret the percentages correctly. Saying that 43% of people with asthma are smokers (correct) is not the same as saying that 43% of smokers have asthma (incorrect; 15% of smokers have asthma).

term 'prevalence rate', this is not a true rate because a rate should include units of time. An example of a true rate is the use of distance travelled *per hour*, i.e. kph or mph, to measure the speed of a car. The time point at which people are counted should, however, always be reported when giving an estimate of prevalence. This is often a fixed point in calendar time, such as 31 December 2007, but it can also be a fixed point in life, for instance, birth or retirement. For example, if 1,000 babies were born alive in one hospital in a given year and, of these, five babies were born with congenital abnormalities, we would say that the prevalence of congenital abnormality *at birth* was 5/1,000 live births in that year. Prevalence can be expressed per 100 people (per cent, %) or per 1,000 (10^3), 10,000 (10^4) or 100,000 (10^5). It doesn't matter as long as it is clear which is being used.

In practice, it would be rare to identify all prevalent cases of disease at one precise point in time; e.g. a blood pressure survey may take weeks or months to conduct, given limited numbers of researchers, amounts of equipment and availability of those being measured. The exact size of the population may also not be known on a given day and this might well be based on an estimate or projection from census data.

Incidence

The **incidence** of disease measures how quickly people are catching the disease and it differs from prevalence because it considers only *new* infections, some-times called *incident cases*, that occurred in a specific time period. During 2007, 1.7 million people in Sub-Saharan Africa or 0.22% of the population were newly diagnosed as HIV-positive. Another way of saying this is that the incidence of HIV infection was 216/100,000 per year (Table 2.2). You will find that people use the term 'incidence' on its own to mean slightly different things – some use it for the *number* of new cases (i.e. 1.7 million), some for the *proportion* of people who are newly infected (i.e. 0.0022 or 0.22%) and some for the *rate* at which new infection has occurred (i.e. 216 new cases per 100,000 people *per year*). To avoid confusion we will describe the latter measure as the **incidence rate**, which, unlike measures of prevalence, is a true rate because it includes a measure of time.

$$\text{Incidence rate} = \frac{\text{Number of people who develop disease in one year}}{\text{Average number of people in the population}} \qquad (2.2)$$

We will look further at how to calculate these measures later, but first let us consider the concept of the 'population at risk' and the relationship between prevalence and the incidence rate.

Population at risk

In the example above it is probably not unreasonable to assume that everyone might be at risk of contracting HIV, although, obviously, some groups will be more 'at risk' than others; but what if the disease of interest were something like cervical cancer? To use the whole population to calculate rates of cancer of the cervix (the neck of the uterus) would be inappropriate, because a man could never develop the disease. We would calculate a *sex-specific* rate by dividing the number of cases by the number of *females* in the population. However, many women will have had a hysterectomy and their uterus will have been removed. They are then no longer at risk of developing cervical cancer and so, strictly speaking, should not be included in counts of the population at risk. In practice, published rates of both cervical and endometrial (uterine) cancer rarely allow for this so it is difficult to compare the rates of these cancers between countries that have very different hysterectomy rates. We discussed above the importance of making sure that different reports used the same definition of disease (i.e. they counted the same thing in the numerator); it is also crucial to ensure that the denominators represent equivalent populations (e.g. they are similar in age, sex distribution, etc.).

The relationship between incidence and prevalence

If two diseases have the same incidence, but one lasts three times longer than the other, then, at any point in time, you are much more likely to find people suffering from the more long-lasting disease. Very crudely (and assuming that people do not move into or out of the area), the relationship between prevalence (P) and the incidence rate (IR) depends on how long the disease persists before cure or death (average duration of disease, D):

$$P \approx \mathrm{IR} \times D \qquad\qquad (2.3)$$

where $\approx$ means approximately equal to. (Box 2.3 shows a more complex version of this formula.)

Box 2.3 More about the relationship among prevalence, incidence and duration

The relationship $P \approx \mathrm{IR} \times D$ is approximately true in what is called a *stationary* population where the number of people entering the population (immigration and birth) balances the number of people leaving (emigration and death). A second requirement is that the prevalence of disease must be low (less than about 10%). This is the case for many diseases, but a more general formula that does not require the disease to be rare is

$$\frac{P}{1 - P} \approx \mathrm{IR} \times D \qquad\qquad (2.4)$$

where P is the prevalence of disease expressed as a proportion and $1 - P$ is the proportion of *non-diseased* people; e.g. if the prevalence (P) is 2% or 0.02 then $1 - P$ is 0.98.

For example, hepatitis A has a relatively high incidence: according to the US Centers for Disease Control and Prevention (CDC), in 2006 there were approximately 32,000 new infections in the USA and approximately one-third of the population had been infected at some time (CDC Division of Viral Hepatitis, 2009). However, because it is an acute infection and people recover fairly quickly, the prevalence of hepatitis A infection at any one point in time would be quite low. In contrast, hepatitis C infection is less common (approximately 19,000 new infections in 2006) but most of those infected develop a chronic infection and so are infected for life. This means that the prevalence of hepatitis C infection is much higher, with between 2.7 and 3.9 million Americans estimated to be infected in 2006.

If a new treatment were developed for a disease, what effect would this have on the prevalence and incidence of the disease?

If the new treatment meant that people were cured more quickly and so were ill for less time then the prevalence would fall. However, if the disease had previously been fatal and the new treatment meant that people lived longer with the disease then the prevalence would increase. In general, a new treatment will not affect the incidence of a disease. The only exception to this rule might be for an infectious disease: if people were ill and thus infectious for less time, they might pass the infection to fewer people and so the incidence would fall.

As you can see, the prevalence of a disease reflects a balance of several factors. If the incidence of a disease increases then the prevalence will also increase; if the duration of sickness changes then the prevalence will change. This means that the prevalence of a disease is generally not the best way to measure the underlying forces driving the occurrence of the disease – we must use the incidence rate for this. Nonetheless, prevalence is useful for measuring diseases that have a gradual onset and long duration such as type-2 diabetes and osteoarthritis, and also for capturing the frequency of congenital malformations at birth. It is also of direct value for describing the overall disease burden of a population and, consequently, is fundamentally important for assessing healthcare needs and planning health services.

Measuring disease occurrence in practice: epidemiological studies

As we discussed above, the occurrence of disease can be quantified by looking at the **prevalence** or the **incidence rate**. We will now consider these further, together with an alternative way of measuring incidence known as **cumulative incidence**. These three fundamental measures form the basis of *descriptive epidemiology*, which seeks to answer the first four of the five core questions that you met in Chapter 1: What (diseases are occurring)? Who (is getting them)? Where? and When? The measures can all be calculated from routinely collected data (as in the HIV example above) or from results of studies conducted specifically to measure the incidence or prevalence of disease, and they are widely used in health reports around the world. We will come back to the use of routine data and for now will concentrate on how we measure the occurrence of disease in an epidemiological study.

To measure the *prevalence* of disease we need to conduct a *survey*, or what is often called a **cross-sectional study**, in which a random sample (or cross-section) of the population is questioned or assessed to ascertain whether they have a particular condition at a given point in time. To measure the *incidence* of disease we need to start with a group (or *cohort*) of people who are currently free of the disease of interest but who are 'at risk' of developing it. We then follow them over time to see who actually develops the disease (a **cohort study**; e.g. the British Doctors Study mentioned in Chapter 1).

When we conduct a research study we can specify exactly who is in the study and can usually collect individual data for all (or most) of those people. We can identify who is 'at risk', calculate quite accurate measures of disease incidence (or prevalence) and also relate the occurrence of disease to its potential causes.

Consider, for example, a study conducted in a hypothetical primary school with 100 pupils. Imagine that, on the first day of the new term, nine children had a cold. Over the next week another seven children developed a cold.

What percentage of children had a cold on the first day of term?

What percentage of the children who didn't have a cold on the first day of term developed one during the next week?

The first measure that you calculated is the **prevalence** of the common cold in this group of children: 9 out of 100 children or 9% had a cold on the first day of term. The second measure is known as the **cumulative incidence** of colds: out of 91 children 'at risk' of developing a cold (i.e. they did not have one already), 7 or 7.7% developed one during the first week of term. The denominator (population at risk) is 91 in this case because 9 of the 100 children already had a cold and were not therefore 'at risk' of catching another at the same time. The cumulative incidence thus measures the proportion, or percentage, of people (children in this case) who were at risk of developing a cold and who did so during the period of the study (one week). Note that it is always important to specify the time period – a cumulative incidence of 5% in 1 year would be very different from a cumulative incidence of 5% in 20 years. The cumulative incidence is sometimes known as the **attack rate**, especially when it refers to a short time period, usually with respect to an outbreak of infectious diseases as in the food poisoning example in Chapter 1.

The above example was simple because the common cold is just that, very common, and we were only interested in the children for one week. Imagine that we were trying to measure the incidence of a much rarer disease such as cancer. We would obviously need a much larger group of people and we would need to follow them for much longer to see who developed the cancer. In this situation it is very difficult to keep track of people and we would inevitably lose some from the study group and not know what happened to them. Another problem is that people will die from other 'competing' causes and so they will no longer be at risk of developing the cancer. In this situation, calculations of the cumulative incidence may be inaccurate (or will become so over time) because we will not know exactly who has developed the disease. In practice, we can calculate cumulative incidence only when we have a clearly defined group of people who are all (or almost all) followed for the whole follow-up period.

When this is not the situation we use a different method to calculate an **incidence rate**. Instead of simply counting the actual *number* of people at risk of disease, we count up the *length of time* they were at risk of disease. Imagine that we followed a group of 1,000 men for 5 years and that during this time 15 of them had a non-fatal heart attack. This gives us a cumulative incidence of 1.5% for the 5-year period. During this period the men have lived a total of $1,000 \times 5 = 5,000$ years of life or **person-years**. We could have obtained the same number of person-years by following a group of 5,000 men for 1 year each, or a group of 500 men for 10 years each. Alternatively, we could have followed some men for one year, some for two years, some for three years, etc., to arrive at the same total of 5,000. We are no longer so focused on the actual number of people who were at risk of the disease, but rather on the total person-time (number of person-years) they were at risk. This not only gives us a much more accurate measure of how quickly disease is occurring among those at risk, but it also gives us much greater flexibility. Assuming that we still saw 15 heart attacks during our 5,000 person-years (py), we could calculate the **incidence rate** (sometimes called the incidence density) as 15 per 5,000 *person-years* or, more usually, 3 per 1,000 or 300/100,000 person-years.

Cumulative incidence (**CI**) measures the *proportion of people* who develop disease *during a specified period*:

$$CI = \frac{\text{Number of people who develop disease in a specified period}}{\substack{\text{Number of } people \text{ at risk of getting the disease} \\ at\ the\ start\ of\ the\ period}} \quad (2.5)$$

The *incidence rate* (IR) measures *how quickly* people are developing a disease:

$$IR = \frac{\text{Number of people who develop disease}}{\substack{\text{Number of } person\text{-}years \text{ when people were at risk} \\ \text{of getting the disease}}} \quad (2.6)$$

Note that, although Equation (2.6) looks slightly different from Equation (2.2), they are measuring the same thing – if you are unsure about this see Box 2.4 for an explanation of why this is true. We will also come back to this under 'Crude incidence and mortality rates' on page 46.

Incidence rates versus cumulative incidence

The distinction between a measure of *cumulative incidence* and an *incidence rate* can be confusing. An analogy that we have found helpful is to think of these measures in terms of driving a car.

- The *incidence rate* is equivalent to the average *speed* of a car at a particular point in time, e.g. 60 km/hour.

Box 2.4 Calculating incidence rates

As you saw above, the 'person-time' method for calculating an incidence rate (Equation (2.6)) is particularly useful in research studies when different people have been followed for different lengths of time. However, at the population level we may be dealing with millions of people and it is clearly not feasible to calculate the person-time that each is at risk. Instead we usually calculate the incidence rate for a single year and work on the assumption that everyone in the population is at risk for the whole of that year (Equation (2.2)). The fundamental concept is, however, the same – if there are 500,000 people in the population and we assume they are all at risk for one year that is the same as 500,000 person-years. The only distinction is that the 'routine rates' calculated using Equation (2.2) are based on population averages, whereas the 'epidemiological rates' calculated using Equation (2.6) are based on adding together carefully measured units of individual person-time to give a precise denominator. The resulting incidence rates are also presented slightly differently: routine incidence rates are usually described per 100,000 *people per year*, whereas in epidemiological studies using individual data they are usually shown per 100,000 *person-years*. You will find that some people differentiate the rates calculated based on person-time by describing them as **incidence density**; however, we, as most others, will refer to both as incidence rates because they are effectively measuring the same thing.

In practice, it will usually only be possible to calculate the incidence rate one way. If data are available for individual people who have been followed for different lengths of time then we have to use Equation (2.6). If we only have summary data for a population then we use Equation (2.2).

- The *cumulative incidence* is analogous to the *distance* travelled by a car during a specified interval of time, e.g. 60 km in one hour.

The *distance* a car travels depends both on its average *speed* and on the length of time it travels for. If a car travels at an average speed of 60 km/hour then it will cover 30 km in 30 minutes, 60 km in one hour and so on. When we consider a time interval of one hour, the total distance travelled (60 km in one hour) looks very similar to the average speed because this is expressed per hour (60 km/hr). Distance and speed are, however, fundamentally different.

In the same way, the incidence rate describes the 'speed' at which new cases of disease are occurring, and therefore reflects what is sometimes called the underlying *force of morbidity*. Cumulative incidence is a measure of the proportion of a group who develop the disease over a particular time and is thus a function both of the underlying incidence rate and of the length of follow-up. If the incidence rate is 10 per 100,000/year then the cumulative incidence will be 10 cases in 100,000 (=0.0001 or 0.01%) in one year, 20 cases in 100,000 (=0.0002 or 0.02%) in two years and so on. As with the car example, when we consider a time interval of one year, a cumulative incidence expressed as 10 per 100,000 people *in one year* looks much like an incidence rate (10 per 100,000 *per year* or *person-years*) because we usually show incidence rates per year. It is important to recognise that, as with distance and speed, the measures are different. A good way to help avoid confusion is to ensure that the cumulative incidence is expressed as a proportion (e.g. 0.0001) or percentage rather than 'per 100,000'.

Example

Imagine that we identified a group of 10 healthy people on 1 January 2000 and that we decided to follow these people for seven years to see who developed a particular disease. Figure 2.2 shows the hypothetical experience of these people: four developed the disease of interest and three of them died, and another three were 'lost to follow-up' (e.g. they moved away or died of some other disease). Let us now look at how we would calculate the different measures of disease occurrence in this group.

Prevalence

Remember that prevalence tells us the proportion of the population who were sick at a particular point in time (Equation (2.1)). For example, on 1 January 2003, two people were sick out of the nine people left in our group on that date (one was lost to follow-up), so

Prevalence = $2 \div 9 = 22\%$

What was the prevalence of the disease on 30 June 2004?

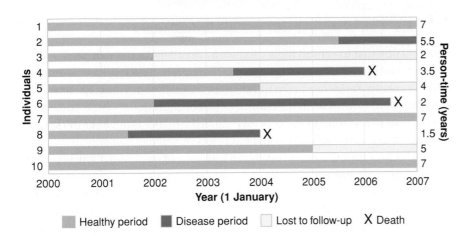

Figure 2.2 A hypothetical follow-up study.

On 30 June 2004 two people were sick but there were only seven people left in the group on that date (one had died and two had been lost to follow-up), so

Prevalence $= 2 \div 7 = 29\%$

Cumulative incidence

This tells us the proportion of a population 'at risk' of developing a disease who actually became ill during a specified time interval (Equation (2.5)). It is also the probability or average *risk* that an individual will develop the disease during the period: if 30% of people in a population develop a disease then each individual has a 30% chance of developing it themselves. It is important to note that this is the average risk for the population; the risk for any individual is either zero (they won't develop the disease) or one[3] (they will). With the exception of some rare genetic diseases such as Huntington's disease where all those who carry the aberrant gene will eventually develop the disease, this individual risk is usually unknown or unknowable, making accurate predictions for individuals in the clinical setting almost impossible.

In the example, four of the 10 people who were at risk at the start of the study developed the disease, but three were lost to follow-up and we do not know whether they developed the disease. This means that we cannot accurately calculate the cumulative incidence at seven years, but a *minimum estimate* would be

CI $= 4 \div 10 = 40\%$ in seven years

This is assuming that none of those lost to follow-up developed the disease. If any of them had developed the disease then the true cumulative incidence would

---

[3] Note that risk can be measured on a scale from 0 to 1, or from 0 to 100%; a risk of 30% is therefore equal to a risk of 0.3.

have been higher than 40%. The *maximum estimate* of the cumulative incidence would assume that all three of the missing people developed the disease:

$$CI = 7 \div 10 = 70\% \text{ in seven years}$$

Note that we could calculate an accurate cumulative incidence at two years – since we do have complete follow-up to that point:

$$CI = 1 \div 10 = 10\% \text{ in two years}$$

One type of study in which the study group is clearly defined and loss to follow-up is usually minimal is a **clinical trial** (see Chapter 4) and this means that the cumulative incidence is an appropriate and common measure of outcome in this type of study. However, the field of clinical epidemiology has developed its own terminology for what we call cumulative incidence (see Box 2.5).

Incidence rate

Although we do not know what happened to three people in the group, we do know that they had not developed the disease before they were lost to follow-up.

We can use this information to help us calculate the incidence rate or what is sometimes called the incidence density (Equation (2.6)). This is the number of new cases of disease (four) divided by the total amount of *person-time* at risk of developing the disease. An individual is at risk of developing the disease until the actual moment when they do develop it (in practice, when they are diagnosed) or until they are lost to follow-up. In this example, individual number one would contribute seven years of person-time; individual number two would contribute five and a half years; individual number three would contribute two years, and so on.

What is the total amount of person-time at risk?

What is the incidence rate for this disease per 100 person-years?

The total amount of person time is

$$7 + 5.5 + 2 + 3.5 + 4 + 2 + 7 + 1.5 + 5 + 7 = 44.5 \text{ person-years}$$

So the incidence rate is

$$4 \text{ cases} \div 44.5 \text{ person-years} = 0.09 \text{ cases/person-year or } 9 \text{ cases/100 person-years}$$

Measuring disease occurrence in practice: using routine data

In practice most of our information about the occurrence of disease comes from routine statistics, collected at a regional, national or international level (we will discuss some of the sources of these data in Chapter 3), and in this format they comprise the core of many published reports. The data are not based on specific information about *individuals* but relate the number of cases of disease (or deaths) in a *population* to the size of that population (often an estimate from a census). This can lead to problems when we try to relate the occurrence of disease to potential causes. For example, if a region has a very high level of unemployment and also has a high incidence of suicide it might be tempting to jump to the conclusion that being unemployed drives people to commit suicide. However, we have no way of knowing from routine statistics whether it is the same people who are unemployed who are also those committing suicide. (This dilemma where we try to extrapolate from an association seen at the population level to draw conclusions about the relation in individuals is often called the **ecological fallacy** and we will discuss it again in Chapter 3.)

A second drawback of routine data relates to the fact that in public health we often want to measure the *incidence* of disease – how quickly are people becoming ill? Unfortunately, it is often difficult to obtain reliable information about incidence because few illnesses are captured reliably in routine statistics. Some diseases, such as HIV infection and cancer, are 'notifiable' in many countries and, therefore, all cases *should* be reported to a central body; however, these examples are the exceptions rather than the rule and such data are not routinely available for most diseases. Furthermore, even where reporting is mandated it does not always occur in practice. When HIV/AIDS first came to world attention and again during the 2003 SARS (severe acute respiratory syndrome) outbreak, some countries suppressed the real numbers of cases for both political and economic reasons.

As a result, many common measures that you will come across will be measures of mortality because death and cause of death are regularly and reliably recorded in many, but certainly not all, countries. Incidence and mortality rates have exactly the same form, but for incidence we count new cases of a disease whereas for mortality we count deaths. Mortality data are obviously uninformative for many diseases that are not usually fatal – things like osteoarthritis, non-melanoma skin cancers, psoriasis and rubella (German measles) to name but a few. But even for those diseases from which a high proportion of cases die, mortality figures might not mirror the underlying incidence of disease, for example if a more effective treatment is introduced. Mortality data can also lag well behind changes in incidence, delaying identification of changes over time that may be important for planning or for providing clues as to the causes of the disease. We will take up these issues in more detail when we discuss the role and uses of surveillance in health planning and evaluation (see Chapter 13).

Crude incidence and mortality rates

As you saw above, when we conduct an epidemiological study we calculate the incidence rate as the number of cases of disease divided by the total *person-time* at risk of disease (where this is summed over all of the individuals in the study). This method is particularly useful when different people have been followed for different lengths of time but at the population level we may be dealing with millions of people and it is clearly not feasible to calculate the person-time that each is at risk. Instead we usually work on the assumption that everyone is at risk for the whole of the year that we are interested in.

When we are working with routine data, therefore, an incidence rate is calculated by dividing the total number of new cases of a specific disease (or the number of deaths) in a specified period, usually one year, by the average number of people in the population during the same period (Equation (2.2)). This is then usually multiplied by 100,000 (10^5) and presented as a rate per 10^5 people per year. The size of the population will, inevitably, change over a period of a year, so ideally we would use the number of people in the population in the middle of the year, the 'mid-interval' population, for our calculations. Depending on the data available, this may be calculated as the average of the size of the population at the start and at the end of the period of interest, or estimated from census data. Incidence rates may be calculated for a broad disease group (e.g. cancer) or a

Table 2.4 Crude mortality rates (per 100,000 per year) for ischaemic heart disease (IHD) in males from selected countries, 1995–1998.

Country	Crude IHD mortality rate (per 10^5/year)
Germany	211
Australia	168
Canada	160
Singapore	118
Spain	116
Japan	50
Brazil	47

(*Data source:* Global Cardiovascular Infobase, www.cvdinfobase.ca, accessed on 23 September 2003.)

more specific disease (e.g. breast cancer). Similarly, mortality rates may include deaths from all causes (sometimes called *all-cause* mortality) or only those from a specific cause. These basic rates are called **crude rates** because they describe the overall incidence or death rate in a population without taking any other features of the population into account (in contrast to **standardised rates** – see below).

Table 2.4 shows crude mortality rates for ischaemic heart disease (IHD) in men in seven countries. We see that Germany, Australia and Canada have high mortality rates, with intermediate rates in Singapore and Spain and low rates in Japan and Brazil. This correctly describes the total burdens that the different health systems have to cope with, but does it give an accurate picture of the level of mortality from IHD in each country? If we were to take this information at face value we would conclude that the death rate for IHD is three to four times higher in Western countries such as Germany, Australia and Canada than in countries like Japan and Brazil. Is that reasonable?

Age-specific incidence and mortality rates

A major disadvantage of crude rates is that they are just that – crude. They do not take into account the fact that different populations have different age structures and that the risk of becoming ill or dying varies with age. Many diseases are more common among older people and the older a person is, the greater their risk of dying. Developed countries like Germany have a high proportion of older people whereas less developed countries like Brazil have a much greater proportion of young people, at a relatively lower risk of dying. Their contrasting population structures are shown in Figure 2.3. In the example above it turns out that we are trying to compare countries with very different age structures, so a

Figure 2.3 Age distribution of the population in Brazil (1995, light bars) and Germany (1998, dark bars). (Drawn from Global Cardiovascular Infobase, www.cvdinfobase.ca, accessed 23 September 2003.)

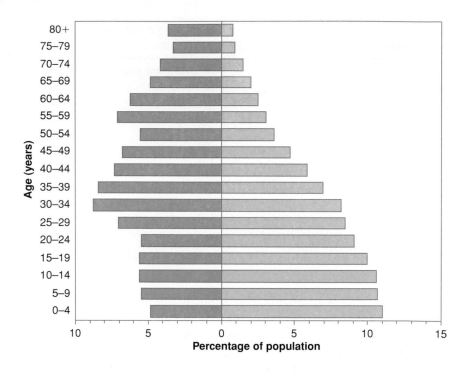

Box 2.6 Cardiovascular diseases simplified

You will find that, when we use examples relating to cardiovascular diseases, the conditions often have different names and abbreviations. Cardiovascular diseases are grouped and described in many different ways, emphasising the need to be sure that you know what the numbers you are looking at represent. The following is a simplified summary of some commonly used terms:

MI: myocardial infarction: heart attack

IHD: ischaemic heart disease: heart attack (MI) or angina

CHD: coronary heart disease: essentially identical to IHD

CVD: cardiovascular disease: includes CHD, stroke and other cardiac and vascular diseases (note that CVD can also be used as an abbreviation for cerebrovascular disease, i.e. stroke and transient ischaemic attack, but we will not use it in this way)

crude comparison of IHD mortality has little meaning if we are trying to assess the comparative 'cardiovascular health' of these countries (see also Box 2.6).

One obvious way to avoid this problem is to calculate separate rates for different age groups (*age-specific rates*). The rate in a particular age group can then be

Table 2.5 Crude and age-specific mortality rates (per 100,000 per year) for ischaemic heart disease in males from selected countries, 1995–1998.

Country	Crude rate (per 10^5/year)	Age-specific rates (per 10^5/year)	
		45–54 years	55–64 years
Germany	211	76	245
Australia	168	68	222
Canada	160	73	239
Singapore	118	100	346
Spain	116	59	156
Japan	50	20	60
Brazil	47	64	183

(*Data source:* Global Cardiovascular Infobase, www.cvdinfobase.ca, accessed on 23 September 2003.)

compared between countries. This process can be extended to calculate separate rates for other groups, for instance men and women (*sex-specific rates*), and for different racial or socioeconomic groups. Table 2.5 extends Table 2.4 to show selected age-specific mortality rates for the seven countries.

If we compare the age-specific rates we can see that in each country the rate is much higher in the older age group. We can also see that, while the crude rates for Singapore and Spain are similar, the age-specific rates are about twice as high in Singapore, which actually has the highest rates of all the countries in both age groups. Brazil has also moved up in the IHD rankings, although it still is doing better than Germany and Australia.

Standardised incidence and mortality rates

If age-specific rates are presented for a large number of different age groups, as well as for both sexes, we end up with a lot of numbers to compare and interpret (we only showed two age groups in Table 2.5 for simplicity). An alternative is to summarise or combine these age-specific rates using a process called standardisation. **Direct standardisation** involves calculating the overall incidence or mortality rate that you would have expected to find in a 'standard' population if it had the same age-specific rates as your study population. (The details of how to do this are shown in Appendix 1.) The same methods can also be used to standardise for other factors that differ between populations that you want to compare, for example sex or race, because disease rates often differ markedly between men and women and those from different ethnic backgrounds.

The age-standardised rates can then be compared across the populations (assuming that the disease is defined in the same way in each) because the

Table 2.6 Crude and age-standardised mortality rates (per 100,000 per year) for ischaemic heart disease in males from selected countries, 1995–1998.

Country	Crude IHD mortality rate (per 10^5/year)	Age-standardised rate (per 10^5/year)
Germany	211	121
Australia	168	111
Canada	160	108
Singapore	118	121
Spain	116	65
Japan	50	29
Brazil	47	60

(*Data source:* Global Cardiovascular Infobase, www.cvdinfobase.ca, accessed on 23 September 2003.)

problem of different age patterns has been removed (Table 2.6). You will notice that, in countries with an older population, the standardised rate is much lower than the crude rate, but in Brazil this pattern is reversed, and the standardised rate is higher than the crude rate because Brazil has a much younger population than the standard population used for this comparison. The age-standardised rates give a more accurate picture of the relative levels of IHD mortality in the seven countries than the crude rates did because they take into account the larger numbers of older people in the more developed countries. It is important to stress, however, that for any individual population the actual rates (crude or age-specific) are of much greater utility for health planning.

A note about standard populations

It is important to add a word of caution at this stage. There are many different 'standard populations' and, in practice, you can age-standardise to *any* population. You will often come across rates that have been standardised to the 'world' population, which reflects the average age structure of the whole world. Other common standard populations reflect the typical age structure of either 'developed' or 'developing' countries. If the aim is to compare rates in different groups within the same country then it is common practice to use the overall age structure of that country as the standard population. To some extent the choice is arbitrary, but it is important to note that if you standardise to two very different populations you will get very different standardised rates, and the relationships between different populations may change. For this reason, it is always important to note what standard population has been used.

For example, when we standardised IHD mortality in Germany to the world standard population we found an age-standardised rate of $121/10^5$ per year. If we

Box 2.7 An over-night doubling of all-cause mortality rates in the USA

Prior to 1999, various American health agencies had used different standard populations, including the 1940 population and the 1970 population, to report vital statistics. This made comparisons between data from different agencies problematic. In 1999 many of these agencies changed their standard population to the projected population in the year 2000 (the Year 2000 Population Standard). In comparison with the earlier populations, the Year 2000 population has fewer people under the age of 35 and more people in the middle and older age groups. Because the Year 2000 population is older and incidence and mortality rates of most diseases increase with age, rates standardised to this population tend to be much higher than those standardised to the 1940 and 1970 standards.

The change dramatically increased age-standardised rates in the USA. The all-cause mortality rate in 1979 was 577/100,000 per year (standardised to the 1940 population) and 1,011/100,000 per year (standardised to the Year 2000 standard population). The comparable difference for the all-cause mortality rate in 1995 was between 504/100,000 per year (1940 standard) and 919/100,000 per year (2000 standard). More reassuringly, in this example at least, the *relative* reduction in mortality between 1979 and 1995 was similar regardless of which standard population was used. Using the 1940 standard, the mortality rate appeared to fall from 577 to 504/100,000 per year, a drop of 13% over the period; using the Year 2000 standard, the rate fell from 1,011 to 919/100,000 per year, a drop of 9% (Anderson and Rosenberg, 1998).

had standardised to the younger 'African' standard population, we would have found an age-standardised rate of only $60/10^5$ per year, whereas if we had standardised to the older 'European' standard population we would have found an age-standardised rate of $198/10^5$ per year. In this example we were comparing populations around the world, so it was appropriate to use the world standard population. If all the countries had been in Europe or Africa then the European or African standard populations might have been more appropriate.

In 2002, the World Health Organization (WHO) proposed a new world standard population to reflect the general ageing of populations around the world. (This and examples of other common standard populations are provided in Appendix 2.) However, what seems like a logical updating of information has major ramifications for anyone looking at time trends in the occurrence of disease because rates cannot usefully be compared if they have been standardised to different populations (see Box 2.7).

Measuring cumulative incidence using routine statistics

Routine statistics may also be used to estimate cumulative incidence. This gives the probability or risk that someone will develop disease (or die) within a given time period, and this time period can be anything from a few days to a lifetime (a lifetime is commonly taken as ages 0 to 74 years). For example, men in Australia have a lifetime cumulative incidence of lung cancer of 4.2% or, in other words, 4.2% of Australian men will develop lung cancer before their 75th birthday (AIHW and AICR 2008). An alternative way to look at the same information is to say that the average *lifetime risk* of lung cancer in Australian men is '1 in 24' or, in other words, 1 in every 24 Australian men will develop lung cancer before their 75th birthday. Note that these measures assume that someone remains 'at risk' of lung cancer until their 75th birthday and they also do not take into account any other factors, such as smoking. Clearly the lifetime risk will be much higher for a smoker than for a non-smoker and for personalising risk, for example in the doctor's surgery, smoking-specific cumulative incidence would be much more informative, but special research studies with individual exposures are needed to provide such data. (The methods for calculating cumulative incidence and lifetime risk for routine data are shown in Appendix 3.)

Other measures commonly used in public health

We will now consider some other measures that are used commonly in public health to assess different aspects of disease burden. Many of these descriptive measures are fundamental to health planning and service provision. They are expressed in a variety of ways – some are ratios, some percentages, i.e. per 100 population, while others are shown per 1,000, 10,000 or 100,000 population. In some cases different people will use the same term to describe a slightly different measure. The definitions that we give are as in *A Dictionary of Epidemiology* (Porta, 2008) and are probably those most commonly used. Whenever you come across these rates it is advisable to check exactly what the numbers being compared are, and what the size of the reference population is – whether the rate refers to 100, 1,000 or 100,000 events or people.

Standardised incidence and mortality ratios

Figure 1.5 in Chapter 1 showed standardised mortality ratios (SMRs) for Indigenous compared to non-Indigenous Australians. These come from an alternative way of standardising rates called **indirect standardisation** (see Appendix 4). In this example the standardisation is for age but the same process is commonly used to adjust for sex and/or to compare data from different time periods. The actual number of deaths 'observed' in a population (e.g. deaths from cancer in Indigenous men) is compared with the number of deaths that would have been 'expected' if the death rates in the Indigenous population had been the same as those for the non-Indigenous population. The standardised mortality ratio (SMR) is calculated by dividing the observed number of deaths (O) by the expected number (E). This measure tells us how much more common death from cancer is in Indigenous people than in the non-Indigenous population (about 1.6 times in this case). We can do exactly the same thing with disease incidence to calculate a standardised incidence ratio (SIR; note that some people call this a standardised morbidity ratio and thus use SMR to describe both standardised mortality and morbidity ratios; we and others use SMR and SIR to distinguish between mortality and incidence.) Standardised incidence ratios are also commonly reported by cancer registries, which are among the few sources of reliable incidence data at the population level.

The SMR and SIR are similar to the relative risk that you met in Chapter 1. Remember also that Snow used observed and expected numbers of deaths to show that cholera mortality in the workhouse near the Broad Street pump was unexpectedly low (Box 1.4). Strictly speaking, they are *measures of association* because they compare disease incidence or mortality in one population with that in a reference population and, as such, would fit more logically into Chapter 5. We have included them here because of the parallels between the processes of direct and indirect standardisation (See Box 2.8 and Table 2.7).

Box 2.8 Direct vs indirect standardisation

It can be hard to get your head around the difference between direct and indirect standardisation. When we standardise for age using **direct standardisation** we calculate the overall *rate* that we would see in a 'standard' population if it had the same age-specific rates of disease as our study population. We can then compare rates that have been directly age-standardised to the same standard population because any age-differences between the original populations have been removed.

In contrast, when we use **indirect standardisation** we calculate the *number of cases* we would have expected to see in our study population if it had the same age-specific rates of disease as a standard population (often the general population). We then compare this expected number of cases to the number of cases that actually occurred in the study population (the 'observed' number) and calculate a standardised incidence (or mortality) ratio by dividing the observed number of cases by the expected number.

Table 2.7 summarises the differences between the two methods; although these are presented in terms of age-standardisation the same issues apply if we are standardising for sex, race or any other factors.

Table 2.7 Direct versus indirect standardisation for age.

	Direct standardisation	Indirect standardisation
Information required	Age-specific rates in *study* population Age distribution of *standard* population	Age-specific rates in *standard* population Age distribution of *study* population Total number of cases (deaths) in *study* population
Measure calculated	Age-standardised incidence (mortality) rate	Standard incidence (mortality) ratio (SIR/SMR)
Advantages and disadvantages	Good for comparing large populations where the age-specific rates are reliable; *less good for small populations because the age-specific rates may be unstable* Allows comparisons between the standardised rates for different populations	Can be used when the age-specific rates in the study population are unknown or unreliable, for example when the population is small. *Two SIRs and SMRs cannot be directly compared because they are both calculated relative to a separate third population*
Uses	Commonly used to compare rates across different countries or between large sub-groups within a country, for example men versus women	Often used to compare incidence or mortality in smaller subgroups of a population, for example veterans from a particular armed conflict, to the general population *Although direct standardisation could be used in this situation, if the subgroup is relatively small the age-specific rates may not be very reliable and indirect standardisation is preferred*

The proportional (or proportionate) mortality ratio (PMR)

This is a measure of the relative importance of a particular cause of death in a given population. A PMR looks like an SMR but it is used when there is insufficient information to calculate an SMR (usually because information is available only about those who have died, so it is not possible to calculate mortality rates). It is calculated by dividing the *proportion* of deaths due to a specific cause in a group of interest by the *proportion* of deaths due to the same cause in a comparison group. A PMR is commonly multiplied by 100, so a PMR of 100 means that the proportions of deaths due to a specific cause are the same in the study and comparison groups, and a PMR of 200 indicates that twice as many of the deaths in the study group are due to the specific cause. Proportional mortality ratios are most commonly used in occupational studies. For example, a study of deaths among electrical workers on construction sites in the USA found that 127 of the

Box 2.9 Rates, ratios and proportions

A **ratio** is simply one number divided by another number; for example, the number of beers drunk in one year divided by the number of people in the population (beers per capita) or the number of cases observed divided by the number of cases expected.

A **proportion** is a special type of ratio in which everything or everyone in the numerator is also counted in the denominator; for example, the number of people who develop disease divided by the total number of people in the population (those with and without disease). A proportion can be expressed as a number between 0 and 1 or as a percentage between 0 and 100%. All proportions are ratios – not all ratios are proportions.

A **rate** should contain some measure of time, for example 60 km *per hour*, 17/100,000 *per year*.

As an example, the **case–fatality ratio** is a proportion and therefore also a ratio, but is not a rate (although it is often described as such) because it does not contain units of time.

total of 31,068 deaths (0.4%) were due to electrocution. This value was almost 12 times higher (PMR = 1,180) than the proportion of such deaths that would be expected in the general US population (Robinson *et al.*, 1999). Proportional mortality ratios have fairly limited utility because they cannot easily be compared across different populations. They are usually calculated only when no population data are readily available and precise mortality rates cannot be calculated.

The case–fatality ratio (CFR)

The CFR (often called the case–fatality *rate*, although, strictly speaking, it is not a rate; see Box 2.9 above) is the proportion of people with a given disease or condition who die from it in a given period. It is a common measure of the short-term severity of an acute disease and allows a direct assessment of the effectiveness of an intervention. For example, the CFR for myocardial infarction (heart attack) is usually measured over a period of 28 days. When deaths occur over a longer time period then it is more appropriate to consider the survival rate (see below). The CFR is usually expressed per 100 cases, i.e. as a percentage. As an example, the overall CFR in the 2003 SARS epidemic was estimated to be 14%–15%, i.e. approximately one in every seven people who contracted SARS died. However, this average ratio hides the fact that, while patients under the age of 25 were unlikely to die (CFR = 1%), approximately half of patients over the age of 65 died (CFR = 50%). (Note that the mortality from SARS occurred so quickly that the particular time period the CFR refers to is generally not specified.)

Survival rate and relative survival rate

As we discussed above, the CFR is an appropriate measure for short-term mortality (a month or so) but is less useful for conditions in which death may occur further down the track. For conditions such as cancer, mortality is often expressed in terms of the proportion of patients who are still alive a specified number of years after diagnosis – the **survival rate**. This proportion is often adjusted to allow for the fact that, depending on the age group being considered, some people would have been expected to die anyway from causes other than their cancer and this is known as the **relative survival rate**. A relative survival rate of 100% thus indicates that mortality does not differ from that experienced by the general population. For example, in developed countries five-year relative survival rates for breast cancer are approximately 75%–80%, compared with only about 15% for lung cancer.

Measures of mortality related to childbirth and early life

In the second half of the twentieth century, organisations such as the World Health Organization started using a number of measures relating to maternal and, in particular, infant mortality as critical indicators of the general health of a community. This allowed comparison between regions and also tracking of improvements in health over time. Table 2.8 shows a number of these measures. (Note that, technically, they are *proportions* rather than true *rates* because they do not have units of time – see Box 2.8; they are, however, commonly described as rates and we will also use this terminology.)

The underlying concept of each rate is the same – it is the ratio of the actual number of deaths that occur in one year to the total population 'at risk of death' in the same year. Because it is not always possible to obtain an accurate figure for the number of people at risk, an approximation is sometimes used. For example, any woman who is pregnant is at risk of maternal death but the number of women who are pregnant in a given year is not routinely recorded, so in practice this is estimated by taking the number of live births in one year. It is also worth noting that the *infant mortality rate* is the number of infant deaths (age 0–1 year) relative to the number of live births in the same year. This means that the children in the numerator (deaths) are not the same as those in the denominator (births) because many of those who die will have been born in the previous year. This is not a problem if the birth rate is fairly stable.

For each rate we have given the most standard definition but, as you will see, there are some variations. For example, the *stillbirth* (or *fetal death*) *rate* should be calculated as the ratio of stillbirths to the number of live births *plus* the number of stillbirths. This is because all of these children (live plus stillbirths) were at risk of being stillborn although not all of them were. This measure is, however,

Table 2.8 Measures of mortality related to childbirth and early life.

Measure	Deaths (numerator)	Population at risk (denominator)	Notes
Maternal mortality rate	Deaths among women from causes related to childbirth in 1 year (the WHO defines this as deaths up to 42 days after birth, but sometimes deaths up to 1 year are included)	Number of live births in the same year	Strictly speaking the denominator should be *all* pregnant women but this information is not recorded directly
Stillbirth or fetal death rate	Number of stillbirths in 1 year where a stillbirth is usually a fetal death after 28 weeks gestation although other time points may also be used (e.g. 20 weeks)	Live births + fetal deaths in the same year	Sometimes calculated as the ratio of the number of fetal deaths to the number of live births (excluding fetal deaths). This is often called the *fetal death ratio*
Perinatal mortality rate	Fetal deaths (>28 weeks) and deaths up to 7 days of life	Live births + fetal deaths in the same year	May be calculated as the ratio of the number of deaths to the number of live births (excluding fetal deaths) and called the *perinatal death ratio* May also include deaths up to 28 days of life
Neonatal mortality rate	Deaths in children aged less than 28 days	Number of live births in the same year	Only live births are included in the denominator because only babies born alive are at risk of dying before the age of 28 days
Post-neonatal mortality rate	Deaths in children from 28 days to 1 year	Number of live births in the same year	Strictly speaking the denominator should exclude children who die before age 28 days because they are no longer at risk.
Infant mortality rate	Deaths in children up to 1 year of age	Number of live births in the same year	Probably the most widely used single indicator of the overall health of a community
Child death rate	Deaths in children aged 1 to 4 years	Number of children aged 1–4 years in the population	An example of an age-specific mortality rate.
Child mortality rate	Deaths in children up to 5 years of age	Number of live births in the same year	An alternative to the child death rate, preferable in countries where it is hard to enumerate the population of young children

Figure 2.4 Infant mortality rates in relation to GDP in 20 countries around the world. (Drawn from: The World Factbook 2009. Washington DC. Central Intelligence Agency, 2009. https://www.cia.gov/library/publications/the-world-factbook/index.html, accessed 16 January 2010.)

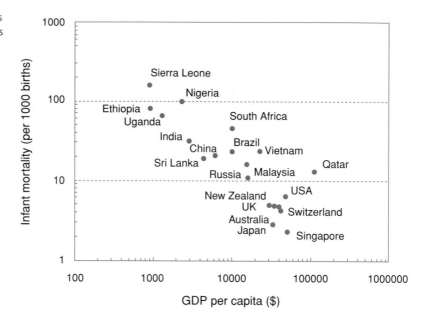

sometimes presented as a *stillbirth* or *fetal death ratio* where only live births are counted in the denominator. The WHO in particular tends to use this variant. Because the number of live births will be less than the number of live births plus stillbirths, the fetal death or stillbirth ratio will always be slightly larger than the stillbirth rate. You will also notice that there is not always a standard definition of what constitutes a case (in this case a death). It just goes to reinforce how important it is to check exactly what the numbers refer to in order to make sure that you are always comparing like with like.

Figure 2.4 shows the enormous variation in infant mortality rates around the world, reflecting the great disadvantages under which many countries still labour. It also shows the very strong inverse correlation between GDP (gross domestic product) and infant mortality – the more wealthy a country the lower the infant mortality rate. In a poor country like Sierra Leone the rate is as high as 154 per 1,000 live births. In other words, more than one in 10 babies die before their first birthday, compared with less than 3 per 1,000 in Japan and Singapore.

It is important to remember that all of these measures just give an average picture for the whole population. Low average rates can often hide much higher rates in some subgroups of the population. This is particularly true in countries that include more than one ethnic group. For example, as you saw in Chapter 1, in Australia the Indigenous population has mortality rates that are several times higher than those of Australians as a whole, and in the USA in 2004 infant mortality was considerably higher among births to non-Hispanic black women

(13.6 per 1,000 live births) than for White or Asian and Pacific Islander mothers (5.7 and 4.7 per 1,000, respectively) (Mathews *et al.*, 2007).

Measuring the 'burden of disease'

In Table 2.6 we saw that age-standardised rates of heart disease were higher in Germany and Singapore than in Spain and Brazil, which, in turn, had higher rates than Japan, but this is only one disease; how does the overall health of these populations compare? The measures that we have looked at so far have focused on either morbidity (incidence) or mortality and many are only really useful for describing a single disease or group of diseases at a time. They can tell us how rates of cancer or mortality from heart disease vary between countries or over time but they are less useful if we want to look at the overall health of a population at a particular point in time and see how it compares with other time periods and/or populations. Although global mortality measures such as the total mortality rate and the infant mortality rate give a broad view of this aspect of the health of a nation or group, they quite obviously tell us nothing about the many states of ill-health short of death. To make comparisons that are more inclusive of other aspects of health we need to use measures that allow us to combine the effects of multiple diseases as well as accounting for their severity and when they occur in life.

To solve this problem several different mortality- and morbidity-related measures have been developed to describe the health of populations. New and more sophisticated variations are continually being introduced as organisations such as the WHO attempt not only to measure disease, but also to take into account related conditions such as pain, disability and loss of income that are associated with ill-health. These measures bring us closer to measuring the overall 'health' of a population according to the WHO definition of health, and are being used increasingly by national and regional health departments for planning and resource allocation.

Life expectancy

A traditional mortality-based measure that accounts for the *timing* of death is **life expectancy**, the average number of years that an individual of a given age is expected to live *if current mortality rates continue*. For example, a boy born in the Russian Federation in 2002 has a life expectancy of 58.4 years, compared with 78.4 years for a boy born in Japan (WHO, 2003). Because it cannot take account of future changes in incidence and/or treatment of diseases, estimates of life expectancy are largely hypothetical. Mortality rates have been falling over time and, until recently, the expectation has been that this trend would continue into

Figure 2.5 Survivorship curve for Australian males and females in 2005–2007. (Drawn from: Australian Bureau of Statistics, 2007.)

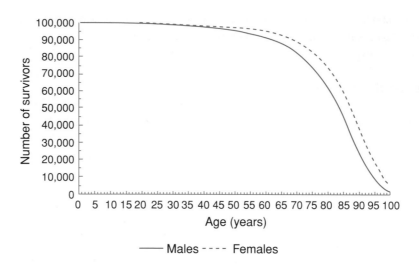

the future. Life expectancy figures therefore almost certainly underestimate the actual number of years someone could expect to live. However, the HIV/AIDS epidemic and other national phenomena, such as that seen for Russian men in Figure 1.2, have already reversed this situation in some countries; and this could become more generally true with the increasing 'obesity epidemic' in many Westernised countries predicted to lead to higher mortality rates and thus lower life expectancy in future (Olshansky *et al.*, 2005).

Life expectancy can be presented for any age, but is used most commonly to describe life expectancy at birth. It is calculated using a 'life-table' similar in principle to that shown in Table 1.4. The starting point is a hypothetical group of newborns (usually 100,000) and age-specific mortality rates are then used to estimate the number that would be expected to die at each year of life. The total number of years of life expected for the entire cohort can then be added up and the life expectancy at birth is this total divided by 100,000. Life expectancy at other ages is estimated by adding up the number of years of life after the age of interest and dividing by the number of people in the cohort who had reached that age (see Appendix 5 for the detailed calculations). If we draw a graph of the number or proportion of people expected to survive to each age we get what is called a survival curve. Figure 2.5 shows the survival curves for Australian men and women in 2005–2007, illustrating the survival advantage that women still have over men.

Potential and expected years of life lost (PYLL and EYLL)

Life expectancy measures what is being achieved and is sometimes described as a measure of **health expectancy**. An alternative approach is to measure what is being lost and this type of indicator is sometimes described as a **health gap** (Lopez *et al.*, 2006 p. 47). One such measure looks not at the number of years someone can expect to live, but instead at the numbers of years of potential life they have lost if they die before a certain age. This age is frequently taken to be 65 although, with increasing numbers of people now living active lives well beyond this age, some reports now consider deaths before 70 to be 'premature' deaths. The number of **potential years of life lost** (PYLL) in a population is calculated by counting the total number of deaths from a specific cause in each age group and then multiplying this by the average number of years of life lost as a result of each of these deaths. For example, taking 65 as the cut-off age, a death from coronary heart disease at age 60 would contribute only 5 potential years of life lost compared with 15 years for a death at age 50. Thus, although there are fewer deaths among younger people, each contributes a greater number of PYLL than the deaths in the elderly.

One advantage this measure has over life expectancy is that it is possible to count the PYLL due to specific causes of death such as cancer or heart disease and thus to target those conditions with the highest PYLL. The years of life lost due to each cause of death can also be summed to give the total years of life lost. The same is not true for health expectancy measures because it is not possible to attribute years of life expectancy to the absence of a specific cause of death. The downside of calculating PYLL is that the choice of the age below which deaths are considered premature is arbitrary and deaths that occur above the specified cut-off age are not counted at all. One way of getting around this is to calculate **expected years of life lost** (EYLL) where the number of years of life lost due to a death at any age is equal to the life expectancy at that age. It is also important to be aware that, unlike life expectancy measures, both PYLL and EYLL depend on the size of the population. Assuming two populations have similar life expectancy and mortality rates, the PYLL lost for the larger population will always be greater than that for the smaller population. It is, however, possible to get around this by calculating average PYLL to facilitate comparisons between populations.

Disability-free life expectancy

As we said at the beginning of this section, it is also important to consider morbidity to create a fuller picture of a population's health. There is little point in working to extend life expectancy if the additional years of life are lived in very poor health. This concept is illustrated by the survival curves shown in Figure 2.6. As in Figure 2.5, the top line shows the proportion of people surviving at each age, but now the lower line shows the smaller proportion of people who are still in full health at each age. The combined areas A and B represent total life expectancy, but only a proportion of that life, the area A, is lived in full health, while area B

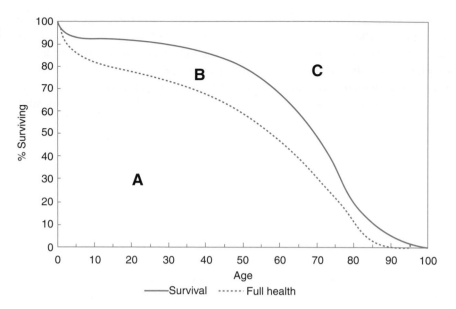

Figure 2.6 Survivorship curves showing years of life lived in full health (A), years lived in less than full health (B) and years of life lost (C). (Adapted from: Murray *et al.*, 2000.)

indicates life lived with some degree of disability. Area C represents the potential years of life lost and the combined areas C and B represent the total health gap – the loss both of years of life and years of health. So how can we measure this?

One solution is to refine the calculations of total life expectancy to calculate **disability-free life expectancy**, which takes into account not only age-specific mortality rates but also the prevalence of disability at that age. This measure effectively adjusts the number of years of life expected for an individual at a given age by the probability that those years will be lived with some degree of disability. One advantage of this measure is that it is relatively simple to calculate, and as a result it is quite widely used. However, it also has some major disadvantages in that, first, an arbitrary decision has to be made as to what level of disability will lead to someone being classified as disabled and, secondly, years of life lived with disability are not counted at all and thus are effectively considered as bad as being dead – a clearly unreasonable situation.

Quality-adjusted life years (QALYs)

The problem of how best to integrate measures of morbidity and mortality also arises in clinical trials. Before introducing a new treatment it is important to know that it will either increase life expectancy, improve quality of life, or both. A treatment that improves both survival and quality of life is clearly worth having but how can we compare two drugs if one increases survival but at the expense of worse quality of life? This challenge led to the development of the concept of a **quality-adjusted life year** (QALY). Quality-adjusted life years weight each

Table 2.9 Life expectancy and health-adjusted life expectancy at birth and age 60 (years).

	Males			Females		
	Life expectancy at birth[a]	Health-adjusted life expectancy		Life expectancy at birth[a]	Health-adjusted life expectancy	
		At birth[a]	At age 60[b]		At birth[a]	At age 60[b]
Australia	79	72	16.9	84	75	19.5
India	63	56	10.8	65	57	11.4
Japan	79	73	17.5	86	78	21.7
Malawi	49	43	9.7	51	44	10.4
Russian Federation	60	55	10.1	73	65	14.2
Switzerland	79	73	17.1	84	76	20.4
United Kingdom	77	71	15.7	82	73	18.1
Unites States of America	76	68	15.3	81	72	17.9

(*Data sources:* [a] Data for 2007 from World Health Organization, 2009; [b] Data for 2002 from World Health Organization, 2003.)

year of life by the perceived quality of that life from a value of one for perfect health down to zero for death. One QALY would thus represent a year of life in perfect health while 0.5 QALY could represent 6 months lived in perfect health or 12 months with 50% disability (or ill-health). The QALYs gained from a new radical treatment that increases life expectancy by 10 years but is associated with major side-effects might thus be lower than those from a less effective drug that increases life expectancy by only 8 years but does not have any major side-effects. It is, however, important to note that these measures are entirely dependent on the magnitude of the weights assigned to different health conditions and this process is necessarily highly subjective.

Health-adjusted life expectancy (HALE)

By combining QALYs with measures of life expectancy we can calculate **health-adjusted life expectancy** (HALE), which is based on life expectancy at birth but includes an adjustment for time spent in poor health. It represents the equivalent number of years an individual can expect to live *in full health*. A health-adjusted life expectancy of 60 years might therefore represent an expectation of 50 years life in full health plus an additional 20 years at 50% or 30 years at 33% of full health.

Table 2.9 shows data on life expectancy and health-adjusted life expectancy for a number of different countries. Notice that healthy life expectancy is consistently 6–8 years less than life expectancy for men and 7–9 years less for women.

This difference is a function both of the expected number of years of life at less than full health and of the extent of disability. Because life expectancy at birth is partly dependent on mortality in the first year of life, it is inevitably much lower in developing countries, which tend to have much higher neonatal and infant mortality rates than developed countries. Once an individual has survived the first few years of life in a developing country, however, their chances of living to old age are then much greater and the difference between developed and developing countries becomes less marked. As an example, see the apparent paradox in Malawi. Healthy life expectancy at birth for a man in 2007 was only 43 years, due largely to the enormous toll that HIV/AIDS has taken on the countries in sub-Saharan Africa; but, if a man makes it to 60, he can then expect about another 10 years of healthy life. Notice also that, while in most countries women can expect to live about 2–5 years longer than men, the high mortality rates among young Russian men (Figure 1.2) mean that the difference in the Russian Federation is 13 years.

Disability-adjusted life years (DALYs)

The concept of a **disability-adjusted life year** or DALY was developed to facilitate attempts to quantify the global burden of disease (World Bank, 1993). Like the expected years of life lost you met earlier, disability-adjusted life years estimate loss of life but they have a major advantage in that they count not only years of life lost completely due to premature death but also years of health lost through disability. As for QALYs, the extent of disability is weighted from zero to one, although the weights go in the opposite direction – from zero for a year spent in perfect health to one for a year lost to death (Lopez *et al.*, 2006, pp. 119–125). These weights were defined by an international panel of health experts. (Note that the actual calculations are somewhat more complicated than this because they also take age into account and consider that productive years lost in mid-life are more important than years lost at very young or old ages.) One DALY can be thought of as one lost year of healthy life. Thus, if a person lives with a moderate disability for 10 years, this might equate to the loss of 5 years of healthy life or five DALYs. Like the measures of potential years of life lost, DALYs are a health gap indicator and have the useful property that they can be calculated separately for different diseases (see Table 2.10) or for different causes of disease such as smoking or unsafe drinking water (Table 2.11). Measurements of DALYs are increasingly used to estimate the burden of various diseases or exposures in different countries, as for example in the World Health Reports produced by the WHO (WHO, 2008), and to identify priorities for health intervention.

The use of measures like DALYs highlights the enormous burden of ill-health due to some common but non-fatal conditions such as unipolar depressive

Table 2.10 The 10 leading causes of mortality and disability-adjusted life-years in the world, 2004 (from WHO, 2008).

Mortality	Deaths (millions)	% of total deaths	Burden of disease	DALYs (millions)	% of total DALYs
Ischaemic heart disease	7.2	12.2	Lower respiratory infections	94.5	6.2
Cerebrovascular disease	5.7	9.7	Diarrhoeal diseases	72.8	4.8
Lower respiratory infections	4.2	7.1	Unipolar depressive disorders	65.5	4.3
Chronic obstructive pulmonary disease	3.0	5.1	Ischaemic heart disease	62.6	4.1
Diarrhoeal diseases	2.2	3.7	HIV/AIDS	58.5	3.8
HIV/AIDS	2.0	3.5	Cerebrovascular disease	46.6	3.1
Tuberculosis	1.5	2.5	Prematurity/low birth weight	44.3	2.9
Trachea, bronchus and lung cancers	1.3	2.3	Birth asphyxia/trauma	41.7	2.7
Road traffic accidents	1.3	2.2	Road traffic accidents	41.2	2.7
Prematurity/low birth weight	1.2	2.0	Neonatal infections and other conditions	40.4	2.7

Table 2.11 The top 10 causes of DALYs in the world, by income level, 2001 (from Lopez *et al.*, 2006).

Risk factor	Low- and middle-income countries DALYs (millions)	% of all DALYs	High-income countries DALYs (millions)	% of all DALYs
Childhood underweight	121	8.7	<0.1	<0.1
High blood pressure	78	5.6	14.0	9.3
Unsafe sex	80	5.8	0.9	0.6
Smoking	54	3.9	19.0	12.7
Alcohol use	49	3.6	7.0	4.4
High cholesterol	43	3.1	9.4	6.3
Unsafe water, sanitation and hygiene	52	3.7	1.8	0.2
Overweight and obesity	32	2.3	11.0	7.2
Indoor smoke from household use of solid fuels	42	3.0	<0.1	<0.1
Low fruit and vegetable intake	33	2.4	4.0	2.7

disorders that do not feature at all on lists derived from mortality-based indicators. It also highlights the enormous burden of ill-health attributable to some entirely preventable risk factors such as smoking and unsafe sex. They can also give a very different sense of priorities for disease control from conventional rates (Figure 2.7 and Box 2.10). Injury, for example, kills proportionally

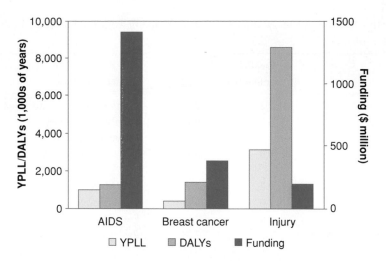

Figure 2.7 Potential years of life lost (PYLL) and disability-adjusted life-years (DALYs) for AIDS, breast cancer and injury in relation to research expenditure by the US National Institutes of Health in 1996. (Drawn from: Gross *et al.*, 1999.)

Box 2.10 Suicide rates: are we winning or losing?

Suicide is a major cause of premature mortality in many countries, but is the situation becoming better or worse? Data from the UK show that

- between 1981 and 1998, suicide rates in men and women aged 15 and over *fell by 18%*;
- between 1981 and 1998, the years of potential life lost due to suicide *increased by 5%*.

How do we interpret these apparently conflicting data? The answer is that the major drop in suicide rates has occurred among the older age groups (45 years and over) and suicide rates in younger men have actually increased over the same time period. Suicide in a younger person leads to greater loss of potential life, so although the overall suicide rates are falling, this average effect hides an increasing loss of life among young men.

These data underline how different measures of health capture different things and can give very different pictures of the health of a population. A politician hoping to demonstrate improvements in mental health could legitimately claim that suicide rates were falling, while an advocate for more funding for mental health could equally legitimately cite the increase in years of life lost.

(Gunnell and Middleton, 2003.)

more young people than other conditions and so makes a major contribution to years of life lost due to premature death and to disability, yet far greater financial resources tend to be given to research into high-profile conditions such as breast cancer and AIDS.

Table 2.12 A summary of measures of disease occurrence.

Measure	Definition	Formula	Units
Prevalence (P)	The *proportion* of the population with disease at a specific point in time	No. people with disease at a given point in time / Total number of people in the population	% or proportion (e.g. 0.01) (or per 1,000, 10,000, 100,000 etc.)
Cumulative incidence (CI)	The *proportion* of people who develop disease during a specified period. Synonyms: *Attack Rate, Experimental* and *Control Event Rate* (in the treated and control groups in a clinical trial)	No. who develop disease in a specified period / No. at risk of the disease at the start of the period	% or proportion (or per 1,000, 10,000, 100,000 etc.)
Incidence rate (IR)	The *rate* at which disease is occurring, measured from individual data in a study. Synonym: *Incidence density*	No. who develop disease in a specified period / No. *person-years* at risk of getting the disease	per 100,000/person-years (or per 1,000, 10,000 person-years etc.)
	The *rate* at which disease is occurring, measured from population data, may be *crude, specific* (e.g. age-specific) or *standardised* (direct standardisation)	No. people who develop disease in one year / Average no. in the population in the same year	per 100,000/year (or per 1,000, 10,000/year etc.)
Standardised incidence or mortality ratio (SIR / SMR)	Compares incidence or mortality to a standard population using *indirect* standardisation	Observed number of cases (deaths) / No. expected for a standard population	A ratio, sometimes a percentage
Proportional mortality ratio (PMR)	Compares the *proportion* of deaths to a standard population (can be used when information is only available for deaths)	Proportion of deaths from a specific cause / Proportion expected for a standard population	A ratio, sometimes a percentage
Case–fatality ratio (CFR)	The proportion of people who die from a disease in a specified (usually short) time period (actually a measure of *cumulative incidence*)	No. who die from disease in a specified period / Total no. with disease	A percentage (or per 1,000, 10,000, 100,000 etc.)

Summary

As you have seen, a plethora of measures are used to try to quantify the health of a population and all of these have their advantages and limitations. Some measure only limited aspects of health but are commonly used because they are easy to calculate, whereas other more complex measures come closer to capturing our ideal notion of 'health' but are much harder to calculate and thus not so easily applied in practice. All measures have their uses and selection of the most appropriate measure for any given situation will depend almost entirely on the question being asked. You should now be able to interpret most measures of disease and health that you come across (the key features of the main incidence and mortality measures are summarised in Table 2.12). It is still important to be very careful when comparing measures of disease across different groups of people because many other factors can complicate the comparisons. We will discuss some of these issues in the following chapters.

Questions

1. For each of the following scenarios, calculate a measure of the incidence of disease and identify what type of measure it is:
   (a) A thousand healthy women were followed for 8 years and 15 developed high blood pressure.
   (b) A large group of elderly men was followed for a total of 5,000 person-years and 75 of the men had a stroke during the duration of the study.
   (c) In a community with a population of 50,000 people, 27 developed diabetes during a 1-year period.
2. Two thousand women aged 55 years were given a health check and 100 were found to have high blood pressure. Ten years later all 2,000 women attended a second check and another 300 women had developed high blood pressure.
   (a) What was the prevalence of high blood pressure in the women (i) at age 55 and (ii) at age 65?
   (b) How many women were 'at risk' of developing high blood pressure at the start of the 10-year period?
   (c) What was the incidence of high blood pressure in these women? Is this a measure of cumulative incidence or an incidence rate?

Assume that, on average, each of the 300 women who developed high blood pressure did so half-way through the 10 year follow-up period.
   (d) Calculate the total number of person-years at risk (of developing high blood pressure) during the 10 years.
   (e) What was the incidence rate of high blood pressure in these women?

3. Community A and community B both have crude mortality rates for ischaemic heart disease of 4 per 1000 population per year. The age-adjusted mortality rate for ischaemic heart disease in community A is 5 per 1000 population and the age-adjusted rate for ischaemic heart disease in community B is 3 per 1000 population. Which of the following is correct?
   (a) community A has a younger population than community B
   (b) community A has an older population than community B
   (c) diagnosis is more accurate in community A
   (d) diagnosis is more accurate in community B.

4. Look back to Table 2.10. What does this tell us about the relative importance of ischaemic heart disease and diarrhoeal diseases as causes of mortality and ill health and explain the patterns you see.

REFERENCES

Agarwal, M. M. and Punnose, J. (2002). Gestational diabetes: implications of variation in diagnostic criteria. *International Journal of Gynecology and Obstetrics*, **78**: 45–46.

Anderson, R. and Rosenberg, H. (1998). Age standardization of death rates: implementation of the Year 2000 standard. *National Vital Statistics Reports*, vol. 47 no. 3, Hyattsville, MD: National Center for Health Statistics.

Australian Bureau of Statistics. (2007). Life Tables Australia: 2005–2007. ABS Publication 3302.*0.55.001*. (http://www.abs.gov.au, accessed on 12 September 2009)

Australian Institute of Health and Welfare (AIHW) and Australian Association of Cancer Registries (AACR). (2008). Cancer in Australia.

CDC (Centers for Disease Control) Division of Viral Hepatitis. (2009). *Disease Burden from Viral Hepatitis A, B, and C in the United States*. (http://www.cdc.gov/hepatitis/PDFs/Disease_burden.pdf, accessed 20 September 2009)

Chan, K.-L., Dumesnil, J. G., Cujec, B. *et al*. for the Investigators of the Multicenter Aspirin Study in Infective Endocarditis. (2003). A randomized trial of aspirin on the risk of embolic events in patients with infective endocarditis. *Journal of the American College of Cardiologists*, **42**: 775–780.

Gross, C. P., Anderson, G. F. and Powe, N. R. (1999). The relation between funding by the National Institutes of Health and the burden of disease. *New England Journal of Medicine*, **340**: 1881–1887.

Gunnell, D. and Middleton, N. (2003). National suicide rates as an indicator of the effect of suicide on premature mortality. *Lancet*, **362**: 961–962.

Lopez, A. D., Mathers, C. D., Ezzati, M. *et al*. (Eds) (2006). *Global burden of disease and risk factors*. World Bank and Oxford University Press.

Mathews, T. J. and Macdorman, M. F. (2007). Infant mortality statistics from the 2004 period linked birth/infant death data set. *National Vital Statistics Reports*, vol. 55 no. 14. Hyattsville, MD: National Center for Health Statistics.

Murray, C. J. L., Salomon, J. A. and Mathers, C. (2000). A critical examination of summary measures of population health. *Bulletin of the World Health Organization*, **78**: 981–994.

Olshansky, S. J., Passaro, D. J., Hershow, R. C. *et al.* (2005). A potential decline in life expectancy in the United States in the 21st century. *New England Journal of Medicine,* **352**: 1138–1145.

Population Reference Bureau. (2007). *2007 World Population Data Sheet.* PRB. (www.prb. org)

Porta, M. (Ed.) (2008). *A Dictionary of Epidemiology,* 5th edn. New York: Oxford University Press.

Robinson, C. F., Petersen, M. and Palu, S. (1999). Mortality patterns among electrical workers employed in the U.S. construction industry, 1982–1987. *American Journal of Industrial Medicine,* **36**: 630–637.

UNAIDS. (2007). *AIDS Epidemic Update December 2007.* Geneva: UNAIDS. (www.unaids. org)

Veenhoven, R. (2002). Commentary: the units of utility. *International Journal of Epidemiology,* **31**: 1144–1146.

WHO (World Health Organization). (2003). *The World Health Report 2003: Shaping the Future.* Geneva: World Health Organization.

WHO (World Health Organization). (2008). *The Global Burden of Disease: 2004 Update.* Geneva: World Health Organization.

WHO (World Health Organization). (2009). *World Health Statistics 2009.* Geneva: World Health Organization.

World Bank. (1993). *Investing in Health: World Development Report 1993.* New York: Oxford University Press.

Who, what, where and when? Descriptive epidemiology

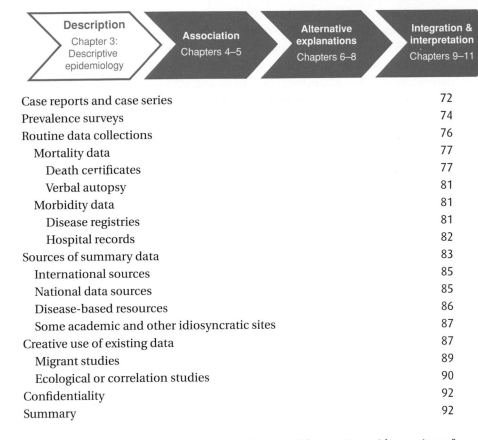

Description
Chapter 3:
Descriptive
epidemiology

Association
Chapters 4–5

Alternative
explanations
Chapters 6–8

Integration &
interpretation
Chapters 9–11

Practical
applications
Chapters 12–15

The rates and measures you have been exploring in Chapter 2 provide a variety of ways of describing the health of populations and thus also enable us to compare patterns of health and disease between populations and over time. This allows us to answer the core questions relating to disease burden that are the essential first step in setting health planning and service priorities. As we discussed in Chapter 1, this **descriptive epidemiology**, concerned as it is with 'person, place and time', attempts to answer the questions 'Who?', 'What?', 'Where?' and 'When?'. This can include anything from a description of disease in a single person (a case report) to the national health surveys conducted in many countries. Most reports of routine population data, including variations in rates of disease in different geographical areas and changing rates of disease over time (time trends), also come under the heading of descriptive epidemiology. But while descriptive studies or reports are essential to identify health problems and may lead to suggestions as to why something has occurred, they cannot usually answer the question 'why?'. Descriptive epidemiology may, however, provide the first ideas about causality and thus generate hypotheses that can then be tested in more formal 'analytic' studies that we will discuss in Chapter 4. As you will come to see, descriptive studies can also play a critical and often underappreciated role in monitoring the effects of large-scale interventions.

In this chapter we will look in more detail at the most common types of descriptive data and where they come from, and will consider some examples of the uses to which they are put. However, before embarking on a data hunt we first need to decide exactly *what* it is we want to know and this can pose a challenge; to make good use of the most relevant descriptive data it is critical to formulate our question as precisely as possible. If, say, we wanted to know about youth suicide, are we interested in the suicide mortality rate, the number of hospitalisations for attempted suicide, or the proportion of teenagers who have considered killing themselves? Mortality data are probably readily available from a number of sources, but the accuracy of the underlying certification of this cause of death is known to be problematic. Hospital admission data are also often quite accessible, but might not capture suicide attempts that are dealt with in the emergency room and not admitted. Furthermore, separating individuals from events can be tricky – are a lot of youths making a single suicide attempt each or are there a smaller number who have made multiple attempts? The resulting policy implications are quite different. In contrast, finding out about the prevalence (or cumulative incidence) of having suicidal thoughts will most probably need a special survey – it is important but you cannot easily 'look it up' in a standard data source.

Case reports and case series

The identification of a new or recurring health problem often begins with a **case report** or **case series**. These are detailed descriptions, usually by a doctor or group of doctors, of one or more cases of a disease that are unusual for some reason. This might be because the disease has not been seen before or the cases may have occurred in individuals who would not normally be expected to develop that disease, or in an area where the disease had not previously been reported or was thought to have been controlled. The cases might also be reported in conjunction with a previous exposure to something that, it is speculated, may have caused the disease.

Box 3.1 Case reports and case series that were instrumental in the early identification of health problems

- The classic description of a series of infants born with congenital cataracts, some with additional cardiac abnormalities, in Australia in 1941. This led Dr N. M. Gregg in Sydney to postulate a causal link between a severe epidemic of rubella (German measles) that had occurred six to nine months before the children were born and the subsequent abnormalities (Gregg, 1941). It is now well known that if a woman develops rubella during pregnancy it may affect her unborn baby.

- A case report published in the UK in 1961 described the development of a pulmonary embolism in a 40-year-old pre-menopausal woman, five weeks after she had started using an oral contraceptive (OC) to treat endometriosis (Jordan, 1961). Because pulmonary embolism is rare in women of that age, the author suggested that it might have been caused by the OC, particularly since it was a novel exposure at that time. A report of one case could not provide conclusive evidence that it was the OC rather than some other characteristic of the patient that led to the embolism – but it did pave the way for more detailed studies. These have consistently shown that there is an association between the use of OCs and the risk of this condition.

- A report of a series of five cases of *Pneumocystis carinii* pneumonia that occurred in young, previously healthy, homosexual men in three Los Angeles hospitals in a six-month period during 1980–81 (CDC, 1981). Until then, this disease had been seen almost exclusively in the elderly, the severely malnourished and those on anti-cancer chemotherapy whose immune systems were suppressed. This cluster of cases in young men suggested that the men were suffering from a previously unknown disease, possibly related to sexual behaviour. We now know this as HIV/AIDS.

The selective nature of these reports and the limited amount of information they contain mean that they provide little evidence of causality and cannot say much about patterns of disease occurrence. However, they can help identify potential health problems such as the acute outbreaks of severe acute respiratory syndrome (SARS), bird flu and swine flu that the world has experienced over the previous decade (we will discuss these further in Chapter 12). They may also stimulate interest in an area, leading on to more detailed studies, and in this regard some have been seminal in advancing knowledge (Box 3.1).

Figure 3.1 Prevalence of
diagnosed diabetes
(self-reported) in the United
States, 2006, by age group and
sex (dark bars, males; light bars,
females). (*Source:* Centers for
Disease Control http://www.
cdc.gov/diabetes/statistics/
prev/national/fig2004.htm,
accessed on 16 January 2010.)

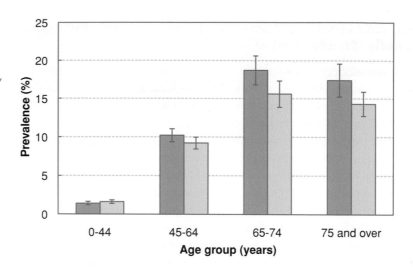

Prevalence surveys

Surveys are conducted to measure the prevalence of a wide variety of aspects of health, including diseases that are not captured by other routine statistics; conditions such as obesity; health-related behaviours such as smoking, sun-exposure and diet; and use of health services. These spot checks on the health of a nation or region are crucial to expanding our understanding of health burdens, needs and services beyond the hospital sector. In recent decades they have become a feature of broad-based community diagnosis and health planning, using a wide range of sampling and data-capture designs. These include telephone and face-to-face interviews, and sometimes very detailed physical examinations, as in the US National Health and Nutrition Examination Surveys (NHANES) (see Box 3.2). However, such undertakings are very expensive so the investigators have increased the value of NHANES by using the data as baseline information for follow-up studies to identify risk factors for subsequent morbidity (requiring further personal contact) and mortality (by linking to centrally held death records in the US National Death Index). Figure 3.1 shows some contemporary data, which will be important for future healthcare planning, drawn from a parallel series of US Health Interview Surveys.

How is the prevalence of diabetes related to age and sex?

What additional data are needed for a comprehensive planning response?

We see that, in 2006, the proportion of diabetics in US men and women rose markedly with age, affecting almost 18% of men and about 15% of women over the age of 64 years. This is a very heavy case load to manage: diabetes is a metabolic disease with many consequences, including heart and kidney damage,

Box 3.2 The US National Health and Nutrition Examination Surveys (NHANES)

NHANES is probably the largest and longest-running national source of objectively measured health and nutrition data. It was born out of the National Health Survey Act of 1956, which provided for the establishment of a continuing National Health Survey to obtain information about the health status of individuals residing in the USA and responsibility for this was given to the National Center for Health Statistics (NCHS). It was originally known as the National Health Examination Survey (NHES) and the first wave was conducted in 1959–62 (see Table 3.1). Subsequent waves focused on children and then adolescents before the NHES was combined with the National Nutrition Surveillance System, which had been established in 1969, to create the current series of NHANES in 1971 and this is still running in 2010. The NHANES populations are carefully selected to reflect the multi-faceted US population, and they have given rich descriptions of many prevalent conditions.

Table 3.1 The US National Health and Examination Surveys.

Survey	Years	Population	Size (approximate)
NHES I	1959–1962	Age 18–79	7,800
NHES II	1963–1965	Age 6–11	7,400
NHES III	1966–1970	Age 12–17	7,500
NHANES I	1971–1975	Age 1–74	32,000
NHANES II	1976–1980	Age <1–74	28,000
Hispanic (H) HANES	1982–1984	Age <1–74	16,000
NHANES III	1988–1994	Age > 2 months	34,000
NHANES Continuous	Every 2 years from 1999–2000 onwards, most recent 2009–2010	Age <1–74	5,000

(Data source: http://www.cdc.gov/nchs/nhanes.htm, accessed 24 January 2010.)

and adequate numbers of doctors, nutritionists and podiatrists must be provided and their care integrated. For a better view of the future healthcare burden we need to know time trends both in diabetes and for its risk factors. This information indicates that a major challenge is coming: the US population is ageing and also becoming more obese (a major risk factor for diabetes), so on both counts the number of cases will continue to rise.

The legend of Figure 3.1 indicates a central quality issue for many prevalence surveys like this: their common reliance on self-reporting. Where reasonably accurate knowledge of disease prevalence is sought a variety of strategies can be employed to improve accuracy. In the above example respondents were asked to report only *doctor-diagnosed* diabetes. For conditions such as cancer or stroke, they may be asked whether they went to hospital or a subset, as in NHANES, may be examined to validate self-reporting for an array of conditions. For some factors, such as medication use, frequency of troublesome symptoms and visits to the doctor, choice of the time span for recall can be critical: use of shorter periods (e.g. 2–4 weeks) increases reliability but will miss less frequent events.

To a large extent, studies such as these are purely descriptive and their aim is primarily to survey a sample of the population in order to determine the prevalence of the factors of interest in the community, often to aid health planning. Sometimes, however, the breadth of information collected allows much more in-depth analysis of the relationships *between* health behaviours and conditions. For example, the Australian National Health Survey is conducted every 3 years and it collects a vast array of information from participants about their health behaviours such as alcohol consumption, smoking and physical activity and about health conditions including diabetes, injury and mental health problems. This allows us to look at the relation between behaviour and health. For example in 2004–5, people who reported high levels of psychological distress were more likely to be physically inactive than those with low levels of distress or, in other words, the prevalence of inactivity was much higher in those with distress (48%) than those without distress (31%) (ABS, 2006). A study like this that looks at the relation between two aspects of health in a 'cross-section' of the population is often described as a **cross-sectional study** and we will discuss these further in Chapter 4.

Routine data collections

Governments, healthcare providers and statistical agencies routinely collect vast amounts of information that we will collectively describe as 'routine' data. These data can often be accessed at two levels: the summary data – often rates in their various forms which you met in Chapter 2 – and the raw counts of individual health events from which the rates are calculated. Since it is the latter that determine the quality and usefulness of the former, we will deal with them first, noting some of their advantages and disadvantages as we go. We will then look at some of the many sources of summary data.

Table 3.2 Some common health data collections and reporting systems.

Data collection or reporting system	Summary data often published	Individual level data available	Source of raw data
Vital statistics	Mortality rates	Date and cause of death, demographics[a]	Death certificates
Disease registries (e.g. cancer registries, injury registers)	Incidence, mortality and survival rates, prevalence	Diagnosis, date and demographics	Pathology reports, testing laboratories, hospital and medical records
Notifiable diseases (e.g. AIDS, SARS, TB, other infectious diseases)	Numbers of cases, incidence	Diagnosis, date and demographics	Laboratories, medical practitioners and hospitals
Hospital administrative systems	None	Diagnosis, date and demographics	Hospital discharge sheets, medical records
Health surveys (morbidity, risk factors, needs, service use etc.)	Special reports	Self-reported health states	Special surveys (often whole population)
Special surveillance systems	Varied	Varied	e.g. 'sentinel' primary care practices or disease registers (UK GP data base), MONICA (international CHD)
Rapid community assessments (health, nutrition)	Varied	Varied	Special surveys (sometimes of targeted groups)

[a] Basic demographic information such as age, sex and last known address.

Table 3.2 summarises some of the most common collection and reporting systems and the sources from which they take their information.

Mortality data

As we noted in Chapter 2, many routine statistics are based on mortality data because they are generally easier to obtain and more reliable than morbidity data – but that does not mean that they are perfect . . .

Death certificates

Death certificates are a widely used primary source of information, and the basis for most reported mortality rates. They often contain additional basic demographic information about an individual, including name, date of birth, ethnicity and gender, as well as the date and cause(s) of death. Figure 3.2 shows an example of a typical form.

Medical Certificate of the Cause of Death

To the Registrar-General

I hereby certify that _____

(name in full)

aged [_____] years, date of birth __/__/__ who usually resided at

_____ Postcode [_____] was attended and last

seen by me on __/__/__ (or by* [Dr. _____] on __/__/__

*if not attended by certifying medical practitioner within 3 months prior to death, insert
name of medical practitioner who last attended deceased and date)

and I am informed that he/she died on __/__/__ at _____

(town, place etc of death)

Cause of Death (print clearly and do not abbreviate)   Duration of
last illness

Disease or condition directly leading to death   1a
*(This means the disease, injury or complication which
caused death – NOT ONLY, for example, the mode of
dying such as 'heart failure', 'asphyxia', etc)*

due to, or as a consequence of

1b

due to, or as a consequence of

Antecedent causes - *morbid conditions, if any*   1c
*giving rise to the above cause, stating the
underlying condition last*

due to, or as a consequence of

1d

Other significant conditions   2
*Contributing to the death, but not related to the
diseases or condition causing it*

Date and type of operation in the last 4 weeks   __/__/__

Was a Coroner consulted before issuing this certificate?

     No, death not subject to the provisions of the Coroners Act [ ]

     Yes, issue of this certificate agreed to by _____, Coroner

Signature of Medical Practitioner _____ Date __/__/__

Initials and Surname (BLOCK Letters) _____

Professional Qualifications _____

Figure 3.2 A typical death certificate.

It is a common legal requirement that a medical practitioner must complete a death certificate for someone who dies. The completion of a death certificate therefore establishes the *fact* that someone has died with virtual certainty. Unfortunately, death certificates are less accurate when the *cause* of death is of interest, rather than the simple fact that death has occurred. This can be a consequence either of misdiagnosis (e.g. if a doctor does not know a person's full medical history) or of mis-specification on the form. The sample certificate shows the challenge of getting the sequence and content right. Look at the instructions on completing the 'cause of death' section: it will often not be easy, and those dying at older ages tend to have a number of coexisting diseases. How should the practitioner sequence the diagnoses of an overweight woman who has had diabetes for 20 years and high blood pressure for 10 years and who dies of pneumonia 1 year after suffering a stroke? Such a scenario is not uncommon, so we can be left with considerable uncertainty about the actual cause of death even on inspection of the original form. Indeed, in research studies where people are followed up for mortality, considerable extra effort often needs to be made in collecting clinical and pathology records in order to ensure accuracy in assigning cause of death. This can never be the case for routine vital statistics collections (it is far too expensive), so reports of mortality rates based on death certificates need to be used circumspectly. Generally only a single cause is extracted from the death certificate for each person who has died, that which is thought to be *underlying* any subsequent conditions. Multiple cause of death coding has recently been introduced in some countries but, while this may alleviate the problem of coding multiple conditions, it introduces another – the question of how to report and use this extra information.

What explanations can you think of for the sudden change in diabetes mortality in the USA over time shown in Figure 3.3 on the next page? Which do you think is most likely?

We saw in Chapter 1 (Figures 1.7 and 1.8) that US death rates for a number of causes have been declining over time, but none as dramatically as seen here in Figure 3.3, where the mortality rate for diabetes appeared to halve between 1948 and 1949 before plateauing at the new level. This *could* be due to a spectacular new treatment (but insulin is still the mainstay, as it was in the 1940s), or to fewer cases of diabetes occurring (but no effective means of preventing diabetes has been identified). So we are forced to consider artefacts in the data as a possible explanation. Here the dramatic shift in diabetes mortality was due to a coding change in the International Classification of Diseases (ICD), such that, when diabetes and coronary heart disease occurred together, diabetes was no longer listed as the underlying cause.

Not surprisingly, some diseases are recorded more accurately on death certificates than others. One that is rapidly fatal is likely to be clear cut, whereas

Figure 3.3 Age-adjusted mortality rates for diabetes by gender in the USA, 1938–1960, Whites only. Figure 3-2, p. 51, from *Methods in Observational Epidemiology*, 2nd edition, by Jennifer L. Kelsey, W. Douglas Thompson and Alfred S. Evans, copyright 1996 by Oxford University Press. Used by permission of Oxford University Press.

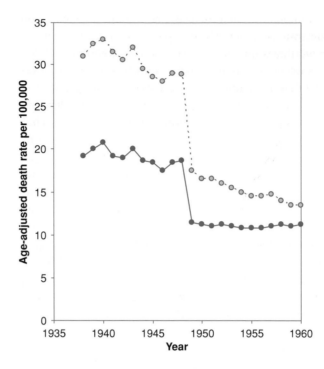

with a long-term disease there is more chance of another illness occurring and being recorded on the death certificate instead. For example, many people like the woman above would not have diabetes recorded anywhere on their death certificates. Similarly, diseases that are easily diagnosed tend to be more accurately recorded than those that require more complex diagnostic procedures: in the absence of an autopsy (and they are now uncommon), death from a motor vehicle accident would clearly be easier to recognise than one from pancreatic cancer. In an Australian study it was found that the overall accuracy of death certificates was only 77% compared with autopsy records, although cancers were accurately reported in 90% of cases (Maclaine *et al.*, 1992). A similarly high concordance for cancers was found in a UK study linking death certificates and hospital records, but chronic diseases such as diabetes and hypertension were correctly listed as an underlying cause only about half of the time (Goldacre, 1993).

Certain diseases may also be under-reported because of a reluctance to record the information. This might be either because of the potential stigma attached to the patient, as in the case of a death from suicide or HIV/AIDS, or because of the possibility that blame might be attached to the physician. The UK research found that conditions generally regarded as 'avoidable' causes of death were frequently omitted from the death certificate; for, example fractured neck of femur (broken hip) in the elderly was recorded in only one-quarter of cases.

Developed countries are now increasingly establishing national registers of deaths, recording both the date and the cause of death as well as key sociodemographic descriptors such as age, sex and last known address. Some of the earliest national death registries were in Scandinavia; for example, Statistics Sweden (www.scb.se) provides life expectancy data back to 1750! The UK National Health Service Central Register was started in 1939 to facilitate the issue of ration books during World War II (www.gro-scotland.gov.uk), while the National Death Index in the USA (www.cdc.gov/nchs) contains information on deaths from 1979 and its Australian counterpart (www.aihw.gov.au/cancer/ndi) has information from 1980. These registries can provide information about numbers of deaths by cause, age, sex, etc., and some also have facilities to allow researchers to obtain death information for specific individuals in their studies.

Verbal autopsy

In many low-income countries mortality rates are high but the vital registration systems are often much less well developed than in high-income countries. In these areas an alternative method used to capture information about causes of death, particularly among children, is the **verbal autopsy**. These 'autopsies' are conducted by a structured interview with the family members about the circumstances of their relative's death. This information is then used to classify the cause of death according to defined rules and criteria.

Morbidity data

Morbidity data provide a much greater challenge than mortality data. The scope of information is enormous and little is captured in a systematic way. As a result it is rarely simple to obtain complete information at a local level, and the problems escalate dramatically when trying to make comparisons between regions or countries. Having said that, attempts are made to record some aspects of morbidity in a routine way and these sources can provide valuable information.

Disease registries

Various disease registries exist (or have existed) to meet local health or research needs, but they cover only a small minority of conditions. For example, when it was noted that mortality from coronary heart disease (CHD) had started to fall in some countries in the late 1960s, it was not obvious what was driving this. Cardiologists of course claimed that better treatment in the newly introduced coronary care units meant that fewer patients were dying (lower case fatality).

It was also possible that the number of new cases (incidence) was falling due to recent changes in smoking and dietary patterns, but no directly relevant data were available to clarify the public health debate. The WHO responded in the early 1980s by encouraging the establishment of a series of registers around the world to capture international trends in CHD incidence (the MONICA programme). These provided a wealth of data on CHD incidence, risk factors and mortality (Tunstall-Pedoe *et al.*, 1999), leading to the conclusion that both falling incidence and better clinical outcomes had contributed to the drop in death rates. However, now that their job is finished, most of the MONICA sites have stopped active monitoring.

Cancer is the only disease group for which good morbidity data are widely and routinely available. Some countries, most notably in Scandinavia, have cancer registries that cover the whole country and have been operating for many decades. In others, such 'population-based' registries are newer and less well-established or, as in the USA, cover only part of the population. However, coverage is generally increasing, and a wealth of data on incidence, mortality and survival is available at regional, national and international levels. In some jurisdictions cancer is a legally notifiable disease, whereas in others (e.g. the UK) comprehensive identification of cases has come about gradually due to a combination of enthusiastic local registries and increasing awareness of the value of good morbidity data for planning and evaluating services. Cancer is an ideal candidate for such monitoring due to its relatively clear-cut diagnosis, which is usually based on a single simple record (a pathology report of histology). Rapid advances in technology now allow much of this information to be transferred electronically from the pathologist to the registry.

Many health authorities also keep registers of notifiable infectious diseases, although their prime purpose is for real-time surveillance to allow rapid response to emerging epidemics. Data for these registers usually come from medical practitioners and pathology laboratories, often under legal compunction. Despite this, and in contrast to cancers, most such diseases are poorly reported. Exceptions are those conditions which are perceived to be more severe, presenting either an acute challenge to a health system (SARS, AIDS) or a long-standing threat, such as tuberculosis. We will come back to discuss *surveillance* in more detail in Chapter 13.

Hospital records

Hospital records can provide useful information on conditions that require hospitalisation, although many hospitals have only recently started to computerise their records and it may be necessary to go through individual files by hand to collect the required information. The available data are usually based on discharge diagnoses as recorded and coded on the patient's record, and should be fairly reliable, although varying degrees of misdiagnosis, mis-recording and mis-coding are inevitable. It is also important to consider whether data obtained from a hospital will be representative of the general population or whether any conclusions will be restricted to the specific individuals from whom the data were obtained. This depends to a large extent both on the disease of interest and on the hospital. For diseases such as heart attacks and many cancers that almost always require hospitalisation, hospital records may provide good information on the levels of disease in the community. For conditions commonly treated outside hospital, however, the hospital-based population will not be typical: rather, it will be biased towards those with more severe disease, or towards those groups of society more likely to be hospitalised. A further limitation occurs where there is no unique patient identifier because aggregate admissions will be greater than the number of people admitted to hospital (because some will go to hospital more than once). Choosing the right numerator for a morbidity rate then becomes a challenge. Finally, most hospital data systems have no information at all regarding the vast majority of community morbidity which is treated by family practitioners or in the home.

Sources of summary data

Although it is sometimes possible to gain access to the individual-level data from the sources described above, for example through record linkage (see Chapter 4) or with informed consent from the individuals concerned, there is a wealth of summary data that is freely available. Also, as you saw in Chapter 2, the raw health data are not particularly informative on their own. Their value comes when they are combined with population data to calculate measures of incidence and prevalence that can then be compared with pre-defined standards or rates in populations in other countries, for different time periods, etc. Traditionally, and this is still the norm, the most used (and useful) measures of health (or, more usually, ill-health) are those collected and reported at national and regional levels for internal planning and evaluation.

The process of tracking down this information has changed dramatically. The World Wide Web now allows instant access to mountains of data that previously mouldered in dusty reports of limited circulation. While there remains a vast array of paper-based resources, many are now mirrored by web-based electronic information. For example, a wide range of information is available through the World Health Organization (WHO) Statistical Information System (WHOSIS, http://www.who.int/whosis/en/index.html). (Note: the web addresses given throughout this chapter and elsewhere in the book are current as of early 2010 and, although most have been stable for some time, web addresses do change.)

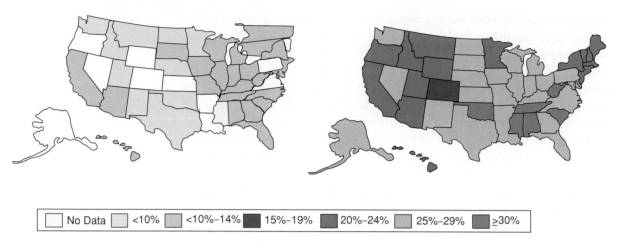

| No Data | <10% | <10%–14% | 15%–19% | 20%–24% | 25%–29% | ≥30% |

Figure 3.4 The prevalence of obesity (body-mass index ≥ 30 kg/m^2) by state in the USA in 1988 and 2008. (Data from the CDC Behavioral Risk Factor Surveillance System, BRFSS, accessed via http://www.cdc.gov/obesity/data/trends.html on 16 January 2010.)

A second change is the advance in computing technology which allows dramatic and informative visualisation of health data. For example, Figure 3.4, taken from the website of the US Centers for Disease Control Behavioral Risk Factors Surveillance System (http://www.cdc.gov/bfrss), shows the enormous increase in the prevalence of obesity across the USA between 1988 and 2008. The new computing flexibility and lesser reliance on hard-copy publications also make it easier to obtain customised data sets from health authorities, although there will often be a price attached. As an example of what is possible, *CDC Wonder* from the US Centers for Disease Control and Prevention (http://wonder.cdc.gov/) allows access to many data portals and was the source of the data on US mortality trends shown in Figures 1.7 and 1.8. Don't get carried away by the technology just yet, though – if you don't know what you are looking at you can misinterpret the results wildly.

As you will see below, there are many sources of data on mortality, morbidity and other factors relevant to health and, inevitably, these are of varying reliability, quality and completeness. This is true not only across different countries (note that our emphasis here is on the better-developed data systems), but also within any country, since all public data sets will have some problems, and some of them will have many. Any comparisons should be made only with a good understanding of the accuracy and completeness of the raw data underlying the summary rates. This section cannot be comprehensive but it should give you a sense of the sorts of material that are available. We have given specific directions to some of the major electronic sources of data from Australia, Canada, New Zealand, the UK and the USA, but most other countries provide similar information and an internet search would lead to them. One thing to remember, however, is that the data will almost certainly have been collected for a reason other than your question of interest and therefore might not be in the ideal form for your purpose. For example, the definition of who is a 'case' might not fit your criteria exactly; the data could have been collected for age groups that do not correspond to those you want to know about, and so on. It is always important to balance these disadvantages against the major advantage of using existing data – someone else has already done the hard work to collect it.

International sources

At an international level, two incredibly rich sources of information are the WHO and the World Bank.

- The WHO publishes the *Weekly Epidemiological Record* and the annual *World Health Report* (amongst other things) and electronic copies of both are available free of charge through the WHO website (http://www.who.int). The WHO Regional Offices (Europe, Africa, etc.) also have their own sites, which are accessible through the main WHO site. They provide access to local data and an array of regional statistics, health reports and information, for example the European 'Health for All' Database which provided the data on mortality in Russia for Figure 1.2 (www.euro.who.int/HFADB).
- The World Bank site (http://www.worldbank.org) provides access to a wide range of health and economic indicators for countries and regions around the world. It includes summary health data along with social, development and environmental statistics.

National data sources

Of particular value for the generalist can be publications that aim to capture the 'healthiness' of a nation or region. These often address contemporary issues via a combination of helpful and readily interpretable data, provide informed comment on implications for disease control, and may include evaluations of the positive and negative features of the health system which contribute to the nation's current 'diagnosis'. Some excellent examples that are accessible on-line (see Box 3.3 for web addresses) include

- *Australia's Health*; a biennial publication from the Australian Institute of Health and Welfare (AIHW);
- *Health, United States*; from the US National Center for Health Statistics (NCHS); and
- *UK Health Statistics Quarterly*; from the Office for National Statistics (ONS) and available through their 'virtual bookshelf'.

Other good sources of national data are the agencies in many countries that publish core health statistics, as well as demographic and other population data.

Box 3.3 E-data – selected health departments and national statistics agencies

Australian Bureau of Statistics (http://www.abs.gov.au)

Australian Institute of Health & Welfare (AIHW) (http://www.aihw.gov.au)

New Zealand Ministry of Health, Health Information Service
   (http://www. nzhis.govt.nz)

Statistics Canada (http://www.statcan.ca)

UK Office of National Statistics (ONS) (http://www.statistics.gov.uk)

US Centers for Disease Control and Prevention (CDC) (http://www.cdc.gov)

US National Center for Health Statistics (NCHS) (http://www.cdc.gov/nchs)

US National Institutes of Health (NIH) (http://www.nih.gov)
   Contains links to the 28 separate institutes, centres and offices that make
   up the NIH, covering areas from child health to ageing; alcoholism to drug
   abuse; and allergy through deafness and eye diseases to cancer, diabetes
   and circulatory diseases.

US Census Bureau (http://www.census.gov)
   Includes a comprehensive listing of other statistical agencies around the
   world.

Box 3.4 E-data – disease-specific sites

Cancer

CANCER*Mondial* at the International Agency for Research on Cancer (IARC)
   (http://www-dep.iarc.fr/)

European Network of Cancer Registries (http://www.encr.com.fr/)

US National Cancer Institute (NCI) (http://www.nci.nih.gov/)

US Surveillance, Epidemiology and End Results (SEER) Program of the NCI
   (http://seer.cancer.gov/)

Infectious diseases

Weekly Epidemiological Record (WER) from the WHO
   (http://www.who.int/wer/en/)

Morbidity and Mortality Weekly Reports (MMWR) from the US CDC
   (http://www.cdc.gov/mmwr/)

Disease-based resources

In addition to the sources listed above and in Box 3.3 there are many sites, both
national and international, dedicated to specific diseases or conditions. Some of
the best-known are listed in Box 3.4.

Some academic and other idiosyncratic sites

Other sites that can provide a helpful starting point for a search include the following:

- The *University of California (San Francisco)* maintains a site that provides access to a wide range of epidemiology and public health-related sites (http://www.epibiostat.ucsf.edu/epidem/epidem.html).
- *Martindale's Public Health Center* has a wide-ranging and eclectic site with many data links (http://www.martindalecenter.com/PHealth.html). (Unfortunately this site no longer includes surf and snow reports!).
- The *American Public Health Association* also has a site with multiple data and other 'public health links' (http://www.apha.org/).
- *SUMSearch* is an internet search tool designed to automate searching for medical evidence (http://sumsearch.uthscsa.edu/).

As the above references imply, today the starting point for a search for health information is the World Wide Web. An incredible array of data is directly accessible through sites such as the WHO website. Additionally many of the sites listed here provide links to a broader set of data-providers worldwide, some of whom will offer a similar set of cross-links, and so on. Many of the figures in this book come directly from readily available electronic sources such as these.

Creative use of existing data

Although, as we said at the start of the chapter, descriptive epidemiology is mainly concerned with 'who, what, where and when', we can also use simple descriptive information to start to link exposures and health outcomes to try to determine 'why' disease occurs. For example, Figure 3.5 on the next page shows trends in lung cancer mortality over time in Hungary, the UK and the USA.

What does this graph tell us about lung cancer? Why might rates have risen in Hungary between 1980 and 1995 but fallen in the UK and USA? Do we need any other information before we can draw any conclusions from this figure?

Figure 3.5 suggests that lung cancer mortality rates in the UK have fallen dramatically since the early 1970s, whereas in the USA they are gradually falling after having peaked in the 1980s. In contrast, the rates in Hungary rose markedly in the 1980s and only started to fall in the late 1990s. However, before we accept that these are real differences we must consider whether there might be an alternative explanation for the observed patterns. Is lung cancer diagnosed in the same way in each country? Have either the method of diagnosis or the criteria for diagnosis changed over time and have they changed differently in the three countries?

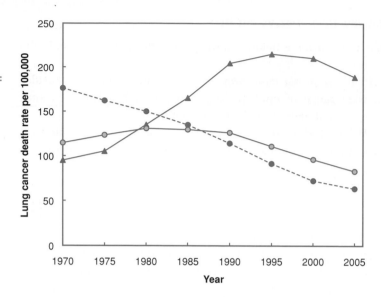

Figure 3.5 Age-standardised annual death rates from lung cancer among men aged 40–69 years in Hungary (▲), the USA (○) and the UK (●). (*Data source*: WHO Mortality Database, accessed via http://www-depdb.iarc.fr/ on 16 January 2010.)

Does lung cancer mortality mirror the incidence of lung cancer (i.e. is lung cancer really more common in Hungary?), or are the mortality rates higher in Hungary simply because treatment is less effective and the case–fatality ratio higher? Are lung cancer mortality rates in the UK and USA falling because the incidence is falling or because treatment has improved? If this is a real effect, does the fall in rates in the Western countries reflect the reduction in cigarette smoking?

Data of this type leave us with many questions but few definitive answers. However, if we can relate them to changes in other factors that might influence mortality they can add support to a hypothesis. For example, by plotting a graph of per-capita cigarette consumption over time and comparing this with lung cancer mortality rates (Figure 3.6), we find that the rise in lung cancer mortality in the USA parallels increasing cigarette sales, but it occurred 20–30 years later. This represents the two to three decades that it takes smoking to cause lung cancer and kill someone. The fact that lung cancer rates started to fall again 20–30 years after the decline in smoking adds further weight to the hypothesis that smoking causes lung cancer: if this fall had not occurred then the hypothesis would have failed a critical test – removal of the cause should reduce the incidence of disease. So, although these data do not prove that smoking causes lung cancer, they add weight to the belief that it could. If we found that an increase in cigarette consumption in Hungary occurred much later than the increases seen in the UK and USA this would strengthen the belief even further.

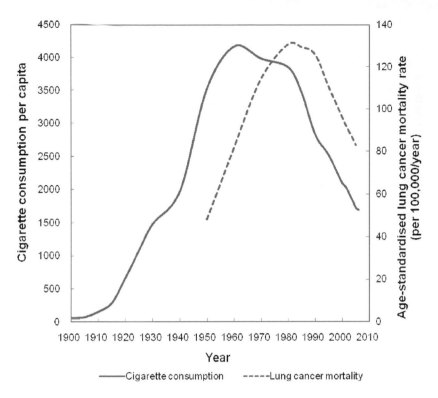

Figure 3.6 Cigarette sales and lung cancer mortality rates in males, age-standardised to the world population. (Cigarette consumption data from www.infoplease.com, lung cancer mortality rates from WHO Mortality Database, accessed via http://www-depdb.iarc.fr/ on 16 January 2010.)

Migrant studies

Another creative use of descriptive data comes from what are often called *migrant studies*. One of the challenges we face when we try to interpret differences in disease rates between countries is separating the effects of nature and nurture. Do Japanese women have very low rates of breast cancer compared with White American women because they are Japanese (i.e. because of a different genetic predisposition) or because they live differently (i.e. have different environmental exposures, such as diet)? For some populations we are fortunate to have what could be called 'natural experiments' when large numbers of people have migrated from a country with a low risk of a particular disease to a high-risk country, or vice versa, which can help to answer these questions. For example, large numbers of Japanese have migrated to Hawaii and California, and their overall rates of some diseases (e.g. breast cancer and coronary heart disease) have changed dramatically within one or two generations, moving away from the low rates in Japan towards the higher rates of the USA. The converse is true for rates of stroke and stomach cancer, which are lower in Japanese people residing in the USA than in those who live in Japan. If these diseases were largely genetic in origin then the rates could not have changed so quickly when the migrants moved to the USA. This strongly implicates the importance of the environment

Figure 3.7 An ecological study comparing the prevalence of serum antibodies to *H. pylori* (a gastric infection) and gastric cancer mortality rates in 46 rural Chinese counties. (From Forman *et al.*, Geographic association of *Helicobacter pylori* antibody prevalence and gastric cancer mortality in rural China. *Int. J. Cancer*, 1990; 46: 608–611, reprinted by permission of John Wiley & Sons.)

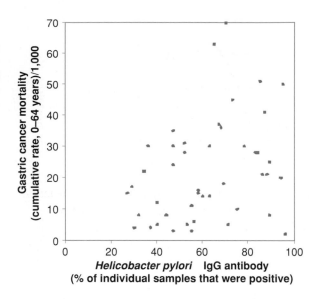

in increasing or decreasing the migrants' risk of disease and has led to enthusiasm for the idea that diet plays an important causal role in these diseases. However, the only specific causal hypothesis that is directly tested by such data is that large-scale international variation in these diseases is not primarily genetic in origin.

Ecological or correlation studies

Figure 3.7 shows the relation or correlation between the prevalence of infection with *Helicobacter pylori* (a bacterium that infects the stomach) and stomach cancer mortality rates in 46 Chinese counties (Forman *et al.*, 1990). In this study, the prevalence of infection was measured as the percentage of the population in the county with antibodies to the bacterium (an indication that they were or had been infected) and the cumulative gastric cancer mortality rate is the rate per 1,000 men and women (summed from birth to age 64). (Note that cumulative mortality is comparable to the cumulative incidence that you met in Chapter 2.) Each spot on the graph represents one of the 46 counties. There is not a perfect association, but the graph indicates that counties with a higher prevalence of *H. pylori* infection also tend to have higher stomach cancer rates and, perhaps more importantly, counties with a low prevalence of *H. pylori* have low stomach cancer rates. This hints that *H. pylori* might play a role in the development of stomach cancer; however, the fact that some counties have a high *H. pylori* prevalence but a low stomach cancer rate suggests that infection alone is not enough to cause cancer. Other factors must also play a role.

Box 3.5 Ecological studies

- In a classic study, Armstrong and Doll (1975) reported the correlation between 27 cancers and a wide range of dietary and other variables in 23 countries. Diet was strongly correlated with several types of cancer, particularly consumption of meat with cancer of the colon. Countries with low per-capita daily consumption of meat had the lowest rates of colon cancer. The findings from this study suggested that dietary factors play a role in the development of cancer and led to a burgeoning of research in this area.
- In 1979, the authors of another study reported a strong inverse association between average per-capita consumption of wine and mortality from ischaemic heart disease (high wine consumption was associated with low IHD mortality) (St Leger *et al.*, 1979). Since then more than 60 ecological, case–control and cohort studies have been conducted and most have shown that *moderate consumption* of wine and other alcohol has a protective effect against heart disease.

This example illustrates the key characteristic of ecological studies – they compare the prevalence of exposure and occurrence of disease in populations or groups of people, not individuals. The points on the graph represent the population prevalence of infection (in this case, taken from special surveys of individuals in each county) and the rate of disease in the population. The focus is on whether counties or populations with a high prevalence of infection also had a high cancer rate. In general, ecological studies are attractive because they are easy to do, especially if the routine data are readily available, but they can be difficult to interpret. The populations being compared may well differ in ways other than their exposure to the factor of interest and it is possible that something else that is related to the exposure is actually responsible for the observed differences in morbidity or mortality (i.e. an apparent relation could be due to **confounding** – see Chapter 8). Another problem with this type of study is that an observed association between variables at the group level might not represent the association at the individual level. In the example above, we have no way of knowing whether the people who developed cancer were actually infected with *H. pylori*. Ascribing characteristics to members of a group that they might not possess as individuals is called an **ecological fallacy**. For these reasons, ecological studies rarely give a strong test of a causal hypothesis but, more often, they help to generate or develop hypotheses. Box 3.5 shows some other ecological studies that have been instrumental in suggesting associations between exposures and disease.

Confidentiality

We cannot end any section on health data without touching on the issue of confidentiality. Clearly, information about an individual's health is private and should not be accessible to anyone else other than their healthcare providers. Much of the available health data is in the form of summary statistics such as rates so that it is impossible to identify specific individuals, and these data can be made freely (or at least readily) available. To gain access to data on individuals it will almost certainly be necessary to sign a confidentiality agreement, have permission from a Human Research Ethics Committee or Institutional Review Board and/or obtain consent from the individual patients and sometimes their physicians as well. Rapidly changing and expanding privacy legislation in many countries is adding to the challenges. While properly highlighting ethical use of data, the increasing emphasis on the principle of autonomy has created tensions between the need to protect personal information on the one hand and the desire for public good, which may require some access to individual data, on the other.

Summary

You have now seen the most common types of descriptive data and where they come from and also some examples of the many ways in which they can be used. These data are core to health planning and, as you will see in later chapters, are also essential for identifying new health problems and monitoring the effects of health interventions. You have also seen that although it cannot provide strong evidence about the causes of disease, creative use of descriptive epidemiology can generate new ideas about causality. These hypotheses then need to be tested in more formal 'analytic' studies and we will move on to discuss these in the next chapter.

REFERENCES

Armstrong, B. and Doll, R. (1975). Environmental factors and cancer incidence and mortality in different countries, with special reference to dietary practices. *International Journal of Cancer*, **15**: 617–631.

ABS (Australian Bureau of Statistics) (2006). Mental health in Australia: a snapshot, 2004–05. Cat no. 4824.*0.55.001*. Downloaded from: http://www.abs.gov.au/AUSSTATS/abs@.nsf/ProductsbyTopic/3AB354FFA0B0A31FCA256F2A007E5075?OpenDocument, 16 September 2009.

CDC (Centres for Disease Control). (1981). *Pneumocystis* pneumonia – Los Angeles. *Morbidity and Mortality Weekly Review*, **30**: 250.

Forman, D., Sitas, F., Newell, D. G., Stacey, A. R., Borcham, J., Peto, R., Campbell, T. C., Li, J. and Chen, J. 1990). Geographic association of *Helicobacter pylori* antibody prevalence and gastric cancer mortality in rural China. *International Journal of Cancer*, **46**: 608–611.

Goldacre, M. J. (1993). Cause-specific mortality: understanding uncertain tips of the disease iceberg. *Journal of Epidemiology and Community Health*, **47**: 491–496.

Gregg, N. M. (1941). Congenital cataract following German measles in the mother. *Transactions of the Ophthalmological Society of Australia*, **3**: 35–46. Reprinted (1991) *Australian and New Zealand Journal of Opthalmology*, **19**: 267–276.

Jordan, W. M. (1961). Pulmonary embolism. *Lancet*, **2**: 1146.

Maclaine, G. D., Macarthur, E. B. and Heathcote, C. R. (1992). A comparison of death certificates and autopsies in the Australian Capital Territory. *Medical Journal of Australia*, **156**: 462–463, 466–468.

St Leger, A. S., Cochrane, A. L. and Moore, F. (1979). Factors associated with cardiac mortality in developed countries with particular reference to the consumption of wine. *Lancet*, **1**: 1017–1020.

Tunstall-Pedoe, H., Kuulasmaa, K., Mahonen, M., *et al.* for the WHO MONICA. (1999). Contribution of trends in survival and coronary event rates to changes in coronary heart disease mortality: 10-year results from 37 WHO MONICA populations. *Lancet*, **353**: 1547–1557.

Healthy research: study designs for public health

Description	Association	Alternative explanations	Integration & interpretation	Practical applications
Chapters 2–3	Chapter 4: Study design	Chapters 6–8	Chapters 9–11	Chapters 12–15

Box 4.1 Oranges and lemons

In 1747, James Lind conducted an experiment to test six different cures for scurvy. While at sea, he identified 12 patients with scurvy whose 'cases were as similar as I could find them' and prescribed a different treatment to each pair of patients. After a few days he found that the two patients fortunate enough to have been prescribed oranges and lemons were almost fully recovered whilst no improvement was seen in the other ten, who had been subjected to various regimens including sea-water, gruel, cider and various elixirs. From this, Lind inferred that inclusion of citrus fruit in the diet of

(*continued*)

Box 4.1 (*continued*)

sailors would not only cure, but also prevent scurvy. Limes or lime juice thus became a part of the diet on ships, earning British sailors their nickname of 'limeys' (Lind, 1753).

When we discussed what epidemiologists do in Chapter 1, we touched on some of the different types of study that we use to collect the information we need to answer questions about health. In Chapter 3 we looked at the *descriptive* studies that provide the 'bread-and-butter' information of public health; in this chapter we will look at the *analytic* studies that are our main tools for identifying the causes of disease and evaluating health interventions. Unlike descriptive epidemiology, analytic studies involve planned comparisons between people with and without disease, or between people with and without exposures thought to cause disease. They try to answer the questions 'Why do some people develop disease?' and 'How strong is the association between exposure and outcome?'. This group of studies includes the **cohort**, **case–control** and **intervention studies** that you met briefly in Chapter 1. Together, descriptive and analytic epidemiology provide information for all stages of health planning, from the identification of problems to the funding of public health solutions and evaluation of whether they really work in practice.

As we discussed in Chapter 1, people talk about many different types of epidemiology but ultimately almost all epidemiology comes back to the same fundamental principles; the only things that differ are the health condition of interest and the factors that might influence that condition. So it is worth bearing in mind that the approaches that we will discuss in this chapter are generic and can be applied across all areas of health. They are equally applicable to studies:

- of treatment, prognosis and patient outcomes (e.g. survival, improved physical function or quality of life) in clinical medicine, dentistry, nursing or any of the allied health professions;
- looking for the genetic and/or non-genetic causes of infectious and chronic diseases;
- of the effects of our occupation or our socioeconomic and physical environment on health;
- aiming to identify factors that influence health behaviours such as smoking, alcohol consumption or whether parents choose to have their children vaccinated; and
- attempting to change these behaviours in order to improve health outcomes ...

And the list could go on. Likewise, the range of exposures or study factors that might influence health – for good or bad – is incredibly broad. The 'exposure' we are interested in could be an environmental factor such as an infectious agent, radiation or some chemical, it could be a behavioural factor like smoking or drinking habits, an intrinsic characteristic of the individual such as sex, age, skin colour or an underlying genetic factor (after all, we are all 'exposed' to our own genes). Furthermore, while most of these are personal exposures that affect us at the individual level, epidemiology is expanding and *social epidemiology* encompasses the additional influences of the broader social environment. At another level, *lifecourse epidemiology* attempts to integrate exposures over an individual's lifetime. While different questions place different demands on the specifics of data collection, all can be addressed via the same suite of research designs, although different designs will be more or less appropriate in different situations. When we discuss the various study designs in this chapter we will do so mainly in the context of 'exposure' and 'disease', but you should be aware of the broader application of the ideas.

It is also important to bear in mind that all of the various study designs that we will discuss have their strengths, but they also have limitations and we will touch briefly on these as we go. We will come back to pick up on some of these limitations when we talk about *bias* in Chapter 7 and look at how to report, read and interpret the results of epidemiological studies in Chapter 9.

Observational studies

If a laboratory scientist wanted to see whether something caused a particular effect they would set up an experiment. This would involve creating two identical test systems under identical conditions, adding the particular factor of interest to one of them and then waiting to see what happened. Any differences between the outcomes in the two systems could then be fairly conclusively attributed to the presence of that factor. The same principles apply in epidemiology – if there is good reason to believe that something might improve health then it is possible to conduct an **intervention study** where the investigator actively intervenes to change something to see what effect this has on disease occurrence. This is what James Lind did in his small, but classic study on scurvy in 1747 (Box 4.1). Such studies include *clinical trials* comparing two (or more) forms of treatment for patients with a disease, as well as *preventive trials*, in which the aim is to intervene to reduce individuals' risk of developing disease in the first place. As with experiments in other sciences, the investigator controls who is exposed and who is not, for example, who is allocated to a new treatment regimen and who receives the old treatment, or who is enrolled in a 'stop smoking' campaign and who is not.

However, when we are dealing with people, things usually are a lot more complicated than this and, as a result, epidemiology is rarely an experimental science. Most of the time an epidemiologist will just go out (after a lot of thought-ful planning) and measure the rate of occurrence of a disease or other health outcome, or will compare patterns of exposure and disease to identify particular exposures or risk factors associated with that disease. This is purely an *observa-tional* role: the researcher does not intervene in any way. They leave nature to take its course, and record what happens, or what happened in the past. These are commonly described as **observational studies**. We will discuss these first and will then come back to consider intervention studies later.

Ecological studies

We mentioned these in Chapter 3 because they compare exposure and disease in populations rather than individuals, but they do attempt to link exposures and outcomes and so could equally well be considered analytic studies. After observing a correlation between rates of infection with the gastric bacterium *H. pylori* and gastric cancer mortality in China as shown in Figure 3.7, the inves-tigators conducted a similar study comparing infection rates and gastric cancer incidence in 17 centres from the USA, Japan and 11 different countries in Europe. From this they were able to estimate that mortality from gastric cancer would be about six times higher in a population where everyone was infected with *H. pylori* than in a population with no infection, i.e. the relative risk of dying from gastric cancer was about six times higher for someone infected with *H. pylori* than for someone who was not infected (The Eurogast Study Group, 1993).

It is, however, always important to remember that communities that differ in one way – for example the prevalence of *H. pylori* infection – probably differ in other ways too. It is therefore impossible to be sure that the factor of interest is what is actually driving their different health outcomes, in this case mortality from gastric cancer.

Cross-sectional studies

In Chapter 3 we discussed the surveys that many countries conduct on a fairly regular basis to measure the prevalence of different health behaviours and health conditions in their population and we showed how these can be used to look at the relationships between behaviour and health. The key factor of these surveys is that they aim to select people in such a way that they are representative of the whole population so that information collected from the study sample can be generalised directly to that population. Studies like this, that set out to look at the relation between an exposure and a health outcome in a 'cross-section' of the population, are called **cross-sectional studies**. As you will see, they have a number of drawbacks compared to other study designs but, because of their

Figure 4.1 The design of a cross-sectional study.

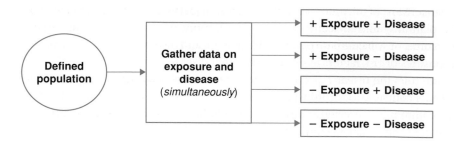

relatively simple design (summarised in Figure 4.1), they are often conducted as an early investigation into the possible causes of ill-health.

For example, a group of researchers in India wanted to estimate the prevalence of and risk factors for suicidal behaviour in young people in Goa. They invited all 16–24-year-olds from two rural and two urban communities to be interviewed for the study and achieved a participation rate of almost 95%. Overall, 3.9% of the 3,662 participants reported some form of suicidal behaviour in the previous three months. Multiple factors were associated with suicidal behaviours, including female gender, not attending school and experience of sexual and recent physical abuse (Pillai *et al.*, 2009).

This cross-sectional study was both *descriptive* in that it defined the scope of the problem (how common is suicidal behaviour), and *analytic* in that it also identified (and measured the prevalence of) a number of possible causal factors. All these data, descriptive and analytic, can be valuable for planning health and social system responses. The key feature of the study is that the young people were not recruited because they had (or had not) exhibited suicidal behaviour or because of their particular histories, but because they were assumed to be typical of young people in Goa.

Cross-sectional studies such as this may be conducted to gather information about many aspects of health and lifestyle and, as in the example above, participants should be recruited without knowledge of either their exposure status (presence or absence of the exposures of interest) or their disease status (presence or absence of the diseases of interest). This is essential to avoid **selection bias** – something that we will come back to discuss in Chapter 7. Information on the outcome (suicidal behaviour in the example above) and the exposures (gender, education, previous abuse, etc.) is usually obtained at the same time. For this reason, it can be difficult to identify which came first – the exposure or the outcome (disease). For example, what would we conclude if we found that people who did not exercise were more likely to have depression than those who exercised regularly? This might suggest that regular exercise prevents depression, but equally it could reflect the fact that people with depression may be less likely to exercise regularly. This problem is a major issue in cross-sectional studies and is sometimes described as 'reverse causality' – does A really cause B or might the reverse be true such that B causes A? Cross-sectional studies can, however, be particularly useful for examining exposures that do not change over time (for example, personal characteristics like sex and blood group) or that occurred many years previously.

Another important thing to note about cross-sectional studies is that they evaluate prevalent cases of disease – those that are already present in the population at the time of the survey. As we discussed in Chapter 2, prevalence is a function both of the incidence and of the duration of a disease. People who have a disease for longer are more likely to be ill at the time of a cross-sectional study than those who are sick for a shorter time. An association between exposure and prevalence of disease can thus reflect not only a link between exposure and the occurrence of new disease, but also a link between exposure and factors that affect survival or persistence of a diseased state.

Thinking back to the study of suicidal behaviour described above:

Is there any problem with the time-directionality of the link between (i) gender, (ii) lifetime sexual abuse and (iii) not attending school and suicidal behaviour?

Are the young adults studied likely to be typical of all young adults in Goa? India?

In this study it is unlikely that there is a problem with the time-directionality of the relationships with gender (as this does not change over time) or sexual abuse as this was recorded over the lifetime and thus is very likely to have preceded the suicidal behaviour which was recorded for the last 3 months only. The relation with not attending school is, however, more problematic as it is possible that young adults with suicidal tendencies may be more likely to miss school than the other way around. In relation to the generalisability of the findings, the results from the study were based on young people from two rural and two urban communities. The participation rates were very high (much higher than would be achieved in most studies in developed countries now), but before generalising the results beyond the study areas we would need to know that the selected communities were representative of all communities in Goa (or India).

Cross-sectional surveys such as the national health surveys conducted in many countries are often carried out at regular intervals – for example the NHANES studies in the USA that we discussed in Chapter 3 (see Box 3.2). They recruit a *different* sample of people for each survey and then study changes in the population prevalence of disease, disability or potential risk factors for disease over time. In this regard they differ from cohort studies, which, as you will see below, follow the *same* group of people over a period of time.

Another type of cross-sectional study that you may come across in the clinical setting is one conducted to evaluate the performance of a diagnostic test – see Box 4.2.

Box 4.2 Diagnostic studies

A study to evaluate the accuracy of a diagnostic test can be thought of as a special type of cross-sectional study in which the data are collected from diagnostic test results or physical examination rather than from interviews or questionnaires. Typically, individuals with symptoms of disease are selected randomly or consecutively from a clinic or hospital to undergo the test of interest (the **index test**). Then independently (and blinded to the results of the index test) the same individuals undergo the best test available to diagnose the disease (the *reference test* or '**gold standard**'). The results of the two tests are then compared and the accuracy of the index test (its **sensitivity** and **specificity**) can be determined (we will discuss the mechanisms of this in Chapter 15). As in all cross-sectional studies, it is important that the people selected are representative of the target population – in this case the patients in a particular setting – in whom the test would be used in real life.

Cohort studies

As we discussed at the start of this section, the best way to test whether something is causally related to health is to see whether people exposed to the factor of interest have different health outcomes from those who are not exposed. Ideally we would conduct an experiment or trial where we could control who was exposed and unexposed but in many cases this would be either unethical (you cannot deliberately expose someone to something thought to be harmful) or impractical. The next best thing is therefore a **cohort study** (sometimes described as a *prospective* or *longitudinal* study) where we follow people forwards (prospectively) over time to see what happens to them. The cohort[1] might be a group of initially healthy people whom we follow to observe the occurrence of disease or a group of patients whom we follow to study their disease outcomes, i.e. their prognosis.

   A classic example of a cohort study is the Framingham Heart Study (Dawber, 1980). It was started in 1948 at a time when heart disease had become the USA's number one killer, and the principal aim was to identify biological and environmental factors that might be contributing to the rapid rise in cardiovascular death and disability. The epidemiological approach was quite novel at the time and it was designed to discover how and why those who developed heart disease differed from those who escaped it. The town of Framingham, Massachusetts, was selected by the US Public Health Service as the study site, and 5,209 healthy

---

[1] In Ancient Rome, a cohort was one of ten divisions of a Roman military legion. It comprised young men of similar age from one region. In service its members were often injured or killed and they were not replaced. The cohort was then disbanded when the term of enlistment was over.

men and women between 30 and 60 years of age were enrolled. Framingham was appealing because it had a stable population and a single medical facility, suggesting that it would be relatively easy to carry out the follow-up. The study was expanded in 1971 when 5,124 children of the original cohort (and their spouses) were recruited for a second study, the Offspring Study.

Before Framingham, the notion that scientists could identify, and individuals could modify, '**risk factors**' (a term coined by the authors of the study) tied to heart disease, stroke and other diseases was not part of standard medical practice. With over 50 years of data collected from residents of Framingham (and the publication of more than 1,000 scientific papers), the Framingham researchers have identified major risk factors associated with heart disease, stroke and other diseases and created a revolution in preventive medicine. The study identified several risk factors associated with increased risks of heart disease including cigarette smoking (1960), high cholesterol levels and high blood pressure (1967), and obesity and low levels of physical activity (1967). These are so commonly accepted today, both by health professionals and by the public, that it is difficult to imagine a time when we did not know about them.

The Framingham Study is quite small by modern standards: the European Investigation into Cancer (EPIC) established in 1995 includes more than half a million individuals from 10 European countries (http://epic.iarc.fr) and the Million Women Study was initiated in the UK in 1996 (The Million Women Study Collaborative Group, 1999). The Framingham study therefore needed particularly long follow-up to accumulate enough endpoints (diagnoses of new disease) to give robust results. A crucial trade-off is that the smaller size and the setting permitted regular detailed physical examination and other 'hands-on' investigations such as the recording of electrocardiograms, giving a rich array of high-quality exposure data that cannot be gathered on a very large scale.

In a cohort study we compare the occurrence of disease in groups of people with and without a particular exposure (Figure 4.2). The participants must be free of the outcome of interest at the start of the follow-up, which makes it easier to be sure that the exposure preceded the outcome. Although if there is a long pre-clinical phase before a disease is diagnosed, as is probably the case for many types of cancer, the apparent exposure–disease sequence can still be wrong and for this reason many cohort studies do not count cases of disease that occur in the first few years of follow-up.

Of all the observational designs, cohort studies generally provide the best information concerning the causes of disease and the most direct and intuitive natural measurements of the risk of developing disease. The other advantage of collecting exposure information before people develop disease is that measurement of exposure is not biased by knowledge of outcome status. It is important to note, however, that if a cohort study has a very long follow-up period and exposure data were only collected at baseline then people may have changed

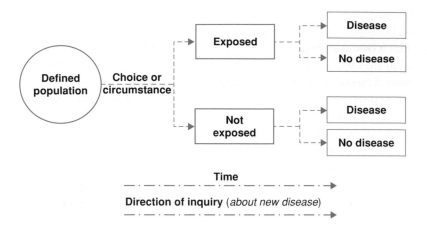

their behaviours over the intervening years. For example, smokers may quit smoking or meat eaters may become vegetarian and it is also an unfortunate fact that many of us will gain weight as we get older. Depending on when the critical period of exposure occurs, this may mean that people are wrongly classified with regard to their exposure (e.g. past smokers as current smokers). This is a problem of **misclassification** and we will discuss it further in Chapter 7. Many cohort studies, for example the US Nurses Health Studies (see Box 4.3), avoid this problem by re-contacting study participants every few years to collect updated exposure information.

Selection of participants is an issue at two points of a cohort study: who is *selected into* the cohort at the start of the study and who is *lost from* the cohort during follow-up. Who is selected into a cohort can influence the generalisability of its findings since they may apply only to the sorts of people who agreed to take part. However, if many people are 'lost to follow-up' such that we don't know if they experienced the health outcome of interest, then the results of the study may be biased. (We will discuss selection bias further in Chapter 7.)

Cohort studies are by nature very time-consuming and expensive. However, the benefit:cost ratio of a well-run cohort study is high, given the enhanced validity over case–control studies and the multitude of associations that can be assessed. For example, over the last decade the Nurses' Health Study has been the basis for between 30 and 50 publications every year (see http://www.channing.harvard.edu/nhs). In principle, a long-term cohort study also has the potential to deliver the public health knowledge of most value, by showing the full array of harms and benefits associated with a given exposure. The British Doctors Study is an outstanding example of this with regard to cigarette smoking because while it, like other studies, shows that there is a potential benefit of cigarette smoking with regard to Parkinson's disease, it also clearly shows the overwhelming

Box 4.3 Some other notable cohort studies

• The British Doctors Study cohort was established in 1951 and followed for more than 50 years, although many of the original 40,701 participants are now dead. It has been of enormous value, particularly in relation to identifying the manifold health consequences of smoking. This is despite the fact that, compared with studies today, only limited exposure data were collected on a very short postal questionnaire mailed to the doctors at 10-year intervals since 1951 (Doll and Hill, 1964).

• The US Nurses' Health Study started in 1976 with 121,964 female nurses aged 30–55, and 5 years of funding. Since then its focus has widened enormously from the oral contraceptive–breast cancer links for which it was first funded (Stampfer *et al.*, 1988) to cover many exposures (including diet) and a multitude of outcomes. It has now accumulated more than 30 years of follow-up and is still going strong. It is very expensive to run, but the scientific and public health yield has been exceptional. The Nurses' Health Study II began in 1989 with 117,000 nurses aged 25–42 (Rockhill *et al.*, 1998) and recruitment has recently started for a Nurses' Health Study III!

• ALSPAC (The Avon Longitudinal Study of Parents and Children) was started in 1990 to determine ways in which an individual's genes combine with environmental pressures to influence health and development over the lifecourse. Comprehensive data have been collected on over 10,000 children and their parents, from early pregnancy until the present. Since the study is based in one geographical area of the UK, linkage to medical and educational records is relatively simple, and hands-on assessments of children and parents using local facilities allows good quality control (Golding *et al.*, 2001).

negative effects of smoking which put control of smoking at the top of the public health agenda.

Historical cohort studies

It is sometimes possible to avoid the long follow-up period common to many cohort studies by establishing a retrospective or **historical cohort**. This requires good records of past exposure for a group of people who can then be traced to determine their current health. Until fairly recently, such studies have been most common in industry or the military where good personnel records exist but they have also been used to study the development of disease in relation to characteristics at birth (e.g. weight and length at birth) because this information can often be obtained retrospectively from birth records. In the absence of close follow-up – the usual situation – they are generally limited to studying mortality or cancer outcomes, given the lack of universal records for other non-fatal end-points. Some interesting and useful variations include the use of college alumni records in the USA to study benefits of physical activity as a young adult (Paffenbarger *et al.*, 1986) and the Boyd Orr Study based on detailed dietary records collected from over 4,000 British children in the 1930s (Frankel *et al.*, 1998).

Now with the increasing opportunities for linking other health records (see Record linkage below), studies of this type are becoming more common and increasingly sophisticated.

Record linkage

Many investigators performing cohort studies enhance their follow-up by using external sources of health data to which they 'link' the identities of their individual cohort members in order to find out about new outcomes, commonly the occurrence of cancer or death as this information is often routinely available from central registries. The matches are made in a variety of ways, including using a common personal identification number as in many Scandinavian countries and the USA (social security number), or through probabilistic approaches based on a variety of personal identifiers (e.g. name, date of birth and address). As health data are increasingly stored in electronic formats, the scope for what is often described as **record linkage** is increasing exponentially and some health jurisdictions are now establishing procedures to link different health-related databases (Kelman *et al.*, 2002). In the Australian states of Western Australia and New South Wales, for example, it is now possible to link information from a wide range of sources including the electoral roll, birth and death records, hospital admissions, emergency presentations, midwives' notifications, cancer registrations and mental health records as well as the national Pharmaceutical (drug prescriptions) and Medicare (tests and procedures) Benefits Schedules. Access to these linked data is, of course, highly controlled to preserve the confidentiality of individual Australians living in these states. However, with appropriate consent from the persons concerned, or a protocol that does not require any personal identifying information (such as names, addresses or dates of birth) to be released, these data can now be accessed and linked to provide valuable information for health researchers and managers alike. For example, by linking data from hospital morbidity and death records, Western Australian researchers were able to show that the presence of other medical conditions (comorbidity), but not advancing age, predicted repeat admission to hospital for adverse drug reactions (Zhang *et al.*, 2009). This information will allow better identification and monitoring of those most at risk of an adverse reaction.

Some studies now rely heavily on record linkage to provide reliable information about an enormous range of potential exposures and health outcomes without having to rely on people's memories for accurate information. For example,

'45 and Up' is a cohort study that is following more than 250,000 men and women aged 45 and older in New South Wales to look at a wide range of health outcomes associated with aging. These range from health conditions to use of health services and quality of life (http://www.45andup.org.au). Although the investigators asked participants to complete a standard health questionnaire when they joined the study, they also asked them to consent to allow the investigators access to their health records to allow linkage to the many health databases listed above (45 and Up Study Collaborators, 2008). This greatly broadens the scope of questions that the study will be able to answer and also has the benefit that there is less reliance on individual memory.

There is also an interesting sub-set of studies that are based entirely on record linkage. They are effectively cohort studies in which both exposure and outcome information comes from electronic records. While they have been used mostly to link health services and outcomes, increasing computerisation of medical information makes more conventional aetiological research possible by this means. As an example, Swedish investigators were able to use the Swedish Inpatient Register to identify a cohort of 29,187 patients hospitalised for type-1 diabetes between 1965 and 1999. They then 'linked' these names to the Swedish Cancer, Total Population, Migration and Death Registers. This told them who had been diagnosed with cancer, the type of cancer and date of diagnosis, and also who had migrated or died from some other cause and so was no longer at risk of being diagnosed with cancer in Sweden. They calculated standardised incidence ratios (SIR) for the cohort compared with the general population and found that diabetes was associated with significantly increased risks of cancer of the stomach (SIR = 2.3), cervix (SIR = 1.6) and uterus (SIR = 2.7) (Zendehdel et al., 2003). Studies like this are essentially the modern version of the historical cohort study we discussed above.

Studies based on linking health (and other) records from a variety of sources do, however, raise a number of issues regarding confidentiality, and current privacy concerns and legislation in some countries have the potential to limit this avenue of research. The 45 and Up Study asks all participants to provide consent for the investigators to collect information from health records, but it is often not possible or practical for researchers to contact all of the individuals concerned to get their permission to access their data. To solve this problem, pure record-linkage studies are conducted without the researchers being given any personal information about the individuals in order to preserve their anonymity. So, for example, the custodians of the relevant databases perform the linkage and remove all identifying information such as names, addresses and dates of birth before giving the linked data to the investigators for analysis. Despite these precautions, however, many health data custodians are still prevented by law from releasing even de-identified information without individual consent. Much effort is being expended to enable a constructive resolution of the tensions between maximising individual autonomy (by protecting against inappropriate access to personal health data) and ensuring that the public good delivered by health research is not compromised (Lawlor and Stone, 2001).

Prognostic or survival studies

As we mentioned above, cohort studies can also be used to see what happens to patients after they are diagnosed with a condition. In this case the cohort would comprise patients with the condition of interest who were at the same point in the course of their illness, e.g. at diagnosis (often called an *inception cohort*) or after completion of their primary treatment. They would then be followed for a fixed period or until they experience the outcome of interest, which might be death, recurrence of the disease or quality of life at a given time point. Studies of this type can identify patient characteristics that predict their outcome, for example demographic factors such as age, gender or socioeconomic status; disease-specific factors such as the severity or stage of disease at diagnosis; genetic factors and the presence of other health conditions (known as co-morbidities). Such characteristics are called *prognostic factors*; they may not actually *cause* the outcome, but must be associated with it strongly enough to *predict* it. Event rates tend to be high, so prognostic studies are usually much smaller than cohort studies of risk factors.

These studies are also increasingly being used to investigate potentially modifiable factors such as diet and lifestyle that might affect patient outcomes. For example, an Australian study found that among a group of 609 women diagnosed with ovarian cancer, a cancer that typically has a high mortality rate, those who ate more vegetables survived for longer than those who ate fewer vegetables (Nagle *et al.*, 2003).

Case–cohort studies

In many cohort studies, all participants provide a wide range of information at the time of recruitment, including answers to detailed dietary questionnaires and blood and urine samples. Because of the large numbers and cost, these resources – especially the biological samples – are often not analysed in detail at the time but are stored for future use. It is then possible to use this information more efficiently by conducting either a **nested case–control study** (see below under case–control studies) or **case–cohort study**. In the case–cohort design a sub-set of participants is selected from the full cohort at baseline. Detailed exposure information can then be retrieved for this subcohort and *all* of the people in the full cohort who develop the disease of interest. This maintains the major advantage of a cohort study in that the exposure data were originally collected before the development of disease, while the much smaller scale reduces effort and cost. It also has the advantage that the subcohort can be used for comparison with multiple different case groups. However, the case–cohort study requires

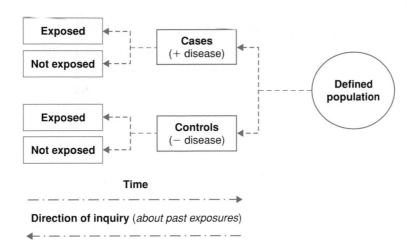

Figure 4.3 The design of a case–control study (adapted from Beaglehole *et al.* (1993) with permission).

a somewhat more sophisticated data analysis than the traditional cohort and nested case–control analyses.

Case–control studies

One drawback of cohort studies is that they can really only be used to study conditions that are relatively common. If we were interested in a very rare disease we would need to follow a large number of people for a very long time to identify many people with the disease. In this situation an alternative study design called a **case–control study** is often used. Instead of identifying people on the basis of their exposure status and waiting to see who develops disease, we effectively start from the end and work backwards (see Figure 4.3). We select people who have developed the disease we are interested in (cases) and a representative sample of people from the same population who do not have that disease (controls) and then ask them about their previous exposures. (Some authors prefer to call the comparison group the 'reference' group and will describe the study as a *case–reference* or *case–referent* study.) For instance, if we wanted to know whether smoking was associated with lung cancer we could compare people with lung cancer and controls without lung cancer to see if they differed in their smoking habits, exactly as Doll and Hill did back in 1950 (see Chapter 1).

A classic case–control study was conducted in Germany in 1961 (Mellin and Katzenstein, 1962). The mothers of children born with unusual limb malformations (cases) were compared with mothers of normal children (controls) with respect to their exposures in pregnancy. Forty-one of the 46 case mothers (89%), but none of 300 control mothers, had taken thalidomide early in their pregnancy. This strongly suggested that thalidomide use early in pregnancy could be

Box 4.4 Case–control studies

- Phenacetin was introduced as an analgesic in 1887 and used extensively until it was suggested that it might be associated with kidney disease. A case–control study involving 554 adults with newly diagnosed kidney disease and 516 matched control subjects selected randomly from the same geographical area was conducted in the USA to investigate this (Sandler *et al.*, 1989). After allowing for the effects of other types of analgesic, the risk of kidney disease was five times higher among daily users of phenacetin and three times higher among daily users of paracetamol (acetaminophen, a metabolite of phenacetin) than it was among infrequent users of these drugs. There was little association between aspirin use and renal disease. Results from this study and others confirmed the risks of phenacetin, which was withdrawn from the market.
- In a case–control study conducted in Tasmania, Australia, the parents of 58 children who had died from SIDS (sudden infant death syndrome) and of 120 control children were interviewed about the sleeping practices of their children. Children who were placed face-down had a four-fold higher risk of SIDS than children placed in other positions. This risk was increased even further if the child slept in a heated room, was tightly wrapped or had recently been ill (Ponsonby *et al.*, 1993). The results of this study and others have led to campaigns aimed at persuading parents to place babies on their backs to sleep in order to reduce rates of SIDS.

responsible for the birth defects. (It should be noted that this study was stimulated by data from an earlier case series.)

Modern case–control studies tend to be much larger, for example the Australian Ovarian Cancer Study included more than 1500 women with ovarian cancer and a similar number of control women. It has confirmed strong inverse associations with pregnancy, breast-feeding and oral contraceptive pill use and risk of ovarian cancer such that women who have several children and/or who use the 'pill' for several years are about half as likely to develop ovarian cancer as nulliparous women or non-pill users (Jordan *et al.*, 2008). A wide range of other possible causes have also been examined within this one study and this is one of the major appeals of the case–control design. Because the focus is usually on a single health outcome, participants can be asked very detailed questions about relevant exposures; this is often not possible in a cohort study, which will usually collect less detailed information on a much wider range of exposures in order to study multiple different outcomes. Box 4.4 gives examples of some other case–control studies which have led to direct health benefits.

Ideally case–control studies include only incident (new) cases of disease as they arise. However, some studies, especially those of very rare diseases, will also include prevalent cases. This makes them rather like cross-sectional studies, with the possible problem of determining a clear time sequence for the exposure–disease relation. (That is, a factor may appear to be related to disease risk simply because it enhances the duration of disease.)

Case–control studies offer a number of advantages over follow-up studies. They are generally quicker and more economical to perform (but are still not a trivial undertaking) and, as we noted above, are good for evaluating rare outcomes. Case–control studies are also good for evaluating many different exposures, all of which can be asked about at the one interview.

The central problem in the design of a case–control study is selection of the control group. Controls should represent the population from which the cases have come such that their exposure prevalence is very similar to that of the whole population. In practice this means that appropriately selected controls should have been identified as cases if they had developed the condition of interest. If the cases form a population-based series (e.g. if all cases from a defined geographical region are included), then the appropriate control group should be representative of that population. **Population controls** can be selected in a number of ways, including from population registers or comprehensive electoral rolls and, in recent times, by sampling residential telephone numbers at random (random-digit dialling). In the ovarian cancer study described above, the controls were selected from the national electoral roll because enrolment to vote is compulsory in Australia; this strategy would not work in countries where voting is not mandatory because electoral rolls would be much less complete. In the UK, selection of controls from the patient lists of the general practitioners (GPs) who referred the cases is often a viable alternative because most of the population is registered with a GP.

Where the case group does not originate from a clearly defined geographical population, a traditional approach to identify controls from the likely source population was to recruit a control from the local neighbourhood of the case, for example someone living in a nearby street. This is time-consuming and expensive, but effective; a modern variant that can be used where telephone numbers are assigned by residential area involves matching telephone numbers with random selection of the last few digits. (The increase in mobile phones may change this.)

Whilst population or neighbourhood controls are ideal, practical reasons mean that **hospital controls** are still used, although not as frequently as in the past. This is usually accomplished by selecting controls from patients admitted to the same hospitals as the cases for conditions other than the one being studied (see e.g. Box 4.5). Although this is a much more efficient and economical process than selecting population controls, it is associated with an obvious major

Box 4.5 Hospital controls: the pros and cons

Tertiary referral clinics may attract patients from an unpredictably wide variety of geographical and social origins. If cases are identified through these clinics it can then be a major challenge to find a group of disease-free controls that represent the same geographical and social backgrounds as the cases. For example, a colonoscopy is needed to diagnose adenoma (polyps) of the large bowel so a colonoscopy clinic is an ideal place to identify cases for a study. If controls are selected at random from the local population there is no guarantee that they would have been picked up as cases if they had adenoma – they might have gone to a different facility. Similarly, we would miss all of those people from outside the local population who would, nonetheless, have travelled to that clinic for treatment. An alternative then is to select controls from among other patients attending the clinic who have a colonoscopy but do *not* have bowel polyps. This solution ensures that the controls will represent the geographical and social distribution of the cases, but it is important to be aware that it might also introduce other biases. For example, if there are characteristics, such as a family history of bowel cancer, that make someone more likely to be referred for colonoscopy then these characteristics will be over-represented in the control group. This example serves to emphasise that epidemiological studies will rarely be perfect – the important thing is to do the best that is possible in a given situation and then to consider the likely effects of any bias (see Chapter 7).

drawback. The controls are themselves ill and thus different from most healthy people in the source population from which the cases come. Indeed, their distribution of risk factors (especially personal habits such as smoking, excessive alcohol consumption, etc.) may well resemble that of the cases rather more than that of the source population, leading to biased results. However, thoughtful use of such designs can still provide good public health information and Box 4.6 shows an example of such a study that has been used for post-marketing drug surveillance (sometimes called pharmacoepidemiology).

An important issue related to the selection of both cases and controls is that they must be chosen *independently of their exposure status*. In a case–control study of oral contraceptive pill use and deep vein thrombosis, for example, whether or not a woman is using the pill should not affect her chances of being recruited as either a case or control. Knowledge of the exposure status of individuals could lead to bias in participant recruitment called **selection bias**. Another type of bias that can occur within case–control studies arises when the information collected from the cases and controls is not comparable. This can occur if an interviewer elicits or interprets exposure information differently when the

Box 4.6 Using hospital controls for pharmacoepidemiology

Hospital controls have been used very successfully to identify harmful side effects of prescription medications in a number of settings. One of the earliest and longest-running pharmacoepidemiology research projects using this design is the Case–Control Surveillance Study run by the Slone Epidemiology Center at Boston University (http://www.bu.edu/slone/Research/Studies/CCS/CCS.htm), which has been going for over 30 years. Its purpose is to systematically evaluate the relationship of medications to the incidence of certain illnesses and to screen for unsuspected drug–disease associations. Since 1983, the main focus of the study has been on various cancers. Patients newly diagnosed with a cancer of interest and who reside in the study area (cases) are recruited from a network of hospitals. Patients from the same area with acute conditions such as appendicitis or chronic conditions such as kidney stones or gallstones diagnosed within the past year are recruited as controls. All patients are interviewed to collect a wide range of information about lifestyle and a medical and lifetime medication history. To date, over 80,000 patients have been interviewed, including over 25,000 with cancer, leading to multiple publications such as a recent report providing reassurance that use of statins to lower cholesterol levels does not increase an individual's risk of cancer (Coogan *et al.*, 2007).

disease status of the individual is known (**interviewer bias**) or because people with disease recall their exposures or experiences more precisely than or otherwise differently from those without disease (**recall bias**). We will revisit bias and other forms of inaccuracy in data collection and discuss the potential impact of these types of error on the results of a study in Chapter 7.

There are several modern variants of the case–control study design, the most common being *nested case–control* and *case-crossover* designs. A third related design is the *case–cohort* study which we discussed under cohort studies above, as it is essentially a different way of analysing cohort data.

Nested case–control studies

The **nested case–control** study is similar in principle to the case-cohort study in that it seeks to combine the cost benefits of a case–control study with the advantages of prospective data collection in a cohort study. It is fundamentally a case–control study that is 'nested' within an existing cohort study. As in the case–cohort study, cases are cohort members who developed the disease of interest, but this time controls are selected from cohort members who were disease-free at the time the cases were diagnosed (i.e. the controls are 'matched' to the cases for follow-up). Nested case–control studies are simpler to analyse than case–cohort studies but require a separate control group to be selected for each case group.

Case–crossover studies

The **case–crossover** design is especially suited to identifying the effects of transient exposures on the risk of an acute-onset disease. Instead of recruiting a separate group of controls, each case is also their own control and their exposure in a defined period prior to the onset of disease is compared with their normal exposure frequency. This innovative design eliminates many of the problems inherent in studies that compare different groups of people and comes closest to the theoretical (but unattainable) ideal, which would be to study an exposed population and then wind back the clock and study exactly the same population again when they had not been exposed.

In the seminal case–crossover study, Maclure (1991) examined the influence of a variety of possible precipitating factors, including sexual activity, on the occurrence of myocardial infarction (MI, or heart attack). He classified cases as exposed if they had been sexually active in the two hours before their MI and then compared this with their usual frequency of sexual activity over a one-year period. He hypothesised that if sexual activity were a risk factor for MI, then more cases would have been sexually active shortly before their MI than would be expected from their usual frequency. After interviewing 300 cases he estimated that sexual activity increased an individual's risk of MI more than two-fold.

Intervention studies

As we discussed above, the ideal way to study whether something is causally related to the occurrence of disease is through an experiment or intervention study although, for practical reasons, this study design is often not a viable option. Box 4.1 gives an example of an early intervention study and the examples in Box 4.7 give a hint of the range of interventions that can be studied experimentally. In each study the investigators 'intervened' to change something in the hope that this would improve the future health of the participants. The participants in the ISIS trials were already sick (patients who had had an MI), and the intervention was intended to improve their duration of survival – aspirin and streptokinase were shown to be very effective. In contrast, the children in the polio vaccine trial were healthy and it was hoped that the vaccine would prevent them from becoming ill. Similarly, it was hoped that vitamin A supplementation would reduce childhood mortality but, in this example, the intervention was given to whole villages rather than individual children.

Box 4.7 Some large-scale intervention studies

- The ISIS (International Studies of Infarct Survival) investigators compared various treatments for myocardial infarction (heart attack), including the use of aspirin and streptokinase in ISIS-2 (ISIS-2 Collaborative Group, 1988). More than 100,000 patients throughout the world were recruited into these studies.
- In the early 1950s, one of the largest epidemiological studies, and almost certainly the largest formal human 'experiment', was conducted in the USA. This was a field trial of polio vaccine in which over 400,000 school children were assigned to receive either the vaccine or a placebo (inactive) injection. The trial clearly demonstrated both the efficacy and the safety of the vaccine, which was then given to millions of children throughout the world (Francis *et al.*, 1955). This has led to a major drop in the incidence of polio not only in industrialised countries but also in many developing countries, which have recently been declared polio-free by the WHO.
- In the US Physicians' Health Study (we have already met the British Doctors and the US Nurses' Health studies!), 22,000 physicians were randomly allocated to take aspirin, in an attempt to reduce cardiovascular morbidity and mortality, and/or capsules of β-carotene, in an attempt to reduce rates of cancer (Hennekens and Eberlein, 1985). After 12 years of follow-up, rates of cancer were very similar in the β-carotene and placebo groups, and, while aspirin was shown to lower the rates of heart attack, so few of these very healthy doctors died that the trial could not determine whether aspirin saved lives from cardiovascular disease.
- A randomised, controlled community trial was conducted to evaluate the effectiveness of vitamin A supplementation to prevent childhood mortality in Indonesia (Sommer *et al.*, 1986). In 229 villages, children aged 1–5 years were given two doses of vitamin A while children in the 221 control villages were not given vitamin A until after the study. Mortality among children in the control villages was 50% higher than that in the villages given vitamin A.

Randomised controlled trials (RCTs)

The best way to evaluate a new treatment is to identify a group of patients with the same condition and then allocate them to receive the various treatments at *random*. A preventive trial differs only in that it involves people who are disease-free but thought to be at risk of developing disease. **Random allocation** (also called **randomisation**[2]) ensures that all of the groups are as similar as possible at the start of the study. (Note that equality of the groups at baseline is highly dependent on group size – with very small groups it is unlikely that the groups will be similar in terms of all important variables that could affect the outcome.) Random allocation is important because if one group were in some way more ill (or less healthy) than the other at the start, this might make this group look worse, even if the intervention really had no effect. (This problem is called **confounding** and we will discuss it in more detail in Chapter 8.) It is because of this aspect of RCTs – the close similarity of the groups in all respects other than the intervention – that they are generally considered to give the best evidence of all epidemiological studies. In a cohort study investigating potentially harmful risk factors, people cannot be randomly allocated to the various study groups and, for example, a group of alcohol drinkers will certainly differ from a group of non-drinkers in more ways than just their alcohol consumption. While we can deal with some of these factors in our analysis, there may also be other important factors that we either do not know about or cannot measure well. The real strength of randomisation is that, on average, it will also balance these other unknown or unmeasured factors across the groups.

From www.CartoonStock.com

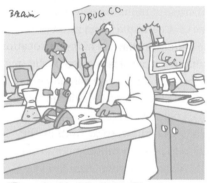

"Do a double-blind test. Give the new drug to rich patients and a placebo to the poor. No sense getting their hopes up. They couldn't afford it even if it works."

Randomised controlled trials also include a **control** or comparison group so that outcomes in the treated group can be compared with those in a group that is not treated. Generally, the patients in the control group either receive no treatment or, preferably, they are given a placebo (something that resembles the real treatment but is not active). If an acceptable standard treatment is available the

---

[2] Note the important distinction between 'random selection', where we select people at random to be in our study but we do not control whether or not they are exposed (unless it is also a RCT), and 'randomisation', where we do control exposure by randomly allocating people to the exposed and non-exposed groups in an intervention study.

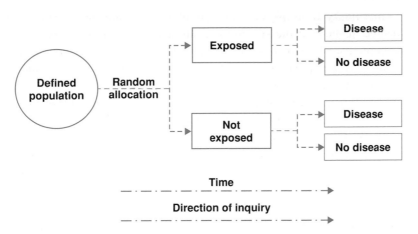

Figure 4.4 The design of a randomised controlled trial.

control group must be given this – it would be unethical to withhold it – and this is compared with the new experimental treatment. Figure 4.4 shows the design features of a simple randomised controlled trial. In practice it is just a special form of the standard prospective cohort study – the only difference being that participants are allocated to the exposed and unexposed groups at random.

Ideally, both the trial investigators and the participants should be unaware of whether the participant is in the active intervention or placebo group, creating a 'double-blind' or 'masked' study. If only the patient is unaware of their allocation, it is a single-blind study. Blinding is important because knowledge of the treatment might affect both the participant's response – quite a few people feel better after taking a placebo simply because they believe it will do them good – and an observer's measurement of outcome. In some situations (e.g. comparing medical treatment with surgery) there may be no feasible way of blinding patients and study personnel to the differences in treatments. Minimising measurement bias in this situation may be best accomplished by bringing in an independent 'blinded' observer whose only involvement is to assess the outcome measure. Blinding of outcome measurements obviously becomes more crucial as the measurement becomes more subjective. When the outcome measure is objective and less dependent on interpretation, as in a biochemical parameter or death, blinding is less important.

Apart from participants and trial investigators, there are many others (e.g. healthcare providers, data collectors, outcome assessors, data analysts) involved in the conduct of a trial who can introduce bias through their knowledge of treatment allocation. For this reason there is a growing tendency to abandon the terms single- and double-blind in favour of a transparent reporting of the blinding status of each group involved in the trial.

As for a cohort study, the other crucial feature of an RCT is good follow-up. It is important to know what has happened to all of the participants in the study.

Community trials are preventive trials in which the intervention is implemented at the community level and are generally conducted when it would be impossible to offer (or evaluate) the intervention at the individual level. An example is the studies of water fluoridation and dental health conducted in various countries. When investigators wanted to study the effects of adding fluoride to the water supply on dental health it was clearly impossible to add fluoride to some people's water and not to others', so whole towns were allocated to receive fluoride in their water or not. The controlled trial of water fluoridation which gave the most striking results was carried out in the towns of Newburgh and Kingston in New York State, USA. After 10 years of fluoridation, the DMF (decayed, missing or filled teeth) score for Newburgh children aged 6–16 was 50% lower than that for children in the unfluoridated town of Kingston (Ast and Schlesinger, 1956). The assumption underlying this result was that, apart from the water, there was no other major difference between the towns that could explain the effect (i.e. there was no confounding). (Note that, although this and other studies clearly showed the benefits of low levels of fluoride on dental health, continuing controversy about the possible adverse effects of fluoride on other organs in the body, particularly the bones, has meant that universal fluoridation of water supplies has not occurred.) Because only two towns were included in this study, in practice it is little different from a non-randomised comparison. Other cluster designs involve larger numbers of groups, so that the random allocation of multiple groups to intervention or no intervention gives more of the benefits of randomisation in terms of balancing out other factors across the groups (e.g. the vitamin A study, Box 4.7).

Crossover trials

Randomised trials can be categorised as either **parallel group** or **crossover** trials. Figure 4.4 shows the design of a parallel group RCT, in which patients are randomly allocated to one of the two groups, which are then followed in parallel. In a crossover design, the participants serve as their own controls (this is analogous to the case–crossover study we described earlier). For example, in a simple two-period crossover study to assess the efficacy of an intervention we would assign each participant to either the intervention or the control (I or C) for a specified period of time and then the alternative for a similar period of time. The order in which each participant receives I and C is randomly assigned. Thus, approximately half of the participants receive the intervention in the sequence I–C and the other half in the sequence C–I. This eliminates any trend from the first period to the second period from the estimate of group differences in response. One of the biggest advantages of this design is that it can produce statistically and clinically valid results with fewer participants than would be required with a parallel design. However, not all interventions are suitable for assessment in this way. If the effects of the intervention during the first period are likely to carry over into the second period then this design is clearly inappropriate, as it is for assessing long-term benefits and harms.

n-of-1 trials

A variant of the crossover trial is the single patient trial, often called an **n-of-1 trial**.[3] An individual patient receives the experimental and control treatments in random order on multiple occasions, with specific outcomes being monitored throughout the trial period. Ideally both the patient and the treating doctor are blinded to the treatment being received and the trial usually ends when it becomes clear that there are (or are not) important differences between the treatments. Although the results of n-of-1 trials are not generalisable to the same extent as those of typical RCTs, they do provide a good guide to individual clinical decisions.

Other intervention designs

The fact that a study is described as a trial or clinical trial does not necessarily mean that it is a randomised trial. Probably the most common non-randomised design in the health setting is one that uses 'historical controls', where health outcomes following the introduction of a new treatment or preventive measure are compared to the outcomes experienced by the same population before the change in practice. For example, in many countries mortality rates from road traffic accidents fell dramatically after the introduction of legislation requiring drivers to wear seat belts. Similarly, patient survival rates might be compared before and after the introduction of a new surgical technique. The main problem with this design is that it does of course assume that the only (or most important) thing that has changed is the new legislation or the type of surgery and that may not be the case. While RCTs remain the gold standard for initial evaluation of new clinical and public health interventions, the effectiveness of these interventions in practice can often only be determined from these very simple 'before and after' comparisons in whole communities or populations. You will see many examples of this throughout the book, and particularly when we discuss prevention in Chapter 14 and screening in Chapter 15.

A word about ethics

We touched on this under Record linkage above but it would be remiss of us to end this discussion of study design without some consideration of the subject of research ethics. Before conducting any research on humans

---

[3] Note 'n' is often used to denote the sample size in a study; an n-of-1 study is thus a study where $n = 1$ person.

Box 4.8 Notable events and documents in the development of modern ethical guidelines

< 1945 German scientists accused of experimenting on human subjects in Nazi concentration camps during World War II; also the beginnings of large-scale research in the USA using groups such as orphans, the mentally handicapped and prisoners

1947 The Nuremberg Code
A list of 10 principles of medical and research ethics developed from the Nuremberg trials in Germany at the end of World War II (see Box 4.9), but largely ignored at the time

1964 The Declaration of Helsinki
Developed at a meeting of the World Medical Association in Helsinki as a statement of ethical principles to provide guidance to physicians and other participants in medical research
(http://ohsr.od.nih.gov/guidelines/helsinki.html)

1966 Beecher's Report
Publication of a report citing 22 post-war studies that were ethically flawed despite being conducted at prestigious institutions and published in the top journals (Beecher, 1966)

1972 Publication of a report from the Tuskegee syphilis study in the USA (1932–1972)
This caused outrage when it became clear that study participants had been misled and deprived of treatment
(http://www.cdc.gov/tuskegee/timeline.htm)

1979 The Belmont Report
A document developed by what was then the United States Department of Health, Education, and Welfare entitled 'Ethical Principles and Guidelines for the Protection of Human Subjects of Research'
(http://ohsr.od.nih.gov/guidelines/belmont.html)

(or animals), most developed countries require the study protocol to be approved by a Human Research Ethics Committee (or Institutional Review Board, IRB, in the USA). This is to ensure that the rights of participants are fully protected in any research study – that they are fully informed of any risks and benefits associated with participation and that the benefits of the research (to the individual or, more often, to society) sufficiently outweigh the potential risks.

Current guidelines for medical research ethics can be traced back more than 50 years to the end of World War II (see Box 4.8) although some of the core concepts go back as far as Hippocrates. They are based on four moral principles:

Box 4.9 The Nuremberg Code, 1947

1. The voluntary consent of the human subject is absolutely essential. This means that the person involved should have legal capacity to give consent; should be so situated as to be able to exercise free power of choice, without the intervention of any element of force, fraud, deceit, duress, over-reaching, or other ulterior form of constraint or coercion; and should have sufficient knowledge and comprehension of the elements of the subject matter involved as to enable him to make an understanding and enlightened decision. This latter element requires that before the acceptance of an affirmative decision by the experimental subject there should be made known to him the nature, duration, and purpose of the experiment; the method and means by which it is to be conducted; all inconveniences and hazards reasonable to be expected; and the effects upon his health or person which may possibly come from his participation in the experiment.

    The duty and responsibility for ascertaining the quality of the consent rests upon each individual who initiates, directs or engages in the experiment. It is a personal duty and responsibility which may not be delegated to another with impunity.
2. The experiment should be such as to yield fruitful results for the good of society, unprocurable by other methods or means of study, and not random and unnecessary in nature.
3. The experiment should be so designed and based on the results of animal experimentation and a knowledge of the natural history of the disease or other problem under study that the anticipated results will justify the performance of the experiment.
4. The experiment should be so conducted as to avoid all unnecessary physical and mental suffering and injury.
5. No experiment should be conducted where there is an *a priori* reason to believe that death or disabling injury will occur; except, perhaps, in those experiments where the experimental physicians also serve as subjects.
6. The degree of risk to be taken should never exceed that determined by the humanitarian importance of the problem to be solved by the experiment.
7. Proper preparations should be made and adequate facilities provided to protect the experimental subject against even remote possibilities of injury, disability, or death.
8. The experiment should be conducted only by scientifically qualified persons. The highest degree of skill and care should be required through all stages of the experiment of those who conduct or engage in the experiment.

(*continued*)

> **Box 4.9** *(continued)*
>
> 9. During the course of the experiment the human subject should be at liberty to bring the experiment to an end if he has reached the physical or mental state where continuation of the experiment seems to him to be impossible.
> 10. During the course of the experiment the scientist in charge must be prepared to terminate the experiment at any stage, if he has probable cause to believe, in the exercise of the good faith, superior skill and careful judgment required of him that a continuation of the experiment is likely to result in injury, disability, or death to the experimental subject.
>
> From *Trials of War Criminals before the Nuremberg Military Tribunals under Control Council Law No. 10, Vol. 2, pp. 181–182.* Washington DC: U.S. Government Printing Office, 1949.

Beneficience – do good;

Non-maleficence – do no harm; in practice this has to be balanced against the principle of beneficience – the potential benefits should outweigh the possible risks;

Respect for autonomy – respect the rights of the individual; this includes the right to privacy and the right to make informed decisions and thus the need for study participants to give their 'informed consent' before enrolling in a study;

Justice – equity, impartiality and fairness.

These principles were first codified in a practical form after the Nuremburg trials of German medical researchers at the end of World War II. The resulting 'Nuremburg Code', which underpins all subsequent codes of health research ethics, is shown in Box 4.9. However, this Code was largely ignored at the time and formal statements outlining requirements for the ethical conduct of research did not start to appear until the late 1970s after continuing reports of disquieting ethical practices such as the Tuskagee Study (see Box 4.8) and the Willowbrook Study (1963–1966) where children in an institution for the mentally handicapped were deliberately infected with hepatitis virus to study the course of the infection (http://iris.uwaterloo.ca/ethics/human/resources/index.htm).

Tensions continue today between the need to protect the rights of individuals (often via strict privacy laws) and the public need for good quality information to improve health. Rigid application of privacy laws can make some forms of epidemiological research almost impossible. As discussed above, this is especially true for record linkage studies where it may be impractical or even impossible to obtain consent from individuals to access their information. The costs of complying with human research guidelines can also drive up the costs of research, with studies often needing to obtain approval from, and report back to, multiple different ethics committees. However, as the historical examples cited above emphasise, we cannot ignore the need for real autonomy in relation to participation in research.

If you are interested in learning more about research ethics the US National Institute of Health (NIH) Office of Extramural Research has developed a free on-line tutorial (http://phrp.nihtraining.com/users/login.php). Although it is designed primarily for NIH grant holders who are subject to US Department of Health and Human Services regulations, the majority of the content is generic and applicable to all.

Summary

Experimental studies like those described above are theoretically the ideal way to look for associations between exposure and disease or health outcome. They do, however, have to be designed, run and reported rigorously to realise this potential in terms of providing convincing evidence concerning causality. Unfortunately, they are often inappropriate (for ethical reasons), not feasible or unaffordable. Furthermore, since they are often conducted in highly selected groups of volunteers, it can be challenging to generalise their findings and we will come back to this problem in Chapter 11. The non-experimental study designs, particularly cohort and case–control studies, are therefore of central importance in public health and, as you will see when we discuss causality in Chapter 10, other designs such as ecological studies can also provide valuable information. The fundamental importance of descriptive studies in monitoring the health of a population and for identifying emerging health problems should already be apparent, and you will see further examples of their essential role in evaluating the effects of population interventions when we discuss prevention in Chapter 14 and screening in Chapter 15. Each design thus has an important role to play and, as you have seen, different designs will be more or less appropriate in different situations. It is also essential to recognise the strengths and limitations of each; we will consider these further in Chapter 7 when we look at some of the sources of bias in epidemiological studies.

Questions

1. Complete Table 4.1 to show the relative strengths and limitations of the main study designs, scoring each one on a scale from 1 = poor (e.g. not good to investigate a rare disease or very expensive) to 5 = excellent (e.g. very good to investigate rare exposure or very quick to do).
2. Look back to Box 4.9 and identify which of the four fundamental moral principles apply to each of the 10 statements in the Nuremburg Code.

Table 4.1 Comparing the strengths and weaknesses of different study designs.

	Ecological	Cross-sectional	Case–control	Cohort	Randomised controlled trial	Nested case–control
Investigation of rare disease or outcome						
Investigation of a rare exposure						
Testing multiple effects of an exposure						
Study of multiple exposures						
Establishing temporality[a]						
Give a direct measure of incidence						
Explore exposures which change over time						
Time required						
Costs						
Ethical problems						

[a] i.e. that the exposure came before the outcome.

REFERENCES

45 and Up Study Collaborators. (2008). Cohort profile: the 45 and Up Study. *International Journal of Epidemiology*, **37**: 941–947.

Ast, D. B. and Schlesinger, E. R. (1956). The conclusion of a ten-year study of water fluoridation. *American Journal of Public Health*, **46**: 265–271.

Beaglehole, R., Bonita, R. and Kjellström, T. (1993). *Basic Epidemiology*. Geneva: World Health Organization.

Beecher, H. K. (1966). Ethics and clinical research. *New England Journal of Medicine*, **274**: 1354–1360.

Coogan, P. F., Rosenberg, L. and Strom, B. L. (2007). Statin use and the risk of 10 cancers. *Epidemiology*, **18**: 213–219.

Dawber, T. R. (1980). *The Framingham Study. The Epidemiology of Atherosclerotic Disease*. Harvard: Harvard University Press.

Doll, R. and Hill, A. B. (1964). Mortality in relation to smoking: ten years' observations of British doctors. *British Medical Journal*, **1**: 1399–1410, 1460–1467.

Francis, Jr T., Korns, R. F., Voight, R. B. *et al.* (1955). An evaluation of the 1954 poliomyelitis vaccine trials: summary report. *American Journal of Public Health*, **45**: 1–65.

Frankel, S., Gunnell, D. J., Peters, T. J., Maynard, M. and Davey, Smith G. (1998). Childhood energy intake and adult mortality from cancer: the Boyd Orr cohort study. *British Medical Journal*, **316**: 499–504.

Golding, J., Pembrey, M., Jones, R. and the ALSPAC Study Team. (2001). ALSPAC – the Avon Longitudinal Study of Parents and Children. I. Study methodology. *Paediatric and Perinatal Epidemiology*, **15**: 74–87.

Hennekens, C. H. and Eberlein, K. (1985). A randomised trial of aspirin and b-carotene among U.S. physicians. *Preventive Medicine*, **14**: 165–168.

ISIS-2 Collaborative Group. (1988). Randomised trial of intravenous streptokinase, oral aspirin, both or neither among 17187 cases of suspected acute myocardial infarction: ISIS-2. *Lancet*, **2**: 349–360.

Jordan, S. J., Green, A. C., Whiteman, D. C. *et al.* (2008). Serous ovarian, fallopian tube and primary peritoneal cancers: a comparative epidemiological analysis. *International Journal of Cancer*, **122**: 1598–1603.

Kelman, C. W., Bass, A. J. and Holman, C. D. J. (2002). Research use of linked data – a best practice protocol. *Australian and New Zealand Journal of Public Health*, **26**: 251–255.

Lawlor D. A. and Stone, T. (2001). Public health and data protection: an inevitable collision or potential for a meeting of minds? *International Journal of Epidemiology*, **30**: 1221–1225.

Lind, J. (1753). *A Treatise of the Scurvy. A Bicentenary Volume*. Edinburgh: Sands, Murray and Cochran.

Maclure, M. (1991). The case–crossover design: a method for studying transient effects on the risk of acute events. *American Journal of Epidemiology*, **133**: 144–153.

Mellin, G. W. and Katzenstein, M. (1962). The saga of thalidomide: neuropathy to embryopathy, with case reports of congenital anomalies. *New England Journal of Medicine*, **267**: 1184–1193, 1238–1244.

Nagle, C. M., Purdie, D. M., Webb, P. M. *et al.* (2003). Dietary influences on survival following ovarian cancer. *International Journal of Cancer*, **106**: 264–269.

Paffenbarger Jr, R. S., Hyde, R. T., Wing, A. L. and Hsieh, C. C. (1986). Physical activity, all-cause mortality, and longevity of college alumni. *New England Journal of Medicine*, **314**: 605–613.

Pillai, A., Andrews, T. and Patel, V. (2009). Violence, psychological distress and the risk of suicidal behaviour in young people in India. *International Journal of Epidemiology*, **38**: 459–469.

Ponsonby, A. L., Dwyer, T., Gibbons, L. E., Cochrane, J. A. and Wang, Y-G. (1993). Factors potentiating the risk of sudden death syndrome associated with the prone position. *New England Journal of Medicine*, **329**: 377–382.

Rockhill, B., Willett, W. C., Hunter, D. J. *et al.* (1998). Physical activity and breast cancer risk in a cohort of young women. *Journal of the National Cancer Institute*, **90**: 1155–1160.

Sandler, D. P., Smith, J. C., Weinberg, C. R. *et al.* (1989). Analgesic use and chronic renal disease. *New England Journal of Medicine*, **320**: 1238–1243.

Sommer, A., Tarwotjo, I., Djunaedi, E. *et al.* (1986). Impact of vitamin A supplementation on childhood mortality. A randomised controlled community trial. *The Lancet*, **327**: 1169–1173.

Stampfer, M. J., Willett, W. C., Colditz, G. A., Speizer, F. E. and Hennekens, C. H. (1988). A prospective study of past use of oral contraceptive agents and risk of cardiovascular diseases. *New England Journal of Medicine*, **319**: 1313–1317.

The EUROGAST Study Group. (1993). An international association between *Helicobacter pylori* infection and gastric cancer. *Lancet*, **341**: 1359–1362.

The Million Women Study Collaborative Group. (1999). The Million Women Study: design and characteristics of the study population. *Breast Cancer Research*, **1**: 73–80.

Zendehdel, K., Nyrén, O., Östenson, C.-G. *et al.* (2003). Cancer incidence in patients with type 1 diabetes: a population-based cohort study in Sweden. *Journal of the National Cancer Institute*, **95**: 1797–1800.

Zhang, M., Holman, C. D. J., Price, S. D. *et al.* (2009). Comorbidity and repeat admission to hospital for adverse drug reactions in older adults: retrospective cohort study. *British Medical Journal*, **338**: a2752 doi: 10.1136/bmj.a2752.

Why? Linking exposure and disease

Description	Association	Alternative explanations	Integration & interpretation	Practical applications
Chapters 2–3	Chapter 5: Measures of association	Chapters 6–8	Chapters 9–11	Chapters 12–15

Box 5.1 Who does all the housework?

His view: Australian men do **three times more** housework today than they did 40 years ago . . .

Her view: Australian men spend 5 minutes a day on laundry now compared to 1.6 minutes 40 years ago – an **extra $3\frac{1}{2}$ minutes a day** . . .

(Maushart, 2003.)

As you learned in Chapter 1, one of the main uses of epidemiology is to identify the causes of disease and this is of fundamental importance in all areas of public health – if we can work out what is causing ill-health then we can work to prevent it. In Chapter 2 we looked at the ways in which we can measure the occurrence of disease and touched on some ways in which we can compare different populations. But while measuring the occurrence of a disease in a population can tell us about the health of that population, it does not directly shed much light on the underlying causes of the disease. To identify the aspects of people or their environment (exposures) that might lead to the onset of disease, we need to *compare* disease occurrence in groups with and without the exposures of interest. In Chapter 4 we looked at some of the study designs that we can use to do this; now we will look more closely at the measures we use to quantify the associations between 'exposures', or potential causes of disease, and the disease itself. By quantifying the association between an exposure and disease we can start to make judgements as to whether the exposure might actually cause the disease (we will discuss causality in more detail in Chapter 10). If we believe that it is causing disease, we can then identify the importance of that exposure in terms of its overall effect on the health of a community.

In this chapter we will look at the ways in which we calculate, use and interpret these 'measures of association', so-called because they describe the association between an exposure and a health outcome. An understanding of these measures will help you to interpret reports regarding the causes of ill-health and the effects of particular exposures or interventions on the burden of illness in a community. Note that, while we will discuss the measures in the context of an 'exposure' and 'disease', they can be used to assess the association between any measure of health status and any potential 'cause'.

Looking for associations

We all know that smoking is a cause of lung cancer but might it also increase the risk of stroke? To answer this question we could compare the incidence of stroke in a group of women who smoke with that in a group of non-smokers.

Table 5.1 displays data from a cohort study in which the investigators followed a large group of women for several years (person-years of observation). They classified the women as never smokers, ex-smokers and current smokers, recorded how many women had a stroke during the follow-up period and calculated the **incidence rate** of stroke in each group.

How many **times more likely** was
 (i) a current smoker to have a stroke than a never smoker and
 (ii) an ex-smoker to have a stroke than a never smoker?

Table 5.1 Stroke incidence rates by smoking category in female nurses.

Smoking category	No. of cases of stroke	Person-years of observation	Incidence rate per 100,000 person-years
Never smoked	70	395,594	17.7
Ex-smoker	65	232,712	27.9
Current smoker	139	280,141	49.6
Total	274	908,447	30.2

(Colditz *et al.*, 1988.)

Compared with non-smokers, how many **extra** strokes were there per 100,000 person-years in

(i) ex-smokers and

(ii) current smokers?

There are two main ways in which we can compare smokers and non-smokers. First, ex-smokers were *1.6 times* (27.9 ÷ 17.7) and current smokers were *2.8 times* (49.6 ÷ 17.7) as likely to have a stroke as never smokers during the follow-up period. An alternative way to look at the data would be to say that, all other things being equal, if the smokers had never smoked we would have expected them to have the same rate of stroke as the never smokers, i.e. 17.7/100,000 person-years. This means that, compared with never smokers, there were an *extra 10.2 strokes per 100,000 person-years* (27.9 − 17.7) in ex-smokers and an *extra 31.9 strokes per 100,000 person-years* (49.6 − 17.7) in current smokers.

What we calculated above were, first, the **rate ratio** and, second, the **rate difference** for the association between smoking and stroke. These measures give us two different ways of quantifying the relation between an exposure and a disease. The **rate ratio** tells us how many times higher the rate of disease is in one group than in another group (e.g. current smokers are almost three times as likely to have a stroke as never smokers). This gives an indication of the *strength* of the association and can help us to decide whether smoking could be a cause of stroke. The **rate difference** tells us how much extra disease occurred in one group compared with another group (e.g. there were an extra 32 strokes per 100,000 person-years among current smokers compared with non-smokers). If we believe that smoking is a cause of stroke then this extra disease can be attributed to the fact that the women had smoked in the past and, theoretically, it would not have occurred if they had never smoked. This information gives some sense of the potential value of a preventive intervention, in this case a programme aimed at stopping women from taking up smoking. (Of course, if such an intervention were successful it would reduce the incidence of many diseases, not just stroke.)

From www.CartoonStock.com

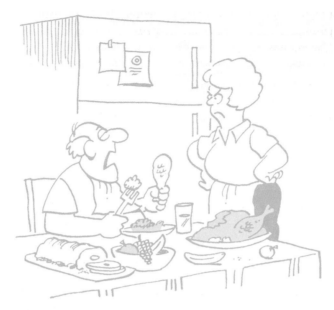

"What do you mean I never help out around the house - Right now I'm cleaning out the fridge!"

It is important to remember that ratio and difference measures give us very different perspectives on a given situation. Look back to Box 5.1 at the start of the chapter. Men would probably prefer to look at the **ratio** or **relative** measure: they do three times more housework now than 40 years ago. In contrast, women would focus on the **difference** or **absolute** measure: men may do three times more laundry now than 40 years ago but they still do an average of only 5 minutes (3.5 minutes extra) per day.

Ratio measures (relative risk)

The cholera was therefore **14 times as fatal** at this period amongst persons having the impure water of the Southwark and Vauxhall Company, as amongst those having the purer water from Thames Ditton (Snow, 1855).

People who ate cold chicken at the youth camp were **almost four times more likely** to become ill than people who did not eat cold chicken (from Table 1.2).

Ratio or relative measures tell us how many times more likely it is that someone who is exposed to something will develop a certain disease or experience a particular health outcome than (or *relative* to) someone who is not exposed. *They do not tell us anything about the actual amount of disease occurring in either group.* They provide information about the *strength* of the association between the exposure and the outcome and, as you will see in Chapter 10, a strong association is more suggestive that the exposure is actually causing the outcome. In the example above, the rate ratio for stroke and current smoking was 2.8. This is a fairly strong association and would add weight to an argument that smoking was actually causing strokes, although it is not as compelling as the much stronger relation between smoking and lung cancer, for which the rate ratio for current smoking is somewhere between 10 and 15.

As the example shows, ratio measures are very easy to calculate – you simply divide the frequency of disease (or of any health outcome) in the group that is exposed to the factor of interest by the frequency in the group that is not exposed to it. This can be done using either of the measures of disease incidence that you met in Chapter 2. If you divide two incidence rates you end up with a **rate ratio** (as for the stroke example above); if you divide two measures of cumulative incidence or risk then it is a **risk ratio**. It is also possible to divide two measures of prevalence to calculate a **prevalence ratio**. Note that you must always divide two measures of the same type – you cannot usefully divide an incidence rate by a measure of cumulative incidence.

Rate ratios

As you saw above, a **rate ratio** is calculated by simply dividing the incidence rate of disease in a group of people exposed to the factor of interest (often denoted by a subscript 'e') by the incidence rate in a group of people who are not exposed to the same factor (denoted by a subscript 'o'):

$$\text{Rate Ratio} = \frac{\text{Incidence Rate in exposed}}{\text{Incidence Rate in unexposed}} = \frac{IR_e}{IR_o} \qquad (5.1)$$

This factor could be a potential cause of disease, it could be a characteristic of a person, such as their age or where they live, or it could be something that influences behaviour. Equally, it could be a preventive measure or, in the clinical context, a drug or other treatment that we hope will reduce the incidence of disease.

Risk ratios

Similarly, the **risk ratio** (also called the **relative risk**) is calculated by dividing the cumulative incidence or risk of disease in an exposed group by the cumulative incidence in an unexposed group:

$$\text{Risk Ratio} = \frac{\text{Cumulative Incidence in exposed}}{\text{Cumulative Incidence in unexposed}} = \frac{CI_e}{CI_o} \qquad (5.2)$$

Table 5.2 The results of a study evaluating the effects of calling patients on influenza immunisation rates.

| | Outcome | | |
Exposure	Immunised	Not immunised	% immunised
Received a call	328	332	50%
No call	288	370	44%
Total	616	702	47%

(Hull *et al.*, 2002.)

In Chapter 2 we considered a randomised trial to evaluate whether taking aspirin would reduce the risk of blood clots in people with infective endocarditis. Look back at Table 2.3 on page 44 and calculate the risk ratio for the association between aspirin and blood clots.

In this trial, the risk ratio was 28.3% ÷ 20.0% = 1.4; those who took aspirin were 1.4 times as likely to develop blood clots as those who did not take aspirin. A risk ratio of 1.0 would mean that there was no difference between the groups, so those taking aspirin were 40% *more likely* to develop blood clots than those not taking aspirin (in the context of clinical epidemiology this may be described as the relative risk increase or RRI). If aspirin had reduced the risk of blood clots then we would have expected to see a risk ratio of less than 1.0. Clearly this intervention did not work the way the investigators had hoped it would.

This approach can be used much more widely than in the search for the causes of disease. As an example, a trial carried out in three general practices in the UK set out to find out whether telephoning patients to offer them an appointment for immunisation against influenza would increase immunisation uptake rates (Hull *et al.*, 2002). In this study, attending for immunisation was the outcome of interest and receiving a telephone call was the exposure. A total of 1,318 patients aged 65 to 74 years were randomly assigned to two groups. Patients in one group ($n = 660$) received a telephone call from the receptionist at their general practice inviting them to make an appointment for immunisation (the intervention or exposed group). Patients in the other group ($n = 658$) were not called (the control or unexposed group). The investigators then waited to see who turned up for immunisation. They found that 328 of the patients who received a phone call attended, as did 288 of those who did not receive a call.

The easiest way to look at these data is in the form of a '2 × 2 table'. These tables are usually set out so that the two columns show the numbers of people with and without the outcome of interest while the rows show the numbers in the exposed and unexposed groups (Table 5.2).

What was the cumulative incidence of immunisation or, in other words, what percentage of patients attended for immunisation in each of the two groups?

How many times more likely were patients to attend if they had received a personal call to make an appointment than if they had not been telephoned?

In the intervention group 50% of patients were immunised, compared with 44% of those in the control group (despite the intervention the immunisation rates were still below the government target of 60%). This means that patients who received an invitation were 1.14 times (50% ÷ 44%) more likely to attend for immunisation. This measure is still a relative risk because it has the same structure – the cumulative incidence (or risk) of a particular health outcome in one group is divided by the cumulative incidence in a second group. In this case the word 'risk' seems less appropriate but the term relative risk is still regularly used.

Prevalence ratios

As you saw when we discussed **prevalence surveys** in Chapter 3 and **cross-sectional studies** in the previous chapter, it is also possible to use measures of prevalence instead of incidence to compare the burden of disease in two groups and in this situation you end up with a **prevalence ratio**:

$$\text{Prevalence Ratio} = \frac{\text{Prevalence in exposed}}{\text{Prevalence in unexposed}} = \frac{P_e}{P_o} \tag{5.3}$$

As we discussed in Chapter 2, measures of prevalence are harder to interpret than measures of incidence and for this reason prevalence ratios are used much less frequently than rate and risk ratios.

A note about relative risks

We noted above that the term **relative risk** is synonymous with **risk ratio**. In practice, it is also commonly used to describe a **rate ratio**, since both the rate ratio and the risk ratio compare the amount of disease in one group *relative* to that in another. If a disease is rare (cumulative incidence or risk less than 1%), then the rate ratio and risk ratio will be almost identical; if it is not so rare then the risk ratio will be closer to 1.0 than the rate ratio although, in practice, there is little difference as long as the cumulative incidence is less than about 10%. The three terms rate ratio, risk ratio and relative risk are also commonly and conveniently abbreviated as RR. When we use the term relative risk it will refer to both the rate ratio and the risk ratio.

It is also worth noting that, although relative risks are also used in the context of clinical trials, several other related measures are also used in the field of clinical epidemiology (Box 5.2).

Box 5.2 Relative risks in clinical epidemiology

In 1998, Botti *et al.* reported a trial of the use of pressure bandages for
patients undergoing coronary angiography. Some of their results are shown
in Table 5.3.

Table 5.3 Use of pressure bandages in patients undergoing coronary
angiography.

Pressure bandages	Total	Number with bleeding	Cumulative incidence or event rate
Yes	519	18	$EER^a = 3.5\%$
No	556	37	$CER^b = 6.7\%$
Total	1075	55	5.0%

[a] EER = experimental event rate or cumulative incidence in the treatment group.
[b] CER = control event rate or cumulative incidence in the comparison group.
(Botti *et al.*, 1998.)

   The relative risk of bleeding among those given pressure bandages
compared with those without is $3.5 \div 6.7 = 0.52$. This tells us that those given
pressure bandages were about half as likely to develop bleeding as those who
were not given bandages. The results of treatment trials are sometimes also
reported as a **relative risk reduction (RRR)**. This is the amount by which the
treatment has reduced the relative risk and it is calculated by subtracting the
relative risk from 1.0. It may then be expressed as a percentage by
multiplying by 100:

Relative risk reduction (RRR) = 1.0 − RR   (5.4)
So the RRR = 1.0 − 0.52 = 0.48 or 48%.

   Alternatively, it can be calculated directly from the cumulative incidence
or event rates among the experimental (EER) and control (CER) groups:

Relative risk reduction (RRR) = (CER − EER) ÷ CER   (5.5)
In this case the RRR = (6.7 – 3.5) ÷ 6.7 = 0.48.

   In other words, use of the pressure bandages has reduced the risk of
bleeding among patients undergoing coronary angiography by 48%.
Obviously, the greater the RRR the better the intervention.
   For studies with a positive association (RR > 1.0) the results are turned
around to give what is logically called the **relative risk increase (RRI)**. In the
aspirin study discussed previously, aspirin increased the risk of bleeding by
40% (RR = 1.4).

(continued)

Box 5.2 (*continued*)

Note that you will see associations described in this way in all fields of epidemiology, e.g. 'The risk of disease was 20% lower among those who exercised more'. It is a simple, informative mode of description that just happens to have been given a separate name in the area of clinical epidemiology.

Standardised incidence and mortality ratios

We discussed these measures in Chapter 2 (pages 52–54) because of the links between direct and indirect standardisation, but they also deserve a mention here since they compare the rate of disease (or death) in two populations and so, in effect, are also measures of relative risk.

Difference measures (attributable risk)

As we noted above, the relative risk tells us nothing about the actual amount of disease that is occurring. If the cumulative incidences or risks of disease in exposed and unexposed groups were 0.5% and 0.1%, respectively, the relative risk would be 5.0. Similarly, if the risks were 50% and 10% the relative risk would also be 5.0. The major difference between these two situations is obvious: the actual amount of disease that is occurring is vastly different – in fact in the second example it is 100 times greater. This vital public health information cannot be obtained from the relative risk.

The approach to measuring the excess amount of disease occurring among those exposed to a potential risk factor is just as intuitive and as simple to calculate as the relative risk. As you saw in the smoking and stroke example at the start of the chapter, we can calculate the *extra* amount of disease that is occurring in the exposed group by simply subtracting the incidence in the unexposed group (IR_o, CI_o or **background risk**) from the incidence in the exposed group (IR_e, CI_e). This can again be done using either of the measures of disease incidence (incidence rate or cumulative incidence) that you met in Chapter 2. If you are subtracting two incidence rates (as in the stroke example) you end up with a **rate difference**, whereas if you are subtracting two measures of cumulative incidence or risk (as in the immunisation example) you have a **risk difference**. These measures are also sometimes described as the **excess rate** and **excess risk** as they measure the extra disease that only occurs in the presence of the exposure. If we think that it is reasonable to assume that the excess disease can be *attributed* to the exposure, i.e. the exposure is causing the disease, then both of these

Figure 5.1 Attributable risks:
the results of a study of smoking
and stroke (drawn from: Colditz
et al., 1988).

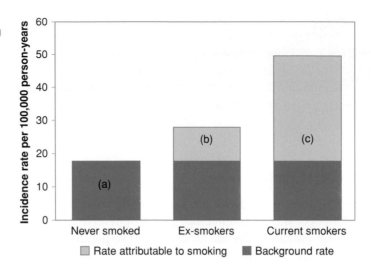

Figure 5.1 Attributable risks: the results of a study of smoking and stroke (drawn from: Colditz *et al.*, 1988).

measures can also be described as the **attributable risk** (in the same way that *relative risk* is used to describe both rate ratios and risk ratios).

Rate differences

Consider the smoking and stroke example again (Table 5.1). Compared with never smokers, there were an extra 10.2 strokes (27.9 – 17.7) per 100,000 person-years in ex-smokers and an extra 31.9 strokes (49.6 – 17.7) per 100,000 person-years in current smokers. These effects are illustrated in Figure 5.1. The left-hand bar (a) shows the incidence rate of stroke in non-smokers. This is often called the background or *reference rate* because it reflects the natural occurrence of the disease in an unexposed population. We expect this to operate on all members of the population regardless of their smoking status, and this is shown for the ex- and current smokers. This lets us visualise directly the extra burden of stroke added by past and present smoking habits. Thus the second bar shows the extra incidence of stroke in ex-smokers (b) that is presumably due to the fact that the women had smoked in the past. Similarly, the third bar shows the far greater added rate of stroke in current smokers (c) that is attributable to their smoking. This extra disease is simply the difference between the rate in the exposed group (smokers) and the rate in the unexposed group (non-smokers). The total rate of disease in exposed individuals is therefore the sum of the background rate (due to other causes) and the additional rate due to the exposure in question.

If the groups differ only in their smoking habit *and if we believe that smoking is actually causing strokes to occur* then we can say that the extra disease in the smokers is attributable to their smoking – if they had not smoked then it would not have occurred.[1] This **rate difference** is also called the **attributable risk** (AR) because it measures the actual amount of disease that can be attributed to a particular exposure:

Rate difference or attributable risk
$$= IR_e - IR$$
$$= \text{Incidence rate in exposed} - \text{Incidence rate in unexposed} \qquad (5.6)$$

Risk differences

Look back to the example of immunisation against influenza in Table 5.2.

What percentage of patients in the intervention group would have been expected to attend for immunisation even if they hadn't received a phone call (background 'risk')?

What extra percentage of patients presumably attended only because they had received a call (i.e. how many attendances could be attributed to the phone call)?

We would have expected 44% of patients in the intervention group to go for immunisation even if the practice receptionists had not called to offer them an appointment. We can therefore say that an extra 6% of patients (50% − 44%) in the intervention group presumably went for immunisation only because they had received a call, i.e. their immunisation can be attributed to this. Here we have calculated a risk difference (as opposed to a rate difference) since we are subtracting cumulative incidences (or risks):

Risk difference or attributable risk
$$= \text{Cumulative incidence in exposed} - \text{Cumulative incidence in unexposed}$$
$$= CI_e - CI_o \qquad (5.7)$$

Attributable fractions (AFs)

A further way to consider attributable risk that can also be informative is as the *proportion* or *percentage* of disease in the exposed group that would not have occurred in the absence of the exposure. This measure is often called the **attributable fraction** or **attributable proportion**, although you will also come across it described as the **attributable risk per cent**. To calculate the attributable fraction you simply divide the attributable risk by the incidence in the exposed

[1] Note that although you will see the attributable risk described as the amount of disease *caused* by the exposure, this is not technically correct because we can never know exactly how many cases are caused by a particular exposure. However, we can usefully use the attributable risk to estimate how much extra disease *occurred* in the presence of the exposure and thus presumably *would not occur* in the absence of that exposure.

group:

$$\text{Attributable Fraction (AF)} = \frac{\text{Attributable Risk}}{\text{Incidence in exposed}}$$

$$\text{or} = \frac{\text{Incidence in exposed} - \text{Incidence in unexposed}}{\text{Incidence in exposed}}$$

Again this can be done using either the incidence rate or the cumulative incidence:

$$\text{Attributable Fraction (AF)} = \frac{\text{AR}}{\text{IR}_e} \quad \text{or} \quad \frac{\text{AR}}{\text{CI}_e} \tag{5.8}$$

$$= \frac{\text{IR}_e - \text{IR}_o}{\text{IR}_e} \quad \text{or} \quad \frac{\text{CI}_e - \text{CI}_o}{\text{CI}_e} \tag{5.9}$$

Consider the smoking and stroke example again. The rate of stroke among current smokers was $49.6/10^5$ person-years and the rate difference or attributable risk was $31.9/10^5$ person-years. The attributable fraction is therefore 0.64 or 64%, i.e. of all the strokes occurring *among current smokers*, about two thirds could be attributed to the fact that the women smoked:

$$\text{Attributable Fraction (AF)} = \frac{49.6 - 17.7}{49.6} = 0.64 = 64\%$$

Interpretation of the attributable risk

The attributable risk tells us how much extra disease actually occurred in the *exposed* group as a result of the exposure. By implication, we can then say that, *if the association is causal*, this is the amount of disease that we could prevent in a comparable group of people in the future *if* we could prevent them from being exposed. This measure is, therefore, of direct use to health planning and policy setting. Note that in the field of clinical epidemiology, what we have called the *attributable risk* is often called the **absolute risk reduction (ARR)** or **absolute risk increase (ARI)** depending on whether the event rate is reduced or increased in the treatment group (See Box 5.3). The ARR and ARI are identical to the attributable risks used elsewhere in epidemiology and are calculated in exactly the same way – the only difference is in the names.

In practice, of course, it is often impossible to remove or prevent an exposure altogether. Someone who smokes cannot go back to being a never-smoker but they can become an ex-smoker. This means that current smokers who stop smoking will not realise the full benefit predicted by the standard attributable risk (which would compare smokers with the unexposed group, in this case never smokers). Rather, the best we could achieve with a 100% effective 'stop smoking'

Box 5.3 Attributable risks in clinical epidemiology

In the trial of the use of pressure bandages for patients undergoing coronary angiography (Table 5.3) and using the terminology of clinical epidemiology (look back to Box 2.5 on page 44 if you are unsure about this) the attributable risk or **absolute risk reduction** (ARR) of bleeding would be

$$ARR = CER - EER = 6.7 - 3.5 = 3.2\% \qquad (5.10)$$

In other words, the use of pressure bandages has prevented bleeding in 3.2% of patients.

Another quite useful way of looking at these data is in terms of the **number needed to treat** (NNT). The NNT is the number of patients who would have to be given the experimental therapy in order to prevent one adverse event (death, complication) from occurring. It is calculated by simply dividing 1.0 by the ARR:

$$NNT = 1 \div ARR \qquad (5.11)$$

In the study of pressure bandages the ARR was 3.2% or 0.032, so

$$NNT = 1 \div 0.032 = 31.3$$

This means that about 32 patients undergoing coronary angiography would need to be given pressure bandages in order to prevent one case of bleeding. (Note that, unlike in most other situations, the NNT should be *rounded up* to the nearest whole number because you cannot treat part of a person.) This gives a good intuitive feel for the treatment benefit, and can aid communication with patients.

campaign would be to reduce the rate of stroke among smokers to the level seen among ex-smokers, a rate difference given by:

$$IR_{current} - IR_{ex} = 49.6 - 27.9 = 21.7 \text{ strokes}/100,000 \text{ person-years}$$

Population attributable risks (PARs)

The attributable risk tells us about the amount of extra disease occurring in the exposed group because of the exposure. An alternative way to look at the burden due to an exposure is to consider *how much disease in the whole community* can be attributed to the exposure. To do this we need to compare the incidence of disease in the whole population or community (some of whom will be exposed and some unexposed) with the amount of disease in an unexposed group (the amount that we would expect if no one had been exposed). In the smoking and

Figure 5.2 Attributable and population attributable risks: the results of a study of smoking and stroke (drawn from: Colditz *et al.*, 1988).

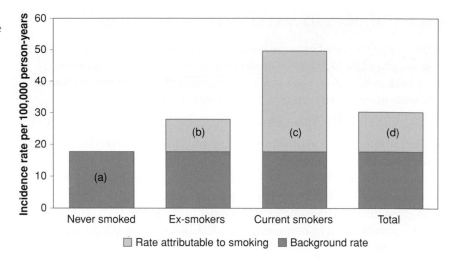

stroke example in Table 5.1 we know that the overall incidence rate of stroke among the women was $30.2/10^5$ person-years.

What would this rate have been if no one had smoked?

How much of the incidence of stroke in the total population is due to the fact that some women smoke or are ex-smokers?

What fraction of the overall rate of stroke in the total population is due to smoking?

If none of the women had smoked the overall rate of stroke in the population would be the same as the rate in never smokers ($17.7/10^5$ person-years). This means that, in the whole population, there are an extra 12.5 cases ($30.2 - 17.7$) per 100,000 person-years that can be attributed to the fact that *some* of the women in the population smoke or are ex-smokers. This is the ***population attributable risk*** (**PAR**) and is depicted (d) in the fourth bar in Figure 5.2.

There are two ways to calculate the PAR. One way, analogous to the calculation of attributable risk (Equations (5.6) and (5.7)), is to subtract the incidence in the unexposed group (IR_0, CI_0) from the incidence in the *whole population* (IR_T, CI_T). As for the attributable risk, this can be done using either incidence rates or cumulative incidence:

$$\text{PAR} = \text{Incidence rate in population} - \text{Incidence rate in unexposed}$$
$$= IR_T - IR_0 \quad \text{or} \quad CI_T - CI_0 \tag{5.12}$$

Clearly the population attributable risk will depend not only on the attributable risk among the exposed, but also on the prevalence of the exposure in the population. An alternative way to calculate the PAR is therefore to multiply the attributable risk by the prevalence of exposure in the population (P_e):

$$PAR = AR \times P_e \qquad\qquad (5.13)$$

Note that, while this is straightforward when there are only two levels of exposure, it is trickier when there are more than two levels, as in the stroke and smoking example. In this situation it is much easier to use Equation (5.12).

Population attributable fractions (PAFs)

As with the attributable risk and attributable fraction, we can also calculate the **population attributable fraction** (or **population attributable risk per cent**) which indicates the proportion of all the strokes that occurred in the population that could potentially have been avoided if no-one had smoked. The formula to calculate the population attributable fraction is analogous to that used for the attributable fraction but with the incidence in the total population used instead of the incidence in the exposed group:

$$\text{Population Attributable Fraction} = \frac{\text{Population Attributable Risk}}{\text{Incidence in total population}} \times 100$$

Population Attributable Fraction

$$= \frac{\text{Incidence in total population} - \text{Incidence in unexposed}}{\text{Incidence in total population}} \times 100$$

Again this can be done using either incidence rates or cumulative incidence:

$$\text{Population Attributable Fraction} = \frac{PAR}{IR_T} \quad \text{or} \quad \frac{PAR}{CI_T} \qquad\qquad (5.14)$$

$$\text{Population Attributable Fraction} = \frac{IR_T - IR_o}{IR_T} \quad \text{or} \quad \frac{CI_T - CI_o}{CI_T} \qquad\qquad (5.15)$$

So, in the stroke example, approximately 41% ($12.5 \div 30.2 = 0.41$) of strokes in the whole population could be attributed to smoking and, in theory, would not have occurred *if no-one had ever smoked.*

Interpretation of the population attributable risk

The PAR is exactly analogous to the attributable risk (AR) but, while the attributable risk tells us how much disease in the *exposed* group can be attributed to the exposure, the population attributable risk tells us how much disease in the *whole population* can be attributed to the exposure. The population attributable risk and population attributable fraction are functions both of the *incidence of disease* due to an exposure and of the *prevalence of the exposure.* An exposure may be associated with a very high attributable risk of a disease such that those exposed have a very high chance of developing it, but if the exposure is rare then this high risk will only affect a small proportion of the population. It will therefore have little impact in a whole community (a low population attributable risk). The population attributable risk is the best way to measure the burden of disease in a whole community that can be attributed to a particular exposure.

As we have noted above for the AR, there is no intervention that we could implement to change a woman who is a current smoker into a never smoker; the most we could do would be to persuade her to stop smoking. If we could do this we could estimate the incidence rate of strokes in the whole group as 23.4 per 100,000 person-years (based on the new mix of never smokers and ex-smokers).[2] This means that, if we could have persuaded all current smokers to give up smoking, we could potentially have prevented 6.8 strokes per 100,000 person-years (PAR = 30.2 − 23.4) or 22.5% of all strokes in the population (PAF = 6.8 ÷ 30.2).

In practice, however, even this is an overly simplistic view. It is very hard to persuade people to stop smoking (or to give up most unhealthy behaviours for that matter) and a more realistic goal might be to look at the health benefits that would follow if we could halve smoking rates. We will come back to this issue and will meet the population attributable risk again when we consider disease prevention in Chapter 14. When thinking about the possibilities for intervention and prevention of disease we should also bear in mind that changing someone's smoking habit will reduce not just their risk of stroke but also their risk of many other diseases, so the public health benefits of a 'stop smoking' campaign are not limited to stroke reduction. While the overall benefits of stopping smoking are clear cut, it is less obvious where an intervention reduces risk of one disease but increases that of another. For example, moderate alcohol consumption can reduce the risk of heart disease but it can also increase the risk of breast cancer. These benefits and risks have to be weighed up and no one would recommend that women should drink more alcohol to prevent heart disease.

At the global level, population attributable risks and population attributable fractions are used to calculate the impacts of various exposures on world health. For example, it has been estimated that in the year 2000 almost five million premature deaths around the world were attributable to smoking (Ezzati and Lopez, 2003). Similarly, organisations like the WHO and World Bank produce regular estimates of the amount of ill-health that can be attributed to various risk factors, for example the World Bank report on the *Global Burden of Disease and*

---

[2] If all the current smokers became ex-smokers at the start of the study their rate of stroke would have been 27.9/105 person-years and about 78 strokes would have occurred in the 280,141 person-years of follow-up. This gives a total of 213 strokes (70 + 65 + 78) in 908,447 person years or a rate of 23.4/105 person-years in the whole population. Note that this assumes that the full benefit is seen immediately after stopping.

Risk Factors (Lopez *et al.*, 2006). You saw an example of this in Table 2.11 on page 65 although it looked somewhat different because, instead of looking at the *incidence* of disease attributable to an exposure, the burden of disease was measured in the disability adjusted life-years or DALYs that you met in Chapter 2. The concept is the same though. Note the variation in the relative importance of some causes depending on the affluence of the population.

A word of caution regarding attributable risks

There are possibly more terms used to describe attributable risks than any other measure in epidemiology. People use different names for the same thing and, what is even more confusing, the same name for different things. This emphasises the importance of never taking things at face value – always take time to check what are being presented. Here the key distinction is whether people are talking about only the exposed group (what we call the attributable risk or, in clinical epidemiology, the absolute risk reduction) or the whole population (what we call the population attributable risk). It is also important to distinguish between absolute differences (what we have called attributable risks) and percentage differences (attributable fractions).[3]

Relative risk versus attributable risk: an example

In the British Doctors Study (discussed in Chapter 1) mortality rates were calculated for deaths both from lung cancer and from coronary heart disease (CHD). These rates, together with the relative risks, attributable risks and attributable fractions, are shown in Table 5.4 on the next page.

Is the association with smoking stronger for lung cancer or CHD?

If everyone stopped smoking, would we prevent more cases of lung cancer or CHD?

In these data there is a very strong *relative* association between smoking and lung cancer (RR = 14), but only a modest link between cigarettes and CHD (RR = 1.6). On its own, this offers powerful support to a belief in smoking as a cause of lung cancer, but leaves quite a few doubts as to whether it has a causal role in the development of CHD (see also Chapter 10). Given that smoking does cause CHD as well as lung cancer (and there is plenty of other evidence to support this), the

---

[3] Strictly speaking, the formulae for the PAF that we have described are only valid when there is no 'confounding' of the exposure of interest (Rockhill *et al.*, 1998) but we show them here to illustrate the underlying concepts. Equation 5.19 on page 147 shows an alternative formula for the PAF that can be used in the presence of confounding. We will discuss confounding in Chapter 8.

Table 5.4 Lung cancer and CHD mortality rates in the British Doctors Study.

Disease	Smoking status	Mortality rate per 10^5 person-years	Relative risk	Attributable risk per 10^5 person-years	Attributable fraction (%)
Lung cancer	Yes	140	14.0	130	93
	No	10			
Coronary heart disease	Yes	669	1.6	256	38
	No	413			

(Doll and Peto, 1976.)

Table 5.5 A comparison of relative and attributable risks.

Measure	Strengths	Uses
Relative risk (RR)	Evaluates the *strength* of an association between exposure and disease	To help identify causes of disease
Attributable risk (AR)	Measures the burden of disease attributable to exposure in the *exposed* group	To assess the magnitude of a public health problem associated with an exposure *among those exposed*
Population attributable risk (PAR)	Measures the burden of disease attributable to exposure in the *population*	To assess the magnitude of a public health problem associated with an exposure *in the whole population*
Attributable fraction (AF)	Identifies the specific exposures that cause most disease *in those who are exposed*	To identify potential targets for prevention
Population attributable fraction (PAF)	Identifies the specific exposures that cause most disease *in a population*	To identify potential targets for prevention

attributable fraction supports the view that smoking is a more important cause of lung cancer than it is of CHD: among smokers 93% of lung cancers but only 38% of CHD can be attributed to smoking. In contrast, the *attributable risks* show that the *public health impact* of smoking is twice as great for CHD mortality as for lung cancer deaths: there are almost 260 additional deaths from CHD in smokers for every 100,000 person-years compared with only 130 from lung cancer. If we look more closely at the actual rates of disease, we see that the background rate of CHD (the rate in non-smokers) is very high, so a large rate difference does not look so impressive when we calculate the RR. In contrast, the background rate of lung cancer is very low, so a much smaller rate difference leads to a very high RR. This example shows very clearly the striking difference in what these measures describe and the different implications of a large relative risk (or attributable fraction) versus a large attributable risk. Table 5.5 summarises some of these differences and the uses of the different measures.

Table 5.6 A case–control study of oral contraceptive (OC) use and ovarian cancer.

	Cases	Controls	Total
Used OC pill	413	1160	1573
Did not use OC pill	206	322	528
Total	619	1482	2101

(Jordan *et al.*, 2008.)

Case–control studies

All of the above measures relate to situations in which we can measure the incidence of disease. This information usually comes from a **cohort study** in which we identify groups of exposed and unexposed individuals who do not have the disease of interest and then follow them over time to see how many develop the disease. As you saw in the previous chapter, in a **case–control study** we usually select only a sample of all possible people without disease as controls. This often means that we can no longer calculate disease incidence, so we need different methods to calculate measures of association in a case–control study.

In the early 2000s a case–control study of ovarian cancer was conducted in Australia. It included the majority of women newly diagnosed with ovarian cancer across the whole of Australia between 2003 and 2005. The controls were a sample of women who did not have ovarian cancer and who were chosen at random from the national electoral roll to give a similar age and state distribution as the cases (we will discuss this process where we 'match' cases and controls further in Chapter 8). The investigators found that 413 of the 619 women with ovarian cancer and 1160 of the 1482 controls had previously used the oral contraceptive (OC) pill (Jordan *et al.*, 2008), as shown in Table 5.5.

What percentage of the OC users have ovarian cancer? Does this reflect the likely incidence of ovarian cancer in OC users?

In this case–control study 26% (413 ÷ 1573) of the OC users have ovarian cancer. It is tempting to interpret this as meaning that the incidence of ovarian cancer among oral contraceptive users was 26% but, even if you don't know anything about ovarian cancer, this should ring some warning bells! The OC pill would never be prescribed if one quarter of the women who used it developed cancer. The numerator (the number of women with cancer) is fine because most of the women with cancer were included, but the denominator (the total population) is wrong because only a tiny proportion of all the women without ovarian cancer

Table 5.7 Calculation of the odds ratio in a case–control study.

	Cases	Controls	Total
Exposed	a	b	$a+b$
Unexposed	c	d	$c+d$
Total	$a+c$	$b+d$	$a+b+c+d$

have been included. This means that, in a case–control study, we cannot calculate the usual measures of disease incidence directly, and so cannot calculate relative risks in the same way.

Relative risk in case–control studies

In a case–control study we calculate another measure of association known as the **odds ratio** (OR). This involves calculating the '*odds*' that a case had used OCs in exactly the same way as odds are calculated in horse racing. Among the cases, 413 women had used the OC pill and 206 had not, so the 'odds' of a case having used the pill are '413 to 206' or $413 \div 206 = 2.00$.

What are the odds that a control had used the OC pill?

Among the controls, 1160 women had used the pill and 322 had not. The odds that a control had used the pill are therefore $1160 \div 322 = 3.60$. We can then calculate the **odds ratio** by dividing the odds that a case had used the pill (i.e. was exposed) by the odds that a control had used the pill. In this example:

Odds ratio (OR) $= 2.00 \div 3.60 = 0.56$

An alternative and simple way to calculate the odds ratio that is often used in practice is as follows. Your data must be arranged in a standard way as shown in Table 5.7 (note that this is the same as the way in which the data are shown in Table 5.6).

The odds that a case used the OC pill $= a \div c$

The odds that a control used the OC pill $= b \div d$

Therefore the ratio of these odds $= (a \div c) \div (b \div d)$

or

$$\text{Odds Ratio} = \frac{a \times d}{b \times c} \tag{5.16}$$

So, for the ovarian cancer data, the OR associated with OC use is

$$\text{Odds Ratio} = \frac{413 \times 322}{1160 \times 206} = 0.56$$

Box 5.4 Rate ratios, risk ratios and odds ratios

Each of the three measures of association is a valid measure in its own right but the relationship among them varies in different situations and depends on how the controls were selected for the study (see Rodrigues and Kirkwood, 1990).

- If they were selected at the *start* of the case-recruitment period and so included anyone who was disease-free at that point in time (regardless of whether they went on to develop disease) then

Odds ratio ≈ Risk ratio

so an OR of 3.0 can be interpreted as meaning that the *risk* of disease in those who were exposed was three times greater than that among those who were not exposed.

- If they were selected at the *same* time as cases were being recruited (i.e. density sampling), as is usually the case in practice, then

Odds ratio ≈ Rate ratio

so an OR of 3.0 can be interpreted as meaning that the *rate* of disease in those who were exposed was three times greater than that among those who were not exposed.

- If they were selected to include only people who were still disease-free at the end of the study then the odds ratio will still provide information about the strength of the association but, if the disease is not rare, it might not be a good estimate of the relative risk. That is, if an OR = 3.0 it tells us that the association is strong but it does *not* necessarily mean that those who were exposed were precisely three times more likely to develop disease than those who were not exposed.

In other words, the odds of a case having used the OC pill is almost half the odds that a control had used the pill. As you will see below, we can interpret this as meaning that a woman who uses the OC pill is almost half as likely to get ovarian cancer as a woman who has not used the pill. But be warned, it is not always possible to interpret an odds ratio in this way – especially if the disease of interest is quite common.

Interpreting odds ratios

How we interpret an odds ratio depends to a large extent on how the control group was recruited for that particular study as in different situations the odds ratio can be a good estimate of either the risk (cumulative incidence) ratio or the incidence rate ratio (see Box 5.4). In many studies the controls are recruited using

what is called **density sampling** and in this situation the odds ratio is a good estimate of the rate ratio. For density sampling, the controls for the study must be
identified during the period when the cases were occurring, *not* at the beginning
or end of the study. In practice this does not make a lot of difference if the disease is rare, but if the disease is common it means that it is possible for someone
to be recruited as a control early in a study and then to be recruited again as a
case if they later develop the disease of interest. Although ovarian cancer is a rare
disease, one woman participated as a control in a case–control study similar to
the one described above but was diagnosed with ovarian cancer a year later. She
then participated in the study a second time as a case. This is not only valid but
essential for true density sampling.

In practice, however, if a disease is rare – and for the purposes of epidemiology
most diseases are rare – then all three measures, the rate ratio, risk ratio and odds
ratio, will be approximately equal and all can be interpreted as a relative risk:

Rate Ratio ≈ Risk Ratio ≈ Odds Ratio

This is often described as the '*rare disease assumption*' and Box 5.5 gives the
mathematical derivation of why this is true for the risk ratio and odds ratio.

Odds ratios in cross-sectional studies

In a cross-sectional study we compare the *prevalence* of disease in different exposure groups and the logical measure to use to do this is the **prevalence ratio** (PR).
However, prevalence ratios are not as easy to work with as odds ratios and, as a
result, you will find that the results of cross-sectional studies are often presented
as odds ratios, sometimes called prevalence odds ratios (POR). As for the cumulative incidence or risk ratio (see Boxes 5.4 and 5.5), the POR will also be a good
estimate of the prevalence ratio in a cross-sectional study *if the outcome is rare*.
However, in many cross-sectional studies the outcome is *not* rare and in this situation the POR will be more extreme (further from the null value of 1.0) than the
prevalence ratio. In other words, if the PR is 2.0 the POR will be > 2.0, likewise if
the PR is 0.8 the POR will be < 0.8. This means that when the outcome is not rare,
a POR of 2.0 suggests there is an association between the exposure and outcome,
but it *cannot* be interpreted as meaning the outcome was twice as common in
the exposed group compared to the unexposed group.

Attributable risk in case–control studies

Because we cannot usually calculate the actual incidence of disease in exposed
and unexposed subjects in a case–control study, we cannot calculate the
attributable risk of disease associated with the exposure. We can, however, estimate the attributable fraction using the following formula:

$$\text{Attributable Fraction (AF)} = \frac{(\text{OR} - 1)}{\text{OR}} \times 100 \tag{5.17}$$

Box 5.5 Why the odds ratio approximates the relative risk for a rare disease

Table 5.8 shows the results of a hypothetical cohort study.

Table 5.8 Results of a hypothetical cohort study.

	Cases	Non-cases	Total	CI (%)
Exposed	75 (a)	9,925 (b)	10,000 ($a + b$)	0.75
Unexposed	25 (c)	9,975 (d)	10,000 ($c + d$)	0.25
Total	100	19,900	20,000	

$$\text{Relative risk} = \frac{CI_e}{CI_o} = \frac{a}{(a+b)} \div \frac{c}{(c+d)} = 0.75\% \div 0.25\% = 3.0$$

However, if the disease is rare then

$a (=75)$ is very small in comparison to $b (= 9,925)$, so $a + b \approx b$

and

$c (=25)$ is very small in comparison to $d (= 9,975)$ so $c + d \approx d$

This means that the

$$\text{Relative risk} = \frac{a}{(a+b)} \div \frac{c}{(c+d)} \approx \frac{a}{b} \div \frac{c}{d} = \frac{a \times d}{b \times c} = \text{Odds Ratio}$$

To show that this is true, imagine we conducted a case–control study in this population with all 100 cases and the same number of controls. Half of the population is exposed and half is unexposed, so we would expect about 50 controls to be exposed and 50 to be unexposed and the

$$\text{Odds ratio} = \frac{75 \times 50}{25 \times 50} = 3.0$$

We can also estimate the population attributable fraction, as follows:

$$\text{Population Attributable Fraction (PAF)} = \frac{P_e \left(\text{OR} - 1\right)}{P_e \left(\text{OR} - 1\right) + 1} \times 100 \qquad (5.18)$$

where P_e is the prevalence of exposure in the population, estimated by measuring the prevalence in the *control* group.

Or, alternatively,

$$\text{Population attributable fraction} = P_{e(cases)} \times \text{AF}$$

$$= P_{e(cases)} \frac{(\text{OR} - 1)}{\text{OR}} \times 100 \qquad (5.19)$$

where $P_{e(cases)}$ is the prevalence of exposure among the *cases*. This version of the equation is perhaps more intuitive than Equation (5.18) because while the AF

Table 5.9 A case–control study of bicycle helmets and head injury.

	Cases	Controls	Total
No helmet (exposed)	67	140	207
Wearing a helmet (unexposed)	31	126	157
Total	98	266	364

(Thomas *et al.*, 1994.)

tells us the proportion of cases in the exposed group that can be attributed to the exposure, when we calculate the PAF we also have to allow for the cases that were not exposed. For example, if 80% of exposed cases were attributable to an exposure but only half of the cases were exposed ($P_{e(cases)} = 0.5$) then in the whole population only 40% of cases (80% × 0.5) would have been attributable to the exposure. Another advantage of Equation (5.19) is that it can also be used in the presence of confounding by using the OR that has been 'adjusted' for the confounders (see Chapter 8).

These measures are the only way of assessing the potential public health importance of an exposure from a case–control study. (Note that these formulae can also be used for follow-up studies by substituting the RR for the OR.)

Another example comes from a study of the effectiveness of bicycle helmets for preventing head injury in children (Thomas *et al.*, 1994). The cases were 98 children who presented to the local children's hospital with bicycle-related head injuries and the controls were 266 children treated for other bicycle-related injuries. In total 207 children, 67 of the cases and 140 controls, were not wearing a helmet at the time of the accident. (Note that we will consider '*not wearing a helmet*' as the exposure in this example.)

What is the OR for the association between not wearing a helmet and head injury?

What percentage of head injuries occurring among the children not wearing a helmet could be attributed to the fact that they were not wearing a helmet (AF)?

What proportion of the control children were not wearing a helmet (P_e)?

What percentage of all bicycle-related head injuries in children could be attributed to not wearing a helmet (PAF)?

Table 5.9 shows the results of the study laid out in a standard 2 × 2 table. The odds ratio for the association between not wearing a bicycle helmet and head injury is

$$\text{OR} = \frac{a \times d}{b \times c} = \frac{67 \times 126}{140 \times 31} = 1.95$$

This indicates that children who do not wear helmets are almost twice as likely to sustain a head injury in a bicycle accident as children who do wear helmets.

The attributable fraction tells us the proportion of head injuries among those not wearing a helmet that could be attributed to the fact that they were not wearing a helmet:

$$AF = \frac{(OR - 1)}{OR} \times 100 = \frac{1.95 - 1}{1.95} \times 100 = 49\%$$

This tells us that 49% of head injuries *among children not wearing helmets* could be attributed to the fact they were not helmeted and were therefore potentially preventable if they had been wearing a helmet.

Out of the 266 controls, 140 or 53% were not wearing a helmet. We can use this information to calculate the population attributable fraction to estimate the proportion of all head injuries that could be attributed to the fact that some children were not wearing a helmet:

$$PAF = \frac{P_e\,(OR - 1)}{P_e\,(OR - 1) + 1} \times 100 = \frac{0.53 \times 0.95}{(0.53 \times 0.95) + 1} \times 100 = \frac{0.5035}{1.5035} \times 100 = 33\%$$

The results suggest that, in the study population, almost one-third of all child head injuries incurred while cycling could be prevented if all children wore bicycle helmets. (Note that it is important not to round off the numbers during calculations like this because this may make the answer inaccurate. Rounding should be used only for communication of the final answer.)

Summary

Box 5.6 gives an example that summarises the calculation and interpretation of the various measures of association that you have just met. It is based on *incidence rates* of type-2 diabetes but the formulae also apply to *cumulative incidence* or risk data – simply substitute CI for IR. In a case–control study it is not usually possible to calculate the AR or PAR but we can use the odds ratio (Equation (5.16)) in place of the RR to calculate the AF and PAF. After working through this example and the questions at the end of the chapter you should feel comfortable calculating and interpreting any of the common measures of association that you come across in the health literature.

Questions

1. In an industry employing 10,000 people, 2,500 were employed in areas where they were exposed to pesticides, while the remaining 7,500 were not exposed. At the beginning of the study, all employees were free of disease. The entire

Box 5.6 An example – obesity and type-2 diabetes

Imagine that 30% of the population in a particular community is overweight, 82.5% of diabetics are overweight and the rate of type-2 diabetes is
- $330/10^5$ person-years in the obese (IR_e)
- $30/10^5$ person-years in the non-obese (IR_o) and
- $120/10^5$ person-years in the whole population (IR_T).

    Then we can calculate the following.

(1) The **rate ratio** or **relative risk** (RR) using Equation (5.1):

$$RR = \frac{IR_e}{IR_o} = \frac{330}{30} = 11.0$$

The **relative risk** tells us that the rate of type-2 diabetes is 11 times higher among people who are obese than among non-obese people.

(2) The **rate difference** or **attributable risk** (AR) using Equation (5.6):

$$AR = IR_e - IR_o = 330 - 30 = 300 \text{ per } 10^5 \text{ person-years}$$

The **attributable risk** tells us that, if obesity is a cause of type-2 diabetes, then, *among obese people*, 300 cases per 10^5 person-years can be attributed to their obesity.

(3) The **attributable fraction** (AF) using Equation (5.9):

$$AF = \frac{(IR_e - IR_o)}{IR_e} \times 100 = \frac{(330 - 30)}{330} \times 100 = 91\%$$

or Equation (5.17) (using the RR instead of the OR):

$$AF = \frac{(RR - 1)}{RR} \times 100 = \frac{(11 - 1)}{11} \times 100 = 91\%$$

The **attributable fraction** tells us that more than 90% of type-2 diabetes in obese people would not occur if they were not overweight.

(4) The **population attributable risk** (PAR) using Equation (5.12):

$$PAR = IR_T - IR_o = 120 - 30 = 90/10^5 \text{ person-years}$$

or using Equation (5.13):

$$PAR = AR \times P_e = 300 \times 0.3 = 90/10^5 \text{ person-years}$$

where P_e = prevalence of exposure in the population = 30% or 0.3.

The **population attributable risk** tells us that, in the **whole population**, 90 cases of type-2 diabetes per 10^5 person-years can be attributed to obesity

(5) The **population attributable fraction** (PAF) using Equation (5.14):

$$PAF = \frac{PAR}{IR_T} \times 100 = (90 \div 120) \times 100 = 75\%$$

(continued)

Box 5.6 (*continued*)

or Equation (5.18) (using the RR instead of OR):

$$\text{PAF} = \frac{P_e\,(\text{RR} - 1)}{P_e\,(\text{RR} - 1) + 1} \times 100 = \frac{0.3 \times (11 - 1)}{(0.3 \times (11 - 1)) + 1} \times 100 = \frac{3}{4} \times 100 = 75\%$$

or Equation (5.19):

$$\text{PAF} = P_{e(\text{cases})} \frac{(\text{RR} - 1)}{\text{RR}} \times 100 = 0.825 \times \frac{(11 - 1)}{11} = 0.825 \times 0.91 \times 100 = 75\%$$

The **population attributable fraction** tells us that 75% of all cases of type-2 diabetes would not occur if no one was grossly overweight.

Note that the estimates of PAF are all identical because we have assumed that there is no confounding (see Chapter 8). In the presence of confounding, Equation (5.19) should be used with the adjusted estimate of the relative risk.

Table 5.10 The results of a hypothetical study of the effects of pesticide exposure.

	Developed disease	Did not develop disease	Total
Exposed to pesticides	40	2,460	2,500
Not exposed	60	7,440	7,500
Total	100	9,900	10,000

population of 10,000 was followed for 10 years to determine whether exposure to pesticides increased the risk of developing a particular disease. For this disease, the findings were as given in Table 5.10.

(a) Calculate the cumulative incidence of the disease in
  (i) the exposed workers,
  (ii) the unexposed workers and
  (iii) all workers combined.
(b) Calculate the relative risk of this disease in those exposed to pesticides. What does this tell us?
(c) How much disease in the exposed workers could be due to their pesticide exposure (attributable risk)?
(d) Calculate the population attributable fraction. What does this tell us?
2. The Family Planning Association in Oxford, England, studied 17,000 women who had been enrolled in a cohort study between 1968 and 1974 to look

at the association between oral contraceptive (OC) use and venous thromboembolism (Vessey *et al.*, 1989). For current users of OCs, person-time was
counted from the time a woman began using OCs. For never or past users,
it was counted from the time a woman enrolled in the study. Woman-years
were counted until venous thromboembolism occurred, the woman was lost-
to-follow-up, or the end of the study.

(a) The incidence rate of venous thromboembolism was 53 per 100,000
woman-years among current OC users and 6 per 100,000 woman-years
among never or past users. Calculate the relative risk of venous thromboembolism for current users compared with never or past users.

(b) The incidence rate of thromboembolism was 62 per 100,000 among users
of OCs containing higher dosages of oestrogen and 39 per 100,000 among
users of lower-dose OCs. Calculate the relative risk of venous thromboembolism for

   (i) low-dose users compared with never or past users and
   (ii) high-dose users compared with never or past users.

(c) What can you conclude about the risk of thromboembolism for users of
OCs containing different doses of oestrogen?

3. Doll and Hill first evaluated the proposition that smoking was a risk factor for
lung cancer in a case–control study (Doll and Hill, 1950). They found that, of
649 men with lung cancer (cases), 647 had smoked at some time, compared
with 622 of the 649 men without lung cancer (controls).

(a) Draw up a clearly labelled and appropriate 2×2 table to show these data.

(b) How many times more likely was a smoker to develop lung cancer than a
non-smoker?

(c) Calculate the proportion of lung cancers attributable to smoking among
(i) *smokers* and (ii) the *whole population*.

(d) What are these measures called and how does their interpretation
differ?

4. The association between decreased duration of sleep and incidence of coronary heart disease (CHD) was studied among women enrolled in the Nurses'
Health Study (Ayas *et al.*, 2003). Among women who reported sleeping 7
or 8 hours per night there were 541 incident cases of CHD during 451,393
person-years of follow-up. Among those who slept for 6 hours per night
there were 267 cases in 175,629 person-years, and among those sleeping 5
or fewer hours per night there were 67 cases during 30,115 person-years of
follow-up.

(a) Calculate the incidence rate of CHD among
    (i) women who reported sleeping 7–8 hours per night,
    (ii) women who reported sleeping for 6 hours per night,
    (iii) women who slept 5 or less hours per night and
    (iv) all women.

(b) How strong is the association between sleep duration and the incidence of CHD?

(c) What percentage of CHD cases could theoretically be prevented if all women slept for 7–8 hours per night?

REFERENCES

Ayas, N. T., White, D. P., Manson, J. E. *et al.* (2003). A prospective study of sleep duration and coronary heart disease in women. *Archives of Internal Medicine*, **163**: 205–209.

Botti, M., Williamson, B., Steen, K., McTaggart, J. and Reid, E. (1998). The effect of pressure bandaging on complications and comfort in patients undergoing coronary angiography: a multicentre randomized trial. *Heart and Lung*, **27**: 360–373.

Colditz, G. A., Bonita, R., Stampfer, M. J. *et al.* (1988). Cigarette smoking and risk of stroke in middle-aged women. *New England Journal of Medicine*, **318**: 937–941.

Doll, R. and Hill, A. B. (1950). Smoking and carcinoma of the lung. *British Medical Journal*, **2**: 739–748.

Doll, R. and Peto, R. (1976). Mortality in relation to smoking: 20 years' observations on male British doctors. *British Medical Journal*, **2**: 1525–1536.

Ezzati, M. and Lopez, A. D. (2003). Estimates of global mortality attributable to smoking in 2000. *Lancet*, **362**: 847–852.

Hull, S., Hagdrup, N., Hart, B., Griffiths, C. and Hennessy, E. (2002). Boosting uptake of influenza immunisation in a randomised controlled trial of telephone appointing in general practice. *British Journal of General Practice*, **52**: 712–716.

Jordan, S. J., Green, A. C., Whiteman, D. C. *et al.* (2008). Serous ovarian, fallopian tube and primary peritoneal cancers: a comparative epidemiological analysis. *International Journal of Cancer*, **122**: 1598–1603.

Lopez, A. D., Mathers, C. D., Ezzati, M. *et al.* (Eds) (2006). *Global burden of disease and risk factors*. World Bank and Oxford University Press.

Maushart, S. (2003). Domesticator: rise of the machines. *The Weekend Australian Magazine*, August 16–17.

Rockhill, B., Newman, B. and Weinberg, C. (1998). Use and mis-use of population attributable fractions. *American Journal of Public Health*, **88**: 15–19; correction in *American Journal of Public Health*, **98**: 2119.

Rodrigues, L. and Kirkwood, B. R. (1990). Case–control designs in the study of common diseases: updates on the demise of the rare disease assumption and the choice of sampling scheme for controls. *International Journal of Epidemiology*, **19**: 205–213.

Snow, J. (1855). *On the Mode of Communication of Cholera*, 2nd edn. London: Churchill. (http://www.ph.ucla.edu/epi/snow/snowbook.html)

Thomas, S., Acton, C., Nixon, J. *et al.* (1994). Effectiveness of bicycle helmets in preventing head injury in children: case–control study. *British Medical Journal*, **308**: 173–176.

Vessey, M. P., Villard-Mackintosh, L., McPherson, K. and Yeates, D. (1989). Mortality among oral contraceptive users: 20 year follow up of women in a cohort study. *British Medical Journal*, **299**: 1487–1491.

Heads or tails: the role of chance

Description	Association	Alternative explanations	Integration & interpretation	Practical applications
Chapters 2–3	Chapters 4–5	Chapter 6: Chance	Chapters 9–11	Chapters 12–15

If the results of a study reveal an interesting association between some exposure and a health outcome, there is a natural tendency to assume that it is real. (Note that we are considering whether two things are *associated*. This does not necessarily imply a causal association. We will discuss approaches to determining causality further in Chapter 10.) However, before we can even contemplate this possibility we have to attempt to rule out other possible explanations for the results. There are three main 'alternative explanations' that we have to consider whenever we analyse epidemiological data or read the reports of others: namely, could the results be due to

* chance
* bias or error or
* confounding?

We will discuss the first of these, **chance**, in this chapter and will cover **bias** and **confounding** in Chapters 7 and 8.

Random sampling error

When we conduct a study or survey it is rarely possible to include the whole of a population so we usually have to rely on a *sample* of that population and trust that this sample will give us an answer that holds true for the general population.

If we select the sample of people wisely and they are truly representative of the target population (the population that we want to study) then we will not introduce any **selection bias** into the study (see Chapter 7). However, if we were to study several different samples of people from the same population it is unlikely that we would find exactly the same answer each time, and unlikely that any of the answers would be exactly the same as the true population value. This is because each sample we take will include slightly different people and their characteristics will tend to vary from those in other samples – just by chance. This is known as **random sampling error**.

Imagine that you were interested in the health effects of obesity and wanted to know the average body-mass index (BMI) of 10-year-old children in your community. If you weighed and measured just one or two children you would not obtain a very good estimate of the average BMI of all children – but the more children you studied, the better your estimate would be. The same is true if we are looking for the association between an 'exposure' and 'outcome', for example the relation between BMI and age. If we only survey a small group of 10-year olds and another small group of 12-year olds we might find that, just by chance, the 10-year olds are bigger than the 12-year olds, but the larger our study, the better or more *precise* our estimate of the true association between age and body-size will be. (We will discuss precision further in Chapter 7.) In general, if we select a small sample of a population then our results are more likely to differ from the true population values than if we had selected a larger sample. The best way to reduce sampling error is thus to increase the size of the study sample as far as is practical. (Of course, there is always a trade-off between study size and cost.)

There are ways in which we can calculate how many people we should include in a study to reduce sampling error to an acceptable level. In an analytic study these calculations involve some knowledge, first, of the likely size of the effect we expect to see and, secondly, of the prevalence of the factor of interest in the population. They also require a decision as to how precisely we wish to measure the effect, i.e. how much sampling error we are prepared to accept in our result. If we are looking for a large effect and the exposure and/or disease are quite common then we do not need a large study to show this. For example, in 1971 a tiny case–control study ($n = 40$) showed that young women who had been exposed in utero to diethylstilboestrol (DES) had an increased risk of developing a rare type of vaginal cancer (clear cell adenocarcinoma) (Herbst *et al.*, 1971). (DES is a synthetic oestrogen that was used between 1940 and 1970 to prevent spontaneous abortion and premature delivery.) In this situation, the frequency of DES use among the mothers of the cases was so high (seven out of eight) and the difference was so large (none of 32 control mothers had used DES) that the investigators needed to study only those 40 women to show that there was a clear association. Unfortunately, in modern epidemiology we are often looking for much smaller effects and our studies have to be much larger than this to detect them with certainty. We will not discuss the statistical methods for performing what are called '*sample size*' or '*power*' calculations further here; the formulae for these can be found in many standard textbooks on medical statistics. We will, however, come back to consider the concept of **power** later in this chapter.

Confidence intervals (CI)

There are two related aspects to consider when looking for associations between exposure and outcome: does an association exist and how strong is the association. As epidemiology is fundamentally about measuring effects we will discuss the second issue first and then come back to the question of whether an association exists.

As you saw above, there will always be some degree of random sampling error in a study and the results we obtain may vary from the truth simply because, by chance, the people who ended up in the study differed in some way from the population norm. To assess the likely effects of this random error we can calculate what is a called a **confidence interval** around our result. This is in effect an explicit admission that the result of a study (typically an OR or RR, also known as the 'point' or 'effect' estimate) is probably not exactly right, but that the real answer is likely to lie somewhere within a given range – the confidence interval. A narrow confidence interval therefore indicates *good precision* or little random sampling error and, conversely, a wide confidence interval indicates *poor precision*.

The most commonly used confidence intervals are 95% intervals (95% CI) and they are often described slightly inaccurately as meaning that we can be '95% confident' that the real value is within the range covered by the confidence interval. What the confidence interval really means is that if we were to repeat the study many times with different samples of people, then 95% of the 95% confidence intervals we calculated would include the true value. Note that this also means that 5% of the time (or 1 in 20 times) the 95% CI would not include the true value and we will never know which times these are. Other percentages can be used, such as 90%, which gives a narrower confidence interval but less certainty that it will contain the true value (we will be wrong about 1 time in 10); and 99%, which will be more likely to contain the true value (we will only be wrong about 1 time in 100) but will give a wider interval.

If we are considering a measure of relative risk, the 'no-effect' or *null value* is 1.0 – a relative risk of 1.0 indicates that there is no difference between the two groups being compared. If both ends of a CI are greater than 1.0 this suggests that there is a positive association between the exposure and outcome; similarly if both ends of the CI are less than 1.0 then it suggests an inverse association. However, if the CI includes the null value, i.e. the lower bound is less than 1.0

and the upper bound is greater than 1.0, then we cannot rule out the possibility that the true relative risk is really 1.0 and thus there is really no association between the exposure and outcome.

To consider a practical example, imagine two studies that have evaluated the association between exposure to air pollution and asthma.

Study 1 finds a relative risk of 1.5 with a 95% confidence interval (CI) of 1.2–1.9.

What does this tell us about the association between air pollution and asthma?

This is a fairly precise estimate. It tells us that people who are exposed to air pollution are about one and a half times as likely (or 50% more likely) to develop asthma than those who are not exposed. It tells us that the risk might be as high as 1.9 times, but that it might be as low as 1.2 times (i.e. a 20% increase) higher in those who are exposed. It also tells us that the relative risk is *unlikely* to be more than 1.9 or less than 1.2 (but it still could be outside these values).

Study 2 finds a relative risk of 2.5 (95% CI 0.9–6.9).

What is the most likely value for the relative risk of asthma in people exposed to air pollution in the second study?

Is it possible that the result could have arisen by chance and there is really no association (i.e. the 'true' population relative risk is 1.0)?

Which of the two studies would give you most concern that air pollution was associated with asthma?

In the second study, the most likely value for the relative risk is 2.5 and the true relative risk could be as high as 6.9. However, the confidence interval is very wide, indicating poor precision, and it also includes the value 1.0 (remembering that an RR of 1.0 suggests no effect), so it is possible that there is really no association and the result of 2.5 arose by chance. Both studies suggest a possible effect of air pollution in inducing asthma. Assuming there is no bias in the results, the first study suggests that there is a real association between air pollution and asthma but the effect is not very great. The second study suggests the relative effect might be larger and thus more important clinically, but because of the wide CI we are left with some uncertainty as to how 'true' that value really is. We should certainly not ignore the results of the second study just because chance is one possible explanation for our findings; after all the real value is just as likely to be close to 6.0 (a very strong association), as it is to be close to 1.0 (no effect). However, we should be cautious, and acknowledge the possibility that it could merely reflect the play of chance. In practice, if we had to make a judgement about the public health effects of air pollution we would want to consider the results of both studies together to increase the precision of our estimate and we will look at ways to do this in more detail in Chapter 11. For now, it is important to remember that

Figure 6.1 Possible outcomes of
an epidemiological study.

STUDY RESULTS (Known)	TRUTH (Unknown)	
	No association	Association
No association	Correct	Type-II error (probability $= \beta$)
Association	Type-I error (probability $= \alpha$)	Correct (probability $= 1 - \beta$) = Power

narrow confidence intervals (indicating good precision) are always more informative than wide confidence intervals (indicating poor precision). We will not
discuss the methods for calculating confidence intervals here but have included
some of the most useful formulae for this in Appendix 7.

Statistics in epidemiology

When we conduct a study to evaluate the relationship between an exposure and
disease we may find an association or we may not. We then have to use the information from the sample of people in the study to infer whether the exposure and
outcome are truly related in the wider population. There are thus four possible
outcomes for any study, as shown in Figure 6.1.

   If there is really no association between the outcome and exposure then we
hope that our study will find just that. Conversely, if the exposure and outcome
are truly associated in the population then we want our study to show this association. What we want to minimise are the situations where our study shows
an apparent relationship between exposure and outcome when the truth is that
there is none (often called a 'type I' or alpha error), or our study says there is no
association when, in truth, there is (a 'type II' or beta error). Unfortunately, in
practice we can never know for sure whether we are right or wrong.

Statistical significance: could an association have arisen by chance?

A confidence interval provides valuable information about the likely *size* of an
effect and, as you saw above, it can also give you some idea about whether a
result might have arisen just by chance – if the confidence interval includes the
null or no-effect value (e.g. 1.0 for a relative risk) then we cannot rule out chance
as a possible explanation. We can also carry out what is known as a **hypothesis
test** to assess this. When we do this we calculate the probability that we would
have seen an effect as strong as (or stronger than) the observed effect *if there*

were really no difference between the groups (the 'null' hypothesis). The results of these statistical tests take the form of a *p*-value (or probability value) and they give us some idea of how likely it is that the groups are truly different and the association is real, or whether the results might just be due to random sampling error or **chance** (in other words, a type I error, α). For example, if a survey of children shows that girls have a higher average BMI than boys, is this likely to be a true difference or could it just be chance that the girls in the study sample happened to have a higher BMI than the boys?

Imagine that the average BMI of the girls in a survey was 2 units higher than the average BMI of the boys and that statistical testing gave a *p*-value of 0.01 associated with this difference. We can say from this that, if the average BMIs of boys and girls were in fact the same (i.e. the *null hypothesis* is true), then we would have only a 0.01 or 1% probability of seeing an apparent difference of 2 units (or more) purely by chance. This is a very low probability, it would occur only 1 in 100 times, thus it seems *unlikely* to be a chance finding, although it still could be. Conventionally, results are considered to be *statistically significant*, i.e. unlikely to have arisen by chance, if the *p*-value is less than 0.05 ($p < 0.05$); in other words, if the probability that the result would have arisen by chance is less than 5% (i.e. the probability that we are making a type I error, α, is less than 0.05). Using this criterion, we would, therefore, conclude that the 2 unit difference in BMI between boys and girls was unlikely to have arisen by chance and that, all else being equal, girls probably do have a higher BMI than boys.

From www.CartoonStock.com

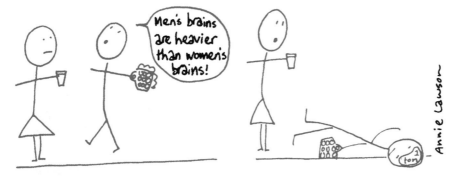

Imagine a study which found that, compared with people who exercised regularly, those who did not exercise had a three-fold higher risk of having a heart attack (RR = 3.0) and that the *p*-value for this association was 0.005.

What would the relative risk be if the risk of having a heart attack were the *same* for people who exercised and those who did not?

Is it likely that a study would give a relative risk of 3.0 ($p = 0.005$) if there were really no association between exercise and heart attack?

If the risk of having a heart attack were the same regardless of how much a person exercised, i.e. there was *no* association between exercising and having a heart attack, then the relative risk would be 1.0. In the example above the study found a relative risk of 3.0, $p = 0.005$. The small p-value suggests that it is very unlikely that the study would have given a relative risk as big as 3.0 if the true relative risk were 1.0. (With a p-value of 0.005, we would expect this to happen only about 5 in 1,000 times.) The observed association between heart attack and exercise is therefore unlikely to have arisen by chance.

Note also the relationship between confidence intervals and p-values. If a 95% CI does *not* contain the 'no-effect' or 'null' value (1.0 for an RR, OR, etc.) then the p-value from a statistical test would be < 0.05. Conversely, if the 95% CI *does* include the no-effect value then $p \geq 0.05$. In the hypothetical asthma studies above, the 95% CI for study 1 does not include the null value. In this situation the corresponding p-value would be less than 0.05 and the result would be termed 'statistically significant'. The result of study 2, on the other hand, would not be statistically significant because the 95% CI includes the value 1.0 so the p-value would be ≥ 0.05.

This form of statistical testing is very common, but it is important to note that the conventional distinction between $p < 0.05$ (statistically significant) and $p \geq 0.05$ (not statistically significant) is purely arbitrary. Hypothesis tests and p-values are tools that can be used to help assess the results of a study, but they should not be used blindly to decide whether or not an association exists (see Box 6.1). They are aids to judgement, not absolute arbiters.

Power: could we have missed a true association?

In addition to considering whether an association might have arisen by chance, we should also consider whether we could have *missed* a true relation by chance. Is it possible that an exposure is linked to an outcome but the study was just too small to detect this reliably (a type II error, β)? Consider again the hypothetical study above that reported a relative risk of 3.0 ($p = 0.005$) for the association between a lack of regular exercise and heart attack. What if the study had been smaller and the p-value was only 0.1? In this situation $p \geq 0.05$ so it is possible that the observed RR of 3.0 has arisen by chance and there is truly no association between lack of exercise and risk of heart attack; but it is also possible that there is really quite a strong association but the study was just too small to detect this with any certainty.

To avoid such a situation it is important to ensure that a study is big enough or, in other words, that it has enough *power* to detect a true association with sufficient precision. The power of a study is the probability that the study will detect an association of a particular size if it truly exists in the general population. (Note: as shown in Figure 6.1, the probability of making a type II error, i.e. saying there

Box 6.1 Why you should not rely only on *p*-values

The convention of describing a result as 'statistically significant' if $p < 0.05$ is now so strongly ingrained that some people tend to believe a result if $p < 0.05$ but not if $p > 0.05$. For example, a relative risk of 2.5 ($p = 0.049$) would, by convention, be called 'statistically significant' because 0.049 is less than 0.05. In contrast, a relative risk of 2.5 ($p = 0.051$) would not be classed as statistically significant because 0.051 is greater than 0.05. However, the relative risk is the same in both cases and $p = 0.049$ is so similar to $p = 0.051$ that it is illogical to believe the first result but not the second. *P*-values are also highly dependent on the size of the study – the bigger the study the smaller the *p*-value (for the same effect size). Imagine a study with 80 cases and 80 controls that found an odds ratio of 1.7 with a *p*-value of 0.11. By convention this result would not be statistically significant and we would say that the association could have arisen by chance. If the same study had been twice as big (160 cases and 160 controls) we would have found the same odds ratio (1.7) but now the *p*-value would have been 0.02, so we would have concluded that the association *was* statistically significant. These problems associated with the blind dependence on *p*-values have led to suggestions from some epidemiologists that *p*-values should not be used at all.

is no association when one truly exists, is often denoted β. The power of a study, i.e. the probability that it will show an association if it exists, is therefore $1 - \beta$.) Imagine that an exposure truly causes a two-fold increase in the risk of disease (of course, we can never know this in practice). If a study has 80% power to detect a relative risk of 2.0 between the exposure and outcome then we can say that 80% of the time, or four times out of five, that study would determine that the exposure and outcome were related. It also means that there is a 20% or one in five chance that we would miss the association. There is no hard and fast rule as to how much power a study should have but, in general, most people would probably want a minimum of 80% power and many would aim for 90%. As discussed above, there are statistical methods to calculate the number of people needed for a study to give a certain level of power.

A major problem in epidemiology is that, for financial or other practical reasons, researchers often cannot conduct as large a study as they would like. However, if they compromise and conduct a small study that shows an association between the exposure and outcome but this is not statistically significant (i.e. poor precision) it is difficult to interpret the results. Is there really an association, i.e. the estimated effect is close to the truth, but the study was just too small to detect this with any certainty? Or was the observed association just due to chance and the truth is that there is no association? The smaller the effect,

Box 6.2 RCTs failed to show a benefit of streptokinase

Between 1959 and 1988, 33 randomised clinical trials were conducted to test whether intravenous streptokinase reduced the risk of death after heart attack. Most of the studies ($n = 25$) found that mortality was lower among the groups given streptokinase but many were small and so their results were not 'statistically significant' (i.e. $p \geq 0.05$). As a result the benefits of streptokinase were not fully appreciated. In 1992, however, a group combined the results of all the individual streptokinase studies using a technique called **meta-analysis** (we will discuss this further in Chapter 11). This showed that streptokinase was associated with more than a 20% reduction in mortality after heart attack and, because of the large sample size, a total of 36,974 patients when all the studies were combined, this effect was now highly statistically significant ($p < 0.001$) (Lau *et al.*, 1992). Importantly, they also found that if the results of just the first eight studies, involving a total of only 2,432 patients, had been combined, the 20% reduction in mortality among those given streptokinase would have been apparent back in 1973. The problem was that individually most of the early studies were simply not big enough to detect this effect with sufficient certainty. As a consequence, their results were rarely statistically significant and so were dismissed. If some of these studies had been bigger (or if more emphasis had been placed on the size of the reduction in mortality and less on statistical significance) the beneficial effects of streptokinase would have been discovered much sooner and thousands of lives could probably have been saved.

the more important it is that we can estimate it precisely in order to distinguish between a real association and chance. This is a major problem in the context of genetic studies when investigators often test many genes and the associations with disease are likely to be weak (RR < 1.5). This makes it very hard to identify which, if any, observed associations are real and, as a result, genetic association studies have to be very large (10s of 1,000s of cases) in order to give sufficient precision. This question is also particularly important in the context of clinical trials when we need to know whether small improvements seen for a new treatment really do represent a benefit that should be passed on to patients (see Box 6.2).

This raises an important ethical issue that most human research and ethics committees would now consider before giving a study approval to proceed. Is the study big enough to detect the effects the investigators are looking for? If the answer is no then it has to be questioned whether the study should be allowed to go ahead.

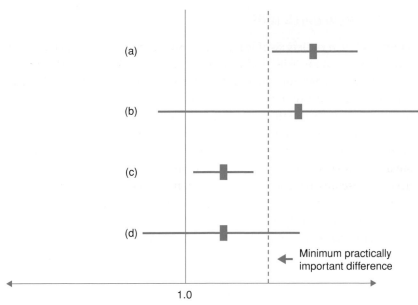

Figure 6.2 Statistical and biological significance: point estimates and confidence intervals from four hypothetical studies.

Statistical versus clinical significance

Randomised controlled trials evaluating the drug finasteride for treatment of lower urinary tract symptoms in men have shown that there is a *statistically significant* improvement in symptom score (a measure of the symptoms experienced) from 2.5 to 2.8 in men treated with finasteride (Hirst and Ward, 2000). However, for men to experience a subjective change in quality of life, their symptom score has to change by at least three points. An increase of 0.3 points, although a 12% improvement, is therefore not *clinically significant.* It is therefore crucial that we also consider how meaningful the result of a study is in practical terms; that is, we should assess the result in terms of its social, preventive, biological or clinical significance.

This is illustrated in Figure 6.2, which shows the results of four hypothetical intervention studies. In study (a) the result is both practically important and statistically significant because the point estimate falls beyond the '*minimum practically important difference*' line and the confidence interval does not include the value 1.0 (in fact, even the lower bound is above the minimum important difference line). The tightness of the confidence interval around the RR also gives reassurance of its precision. In study (b) the result is again practically important but not statistically significant, since the confidence interval is wide and does include 1.0. The width of the confidence interval suggests that the study was small, leaving imprecision and therefore some uncertainty about the role of chance. The finding could be important but we really need more data for a confident judgement. In contrast, the results shown for (c) are statistically significant but not important, as in the finasteride example above. The narrow confidence interval tells us that our estimate is fairly precise (i.e. there are plenty of data). Finally, the results of study (d) are neither statistically significant nor practically important. This study provides little useful evidence about the benefit of the intervention – the very wide confidence interval that spans well across the null shows that this is a very poor test of the original hypothesis.

In summary, *statistical significance* is evident on looking at the *p*-values from appropriate statistical tests and from the confidence intervals around the point estimates; and the extra information the latter give as to the *precision* of an effect estimate is valuable. In health research where we are looking to improve outcomes through preventive, clinical or other interventions, we may have a fair idea of how big an effect needs to be for it to be *clinically or practically significant*. This might be a certain percentage improvement (i.e. a relative effect) or an absolute increase (as in the finasteride example above) and this might also have to be weighed against any adverse effects of the therapy (see also Box 6.3). In observational (aetiological) epidemiology, however, there is no clear rule as to how big an effect should be for it to be meaningful. A relative risk greater than 2.0 would probably be considered fairly strong and thus, by implication, *practically significant*. An RR less than this would not, however, immediately be dismissed because, as you saw in the example of smoking and coronary heart disease in Table 5.4, a modest *relative risk* may still lead to a high *absolute* or *attributable risk*.

A final word about confidence intervals and *p*-values

It is easy to get fixated on *p*-values and to implicitly believe an association is real if $p < 0.05$ and to assume it is not real (i.e. it is due to chance) if $p \geq 0.05$. But it is important to remember that confidence intervals are much more informative than *p*-values. The width of a confidence interval gives an indication of the precision of the estimate and the two bounds tell you both how weak the association might be and also how strong it might be. It is also important to understand that the true value of an association is most likely to be somewhere near the point estimate in the middle of a confidence interval; it is much less likely to be near the ends of the interval and even less likely to be outside it completely. Thus if an OR = 2.5 with a 95% CI from 0.9 to 7.3, then the real effect is much more likely to be close to 2.5 than it is to be close to 1.0; furthermore it is just as likely to be close to 6.0 or 7.0 as it is to be as low as 1.0.

In contrast, a *p*-value simply gives an indication of whether an observed association could be 'due to chance' and there might really be no effect (i.e. the true RR or OR is 1.0). It effectively focuses on the end of the confidence interval that is closest to the null (does this or does it not include the null value?) and ignores the other end completely. For these reasons, the epidemiological and wider health literature has seen a shift away from using *p*-values in recent years towards reporting confidence intervals because of the additional information they provide and to reduce the dependence on '$p < 0.05$' which, as you have seen, can be misleading or mean that important results are missed.

Summary

In any study there will always be an element of chance as to who is studied and who is not – this type of random error is called *sampling error*. As you have seen, statistical methods have been developed to assess the amount of sampling error that is likely to be present in any particular study but it is easy to be seduced by statistics and important to be able to interpret the results of a study practically, regardless of what the investigator might claim. It is, however, important to reiterate that if we do not select the study participants carefully and they are not representative of the wider population (i.e. they differ from the target population in a *systematic* way) then we will introduce *selection bias* into the study. This is a completely separate issue from the problem of random sampling error that we considered above and we will discuss it in more detail in the next chapter.

Questions

1. The authors of a study report a RR of 1.8 (95% CI 1.6–2.0) for the association between alcohol intake and cancer. The authors of a second study report an

OR of 1.8 (95% CI 0.7–3.5) for the association between caffeine intake and the same cancer. What do the results of these studies tell us (i) about the studies and (ii) about risk factors for the cancer?

2. What is the best way to reduce sampling error in a study?
    (a) Select people from the population at random.
    (b) Increase the size of the study.
    (c) Calculate a 95% confidence interval for the results.
    (d) Use a more reliable instrument to measure exposure.

3. A randomised, placebo-controlled trial was conducted in Indonesia to study the effects of vitamin A for treating children with measles. The investigators reported a confidence interval for the relative risk of 0.26 to 0.94. Which of the following statements are true?
    (a) Because the confidence interval does not include the value 'zero' we can say the result is statistically significant.
    (b) Because the confidence interval does not include the value 'zero' we can say the result is not statistically significant.
    (c) Because the confidence interval does not include the value 'one' we can say the result is statistically significant.
    (d) Because the confidence interval does not include the value 'one' we can say the result is clinically significant.

4. What is the difference between statistical significance and clinical significance?

REFERENCES

Fojo, T. and Grady, C. (2009). How much is life worth: Cetuximab, non-small cell lung cancer, and the $440 billion question. *Journal of the National Cancer Institute*, **101**: 1044–1048.

Herbst, A. L., Ulfelder, H. and Poskanzer, D. C. (1971). Adenocarcinoma of the vagina. Association of maternal stilbestrol therapy with tumor appearance in young women. *New England Journal of Medicine*, **284**: 878–881.

Hirst, G. H. L. and Ward, J. E. (2000). Clinical practice guidelines: reality bites. *Medical Journal of Australia*, **172**: 287–291.

Lau, J., Antman, E. M., Jimenez-Silva, J. *et al.* (1992). Cumulative meta-analysis of therapeutic trials for myocardial infarction. *New England Journal of Medicine*, **327**: 248–254.

All that glitters is not gold: the problem of error

Description		Association		Alternative explanations		Integration & interpretation		Practical applications
Chapters 2–3		Chapters 4–5		Chapter 7: Error		Chapters 9–11		Chapters 12–15

Box 7.1 Bigger isn't always better!

In the run-up to the 1936 presidential election in America, the *Literary Digest* conducted a poll of more than two million voters and confidently predicted that the Republican candidate, Alf Landon, would win. On the day it was the Democrat candidate, Franklin D. Roosevelt, who won a landslide victory. The *Digest* had correctly predicted the winner of the previous five elections, so what went wrong in 1936?

The *Digest* sent polling papers to households listed in telephone directories and car registration records. In 1936, however, telephone and car ownership was more common among more affluent households and these were the people who were also more likely to vote Republican. The generally less affluent Democrat voters were thus under-represented in the sample of voters polled. In contrast, a young George Gallup conducted a much smaller poll of a few thousand representative voters and correctly predicted the Roosevelt win. As a result of this fiasco the *Digest* folded but Gallup polls are still conducted today.

We saw in Chapter 6 that larger studies are less likely to get the wrong results due to chance (or random sampling error) than smaller studies; however, the example in Box 7.1 shows that a large sample size is not sufficient to ensure we get the right results. The enormous presidential poll conducted by the *Literary Digest* didn't get the right answer because it included the 'wrong' people, i.e. they were not representative of everybody in the voting population. Furthermore, in epidemiology we frequently rely on records that have been collected for some other purpose, and we have already discussed some of the problems inherent in this in Chapter 3. Even when the data we use have been collected specifically for our research they are unlikely to be completely free of error. We often have to rely on people's memories, but how accurate are they? And biological measurements such as blood pressure and weight are often subject to natural variation as well as being affected by the performance of the measurement system that we use.

People live complicated lives and, unlike laboratory scientists who can control all aspects of their experiments, epidemiologists have to work with that complexity. As a result, no epidemiological study will ever be perfect. Even an apparently straightforward survey of, say, alcohol consumption in a community can be fraught with problems. Who should be included in the survey? How do you measure alcohol consumption reliably? All we can do when we conduct a study is aim to *minimise* error as far as possible, and then *assess the practical effects* of any unavoidable error. An important aspect of epidemiology is, therefore, the ability to recognise potential sources of error and, more importantly, to assess the likely effects of any error, both in your own work and in the work of others.

In this chapter we will point out some of the most common sources of such error in epidemiological studies and how these can best be avoided. We also want to emphasise from the outset that some degree of error is inevitable and that this need not invalidate the results of a study.

Sources of error in epidemiological studies

In an epidemiological study we usually want to measure the proportion of people with a particular characteristic or identify the association between an exposure and an outcome. To do this we have to recruit individuals into the study, measure their exposure and/or outcome status and then, if appropriate, calculate a measure of association between the exposure and outcome. We also want the results we obtain to be as close to the truth as possible. (Note that, although we will discuss error in the context of exposure and disease, when we talk about an exposure we mean anything from a gene to a particular behaviour, and the outcome need not be a disease but could be any health-related state.)

As you will discover, there are dozens of different names that have been given to the kinds of error that can occur in epidemiological studies. Fortunately, in practice, all types of error can be classified into one of two main areas: they relate either to the **selection** of participants for study or comparison, or to the **measurement** of exposure and/or outcome. These errors can in turn be either **random** or **systematic**. Random error or poor precision is the divergence, by chance alone, of a measurement from the true value. Systematic error occurs when measurements differ from the truth in a systematic way.

We will now discuss the main types of both selection and measurement error in more detail and will also consider the effects that they may have on the results of a study. Remember that in practice it is impossible to eliminate all error and the most important thing is therefore to consider the likely practical effects of any remaining error.

Selection bias

Depending on how we select subjects for our study, and how many we select, we can introduce both random and systematic sampling errors into our study. As you saw in the previous chapter, even if the people selected for a study are generally representative of the population that we wish to learn about (the target population), we may still get the wrong result just because of *random* sampling error, i.e. by chance, and this is especially likely when we take only a small sample. In contrast, the example in Box 7.1 shows how the results of even a large study can be biased if the sample of people selected for the study *systematically* differ from the population that we wish to learn about in some way.

Selection bias occurs when there is a systematic difference between the people who are included in a study and those who are not, or when study and comparison groups are selected inappropriately or using different criteria. Unlike random sampling error, we cannot reduce selection bias by simply increasing the size of the study sample – the problem persists no matter how large the sample. Nor are there simple statistical techniques to assess the amount or direction of systematic error in a study, so it is not always easy to know what effect it might have on the results.

The issue of selection bias is a major problem in simple descriptive studies such as prevalence surveys. If the sample of people included in the survey is not representative of the wider population the results of the survey can be very wrong, as the *Literary Digest* found in their biased opinion poll which under-represented the views of poorer Americans. It is also a problem in analytic studies because it can lead to inappropriate comparisons and hence biased measures of association (OR, RR, AR or PAR). It is a particular concern in case–control studies because the participants are recruited as two separate groups and it can be difficult to ensure that the final control group makes an appropriate comparison group for the cases. A similar problem can arise in cohort studies when the exposed and unexposed groups are recruited separately, for example when the exposed group comprises workers in a particular occupation or military group and a separate unexposed group has to be identified for comparison.

In a case–control study, it is important to have a clear definition of the population group that you want to study (the target population). This need not be everybody, but could be a specific subgroup of the whole population. Cases and controls should then be selected from the same identifiable group. Ideally all cases in a defined population would be included, but if only a sample is used they should be truly representative of all cases arising in the population. The controls too should then be selected to be representative of this population. (We discussed options for control selection in Chapter 4.)

In cohort studies such as the Framingham and Nurses' Health studies that we discussed in Chapter 4 we usually recruit a single group of participants and then classify them according to their exposure. In this situation, the question of how individuals were recruited is usually less important in terms of the validity of the study results (what is often called **internal validity**). However, it can influence the generalisability or **external validity** of the findings since they may apply only to the sorts of people who took part. In some situations, however, selection bias (at the point of recruitment) can also influence the effect estimates. As an example, consider a cohort study examining the effect of children's socioeconomic status (SES) on their risk of injury. If the families of lowest SES are more likely to refuse to participate, then this group may be under-represented in the total cohort. In this situation, measurement of the risk of injury within the low SES group and comparisons with those of higher socioeconomic status should still be accurate;

the low SES group will just be smaller than it might have been had more low SES families participated. If, however, those families of lower SES who refuse to take part are also those whose children are at highest risk of injury, then the study will underestimate the true amount of injury in this group. It will then also underestimate the effect of low SES on injury risk because the really high-risk children in that group were not included.

As for cohort studies, selection bias at recruitment and exposure assignment is not usually a major issue for internal validity in clinical trials, although it can occur if the allocation process is predictable and the decision whether or not to enter a person into the trial is influenced by the expected treatment assignment. For example, if alternate patients are assigned to receive active drug or placebo, a physician may decide not to enter sicker patients into the trial if he or she thought they were not going to be given the active drug. This selection bias *will* affect the internal validity of the study and is another reason why the allocation process should be truly random and ideally neither the investigators nor the participant should know what group the participant is in (see Chapter 4).

For both cohort and intervention studies the more important issue is to avoid or minimise selective losses from the cohort or study group. Regardless of the length of the follow-up period, one of the most important criteria for a high-quality study is to ensure complete *follow-up* of all participants. The more people who are 'lost to follow-up' with unknown health status, the more likely it is that the results will be biased.

Sources of selection bias

Some common ways in which selection bias can arise include the following.

Volunteers

It is well known that people who volunteer to participate in surveys and studies (i.e. they spontaneously offer their involvement rather than being selected in a formal sampling scheme) are different from those who do not volunteer. In particular, volunteers are often more health-conscious and, as a result, volunteer groups will often contain a lower proportion of, say, smokers than the general population. Advertisements calling for volunteers for a survey or study may also attract people who have a personal interest in the area of the study. The prevalence of various diseases or behaviours in a volunteer group may thus be very different from that in the underlying population because of this self-selection into the study. This means that volunteer groups are completely unsuitable for surveys conducted to measure the prevalence of either health behaviours or diseases in the population and they are also likely to introduce bias into studies looking for associations between exposures and health outcomes. For this reason, epidemiological research rarely uses groups of volunteers and, if it does, it is advisable to pay close attention to whether the use of volunteers may have biased the results in some way.

Imagine a survey about a sensitive area such as sexual behaviour where participants were recruited via advertisements in women's magazines. How representative do you think the results would be of all women?

There are two potential problems with this type of recruitment. First, different magazines target different types of women so it is likely that the readers of one particular magazine will not be representative of all women. It is also likely that the women who choose to respond to a survey of this type will differ markedly from those who do not respond, for example they may well be more confident and out-going and thus more likely to engage in less conventional sexual behaviours. This exact issue plagued Kinsey, who conducted some of the earliest work on sexual behaviour in the mid 1900s (Kinsey, 1948). He reported high levels of unconventional sexual behaviours in his study groups but was roundly criticised for using samples of volunteers, prisoners and male prostitutes, thus raising concerns about the reliability of his results. At the time, others demonstrated that women who agreed to take part in a survey of sexual habits were much more likely to have high levels of self-esteem than non-participants, and that women with a high self-esteem score reported very different sexual behaviours from those with low self-esteem scores (Maslow and Sakoda, 1952). Although Kinsey attempted to address the criticisms of his studies, the concerns remained and his results still cause controversy today. (Kinsey's life and work were dramatised in the 2005 Hollywood movie 'Kinsey: let's talk about sex'.)

Low response rates

What might be thought of as a type of volunteer bias, and one that again is a particular problem in surveys and case–control studies, is the problem of low response rates. People who have a particular disease are often highly motivated to take part in research into that disease. Controls, however, have no such motivation to participate and investigators are finding it increasingly hard to persuade healthy people to take part in research. Even if potential controls for a study are selected at random, if some do not agree to take part then the remaining group may no longer be a true random sample of the population and the results may be biased. Box 7.2 shows an example from a study looking at passive smoking and heart attack where the authors assessed and reported the likely existence and extent of error in their estimates of smoking rates in the control group. This degree of thoroughness is commendable but, unfortunately, rarely seen due to logistical constraints. Note also how this information can be used to make a tentative practical assessment of the likely bias this error may have introduced into the estimate of the effect of passive smoking on heart disease.

Box 7.2 Differences between responders and non-responders

In a case–control study of the effects of passive smoking on the risk of heart attack or coronary death, the investigators put a lot of effort into trying to achieve a high response rate from controls. Potential controls were initially invited to attend a study centre where they would have blood collected and physical measurements taken as well as completing a risk factor questionnaire. Participants who did not respond to this invitation were sent a shorter questionnaire to complete at home and some people who still did not respond were then visited and interviewed at their homes. There were thus three types of people among the control group: the willing volunteers who replied to the initial invitation, the slightly less willing who replied to the shorter home questionnaire and the even more reluctant who agreed to take part only when visited by an interviewer. The investigators then compared the prevalence of smoking in these three groups (Table 7.1).

Table 7.1 Prevalence of smoking increases with increasing reluctance to take part in a study.

Ease of recruitment	Never smoker (%)	Ex-smokers (%)	Current smokers (%)
Men (age 35–69 years)			
Full participation (willing)	35	40	24
Short questionnaire (less willing)	30	42	28
Home interview (reluctant)	29	42	29
Women (age 35–69 years)			
Full participation (willing)	67	19	14
Short questionnaire (less willing)	66	13	21
Home interview (reluctant)	53	16	31

(Dobson *et al.*, 1991.)

The harder it was to persuade someone to take part in the study, the more likely they were to be a current smoker, especially for women. This suggests that those who refused completely probably had even higher smoking rates. The measured prevalence of smoking in the control group is therefore likely to be an *underestimate* of the true level of smoking in the whole population. Using the study data, the calculated odds ratio for the association between smoking and heart disease in men was 2.3. However, if the *true* proportion of current smokers in the population was actually 3% higher and the proportion of non-smokers 3% lower than in the study controls, then the *true* odds ratio would have been lower, about 1.8. The study would thus have overestimated the strength of the association.

Ascertainment or detection bias

This can occur if an individual's chance of being diagnosed as having a particular disease is related to whether they have been 'exposed' to the factor of interest. An example of this type of bias was seen in early studies of the risk of oral contraceptive (OC) use causing thromboembolism (a condition in which a blood clot develops in the legs and subsequently breaks off and moves to another part of the body, often the lungs). Doctors who were aware of the potential for this risk were more likely to hospitalise women with symptoms suspicious of thromboembolism if they were taking OCs. Early case–control studies, which were hospital-based, then overestimated the risk of thromboembolism associated with OC use. This was because the cases were more likely to be on OCs simply because of the way in which they were selected to be sent to hospital, since in the minds of their doctors this partly determined their diagnosis.

The healthy-worker effect

This is a well-documented type of selection bias that can occur in occupational studies. People who are working have to be healthy enough to do their job, so they tend to be more robust than the general population, which necessarily includes those who are disabled or seriously ill and hence unable to work. As a result, if occupational groups are compared with the general population – which is not uncommon in cohort studies of occupational hazards – they will almost always appear to be healthier overall. Comparisons within a workplace can also be flawed because different types of job often attract different types of people as well as requiring different levels of fitness. Imagine a study of the effects of heavy physical work on the occurrence of heart disease in which the investigators compared a group of manual labourers with a group of people of similar socioeconomic status who had desk jobs. In this situation, people who had heart disease might be incapable of doing a manual job and therefore more likely to hold a desk job. The frequency of heart disease would thus appear to be higher in those with desk jobs, falsely suggesting that heavy work was protective against heart disease. Similar problems can arise in other groups where members are selected on the basis of physical capability, e.g. the armed forces (see Box 7.3).

Loss to follow-up

In a case–control study the main concern with subject selection is with regard to who is included in the study. In a cohort study or a clinical trial, selection bias can arise if those who *remain* in a study are different from those who do not, i.e. the issue is selection *out* of the study population rather than selection *in*. This can be a particular problem if more people are 'lost to follow-up' in one exposure group than another and if loss is also related to the outcome of interest. For example, imagine a randomised clinical trial comparing a new drug with the current standard treatment. If the sickest people in the intervention group withdrew

Box 7.3 Veterans' health

There is concern that men and women who saw active service in conflicts such as the Vietnam War have worse health than those who did not. Studies that have compared mortality rates among Vietnam veterans with those in the general population are hampered by the fact that the veterans had to pass a stringent medical examination at the time of their enlistment and so, at that time, were much more healthy than the average person. An analysis of mortality rates among male Australian Vietnam veterans found that, up until 1979, mortality among the veterans was actually 18% lower than in the general population (Table 7.2). It is highly unlikely that service in Vietnam would reduce a man's subsequent risk of death, so this inverse association is likely to be due entirely to the healthy-worker effect. It is impossible to say how large this effect might be and to assess whether it could actually be masking an underlying increase in mortality in the veterans.

Table 7.2 Standardised mortality ratios (SMRs) and 95% confidence intervals (CIs) for selected causes of death among male Australian Vietnam Veterans.

Cause of death and time period		SMR	(95% CI)
All causes:	1963–1979	0.82	(0.77–0.87)
	1980–1990	0.95	(0.90–0.99)
	1991–2001	0.99	(0.96–1.02)
Lung cancer:	1963–1979	0.59	(0.32–0.90)
	1980–1990	1.25	(1.05–1.45)
	1991–2001	1.21	(1.08–1.33)

(Wilson *et al.*, 2005.)

In the years from 1980 to 2001, overall mortality among the veterans was similar to that in the general population; however, cancer mortality was more than 20% higher among the veterans. With the increasing time interval since enlistment, the healthy-worker effect will have been wearing off for most causes and it now appears that the veterans do have higher rates of cancer death compared with the general population. The question of veterans' health is now a major issue in many countries.

from the trial, the people remaining in the intervention group would be healthier than those in the standard treatment group and the new drug would appear to be more beneficial than it really was. The opposite situation would occur if people who were doing well were less likely to return for assessments and thus were more likely to be lost to follow-up. In a cohort study, participants with socially stigmatised behaviours (which these days can include smoking cigarettes) may be less easy to follow up and more likely to develop the health conditions being studied.

Control of selection bias

The question of selection bias has to be considered and then eliminated or minimised in the design and conduct of a study. Any error introduced here that leads to inappropriate comparisons is intractable and cannot be removed in the data analysis although, as shown in the example in Box 7.2, it is sometimes possible to estimate the effects of any such bias. As we have seen, in a case–control study the critical issues are defining the case group clearly, selecting an appropriate control group and then ensuring high participation rates among both cases and controls. In a cohort study or trial it is important to have measures to maximise retention of people within the study and, if possible, to follow up those who drop out of the study. For example, studies with cancer incidence or mortality as an outcome can often use population-based cancer or death registers to obtain this information even for people who have dropped out of the study or been lost to active follow-up.

A good study will have clearly defined *eligibility criteria* that can be used to determine whether specific cases are included. For example, in a study of myocardial infarction, specific criteria developed by the World Health Organization might be used to define a case or, in a study of cancer, only those patients with histologically confirmed cancer might be eligible. Additional eligibility criteria might require people to fall within a certain age range (e.g. children are usually excluded from studies of adult diseases), reside in a defined area or be admitted to specific hospitals. Box 7.4 gives typical eligibility and exclusion criteria for a study of ovarian cancer.

Note that the eligibility criteria describe the target population, i.e. all women who are *eligible* to take part in the study. For practical reasons some eligible women might later be *excluded* from the study. It is important to note that if large numbers of women are excluded, regardless of how good the reasons for this, then the resulting study sample might no longer be representative of the whole population. For example, the exclusion of very sick women might mean that cases of advanced cancer are under-represented in the study group. If advanced cancers differ somehow from early cancers in terms of their aetiology then this might affect the overall results.

Once a study has been conducted, all we can do is consider whether any possible selection bias is likely to have made the association appear stronger (further from the null or 'no effect' value) or weaker (closer to the null) than it really is (see below). Any such consideration can, however, only be based on informed guesswork, and the results of any case–control study with low participation rates (particularly among controls) or of a cohort study or trial with high loss to

Box 7.4 Eligibility and exclusion criteria

Eligibility criteria for cases for a study of ovarian cancer could be as follows:

- A *histologically confirmed diagnosis*: the cancer must be confirmed by a pathologist.
- *Incident*: the woman must have no previous history of ovarian cancer.
- *Primary* ovarian cancer: the cancer must originate in the ovary; metastases (cancers that have spread from another anatomical site) would thus be excluded.
- *Age 18–79*: studies often exclude children for practical reasons and in this case ovarian cancer is very rare in children. Older adults are also commonly excluded, particularly if exposure information is to be collected by questionnaire or interview because the problems of recall increase with age.
- *Resident in a specific geographical area*: women who just happen to be diagnosed with ovarian cancer while visiting that region will be excluded.

Comparable eligibility criteria for the *controls* might then be the following:

- Women aged 18–79
- Resident in the same specific geographical area
- No previous history of ovarian cancer; and
- No history of bilateral oophorectomy (i.e. they must have at least one ovary and so be at risk of developing ovarian cancer).

Exclusion criteria might include the following:

- Women who are unable to give informed consent (for example they have dementia)
- Women who are too sick to participate (this decision might be made by the treating doctor); and
- Women who do not speak English (if the main study documents are all in English it might not be financially viable to translate them into other languages).

follow-up are likely to be viewed with suspicion because of the possibility that some unaccounted-for bias could explain the results.

Assessment of the likely effects of selection bias on the results of a study

In practice, participation rates in studies are rarely 100% and the important thing is to assess the likely extent of any bias and the potential impact, if any, of this on the results of the study. Figure 7.1 summarises the issues regarding selection bias that we have covered above and also the effects of random sampling error or

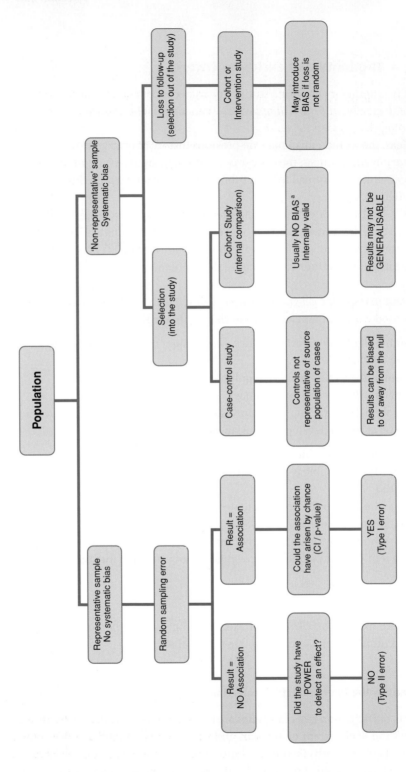

^a The same cannot be said for cohorts with an external comparison group where factors like the healthy worker effect can introduce bias at this stage

Figure 7.1 Random and systematic selection error and their consequences for effect estimation.

chance that we discussed in the previous chapter. The most important consideration is whether it is possible that an observed association is entirely due to error, or would it still exist (and perhaps be even stronger) if the error could be eliminated? Conversely, if a study shows no association, could this be because a real effect has been masked because of the way the subjects were selected (bias) or because the study was just not big enough to show a clear association (chance)? Unfortunately, while we can quantify the effects of random sampling error or chance, questions as to the possible presence and effects of any bias are often difficult to answer – if people did not agree to take part in a study then there is usually no information about them.

External comparisons

Although it might not be possible to obtain information about the non-responders in a study, we may have some knowledge of the wider target population, allowing us to check for differences between it and the actual study population. For example, many countries have cancer registries, so in a case–control study of cancer we might be able to find some basic information such as the age and stage (extent of disease) distribution of all cancer patients diagnosed in a particular region at the time of the study. By comparing the cases who took part in the study with these routine statistics we can see whether the people who did not take part differ in some way from those who did, e.g. they might tend to be older and sicker. Similarly, it may be possible to extract information about possible risk factors such as smoking and alcohol consumption from a national health survey. If so, we can then compare, say, the smoking habits of the study population with those of the general population. If there are fewer smokers among the controls in a case–control study than in the general population, then the study may have overestimated the strength of the association between smoking and disease. For example, a recent study observed an odds ratio of 1.6 (95% CI 1.2–2.2) for the association between current smoking and risk of ovarian cancer, but it was found that the proportion of current smokers in the control group was lower than would be expected from national statistics (13% vs 19%) (Pandeya, 2009). By imputing (estimating) smoking status for the non-participating controls based on the assumption that the total control group should have had a similar prevalence of smoking to the general population, it was estimated that the true odds ratio would have been approximately 1.1 (95% CI 0.8–1.4). Thus non-participation had biased the odds ratio upwards, making it seem as if smoking was associated with ovarian cancer when, in all probability, there is really no association.

Sensitivity analysis

Even without such external data it is still possible to estimate the influence of bias on the results of a study by conducting what is known as a 'sensitivity analysis'

Box 7.5 The worst-case scenario

Imagine a study that compared a new anti-arrhythmic drug (drug A) with an older drug (drug B) for the prevention of sudden death. The results of this hypothetical study are given in Table 7.3.

Table 7.3 Results of hypothetical study comparing two anti-arrhythmic drugs.

Drugs	Number of patients randomised	Number of sudden deaths	Mortality per 100 people
Drug A	860	36	4.2
Drug B	842	72	8.6

From these results, drug A appears to reduce the risk of sudden death by about half (RR = 4.2 ÷ 8.6 = 0.49) compared with drug B. However, what if we find that some patients were lost to follow-up: 32 from group A and 16 from group B? The worst-case scenario (if we are hoping to find evidence in favour of drug A) would be if all the patients lost from group A had actually died from an arrhythmia while all those lost from group B were alive and feeling so well that they had decided not to return for follow-up. We can then recalculate the mortality for drug A on the basis of this scenario (the mortality for drug B will not change):

Mortality in group A if the 32 patients lost to follow-up died due to an arrhythmia = (36 + 32) ÷ 860 = 7.9 per 100 people

Drug A is still found to give a benefit compared with drug B, although the reduction in risk of mortality is now less than 10%. In practice it is highly unlikely that all participants lost to follow-up from group A had met an untimely arrhythmia-related death whereas none of those taking drug B had. The true reduction in risk for drug A is therefore likely to be greater than 10% and in this situation we might be happy to conclude that, even in the presence of the loss to follow-up, drug A was more useful than drug B.

(see Box 7.5). If there is loss to follow-up in a cohort study or clinical trial, then imagine the worst-case scenario i.e. that everyone lost from one group developed the outcome of interest and nobody lost from the other group did. How would that have affected the results of the study? What if the loss had been the other way around or if only half of the people lost had developed disease? How bad would the loss have to have been to explain the whole association? If there is still an association after such worst-case assumptions then the observed result cannot be an artefact due entirely to bias. (Note that this does not imply that the association is real; it could also be due to measurement error, which we discuss below, or confounding (see Chapter 8).)

Measurement or information error

We will now turn our attention to possible sources and effects of error in the information we collect from or about people. Few measures of exposure will be perfect and there may also be errors in the measurement of outcome, leading to **misclassification** of participants with respect to their exposure status and/or outcome (disease); i.e. someone may be labelled as 'exposed' (or as a 'case') when they were actually 'unexposed' (or a 'non-case'). This can then lead to bias in the results of the study. Some error can and will creep in whenever we measure or collect information from or about study participants and, as in the process of subject selection, this error (and any resulting misclassification) can be either random or systematic.

From www.CartoonStock.com

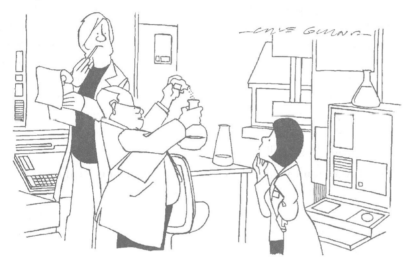

"...then we add a smidgin of this – that's less than a dollop, but more than a pinch..."

Random error

If you were to weigh yourself several times on the same set of scales, how similar would the results be? If there is little variation between the results we say that the measuring device is **precise**. If there is a lot of variation between the results then the precision is poor or, conversely, we have a lot of **random error**. Some measuring instruments will be better than others and although we would not expect to obtain exactly the same result every time, we would hope that if were measuring the same thing the results would all be close. If, for example, we measured someone's systolic blood pressure and the reading was 140 millimetres of mercury (mmHg), then, ideally, if we measured it again and again the results would all be close to this value – perhaps ranging from 137 to 143 mmHg. This would indicate that the measuring device was quite *precise*, i.e. it always gives approximately the same answer when measuring the same thing. But note that it tells us nothing about the **accuracy** of the measurement, i.e. whether the person's systolic blood pressure really is 140 mmHg.

Many biological parameters, including blood pressure, vary on a day-to-day, hour-to-hour and even minute-to-minute basis. Assuming that we always measure blood pressure under standard conditions and our participant has not, for example, just run up a flight of stairs, then any variation should again be largely random. Depending on when we take our measurements, we will obtain different readings that will vary around the patient's usual blood pressure. We will overestimate some people's blood pressure and we will underestimate it for others.

We can reduce random error and thus increase the precision of our measurements by taking repeated measurements on one subject, preferably on different occasions, and using the average value in the study. The more measurements we take, the more precise our answer will be. Note that this is analogous to our discussion of *precision* in the context of random sampling error or chance in the previous chapter. As you saw there, we can calculate a confidence interval to quantify random sampling error: a bigger study has less error and gives a narrower confidence interval and thus a more precise estimate.

Systematic error

Given a measuring instrument was not 100% precise, we would expect some results to be a bit too high and some a bit too low, but we would still hope that the *average* results would be close to the true value. In other words, we want the device to be *accurate*. Consider the measurement of blood pressure again. If we use a sphygmomanometer that has not been calibrated for a year it might consistently read 10 mmHg too high. The person with a blood pressure of 140 mmHg would now appear to have a blood pressure of 150 mmHg. The precision of the measurements may be unchanged but, if we were to make several measurements on each person and average them, we would find that the average value was always 10 mmHg too high. In this situation our measurements might be precise but they are not accurate because we are systematically recording everybody's blood pressure as 10 mmHg greater than it should be. We have, therefore, introduced **systematic error** or **bias** into our measurements. Unlike random error, systematic error cannot be reduced by taking repeated measurements.

We can summarise the effects of systematic and random error, or their inverse accuracy and precision, by analogy with target shooting (Figure 7.2). If someone is a good shot and they are using a gun with the sights properly aligned, their shots will tend to cluster closely around the bull's-eye in the centre (situation (a)). The shots are therefore both accurate (close to the centre) and precise (close to each other). But if the sights on the gun are not aligned correctly, it will

(a) (b) (c) (d)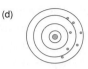

Accurate and precise	Precise, not accurate	Accurate, not precise	Neither accurate, nor precise
Little systematic or	Systematic error but	Random error but	Random and
random error	little random error	little systematic error	systematic error

Figure 7.2 Accuracy and precision (systematic and random error).

not be so accurate and the shooter might always hit a spot to the right of the centre (situation (b)). The results are still precise because they are tightly clustered around this point, but they are no longer accurate because they are consistently falling too far to the right. We have introduced a *systematic error*. If a less experienced shooter were to use the first gun then their shots would be more spread out, but they should still land around the bull's-eye (situation (c)). In this situation we have good accuracy because, on average, the shots are centred around the bull's-eye, but the shots are very spread out so we have more *random error* and thus less precision. Finally, an inexperienced shooter with a faulty gun would both miss the centre of the target and cover a wide area (situation (d)). In this situation we have neither accuracy nor precision. This visualisation shows how we can conceptualise the separate effects of accuracy and precision, i.e. systematic and random error.

The effects of measurement error

The effects of both biological variation and measurement error mean that measurements will never be perfect – even if there is no systematic error there will always be some degree of random error. If something is measured on a continuous scale (for example weight in kilograms or height in centimetres) then random error alone will not lead to any bias in estimates of the *average* weight or height of the study population. This is because, although the weight of some people will be overestimated and the weight of others underestimated, if these errors are truly random, the overestimates and underestimates should cancel each other out when we calculate the average weight. However, problems arise in the presence of systematic error. If people systematically underestimate their weight then their average weight will be an underestimate of the true average for the population.

If instead of measuring something on a continuous scale we want to classify people into groups, for example normal and overweight, then both random *and* systematic errors will lead to **misclassification** of people into the wrong groups. Some normal-weight people will be wrongly labelled as overweight and vice versa. As you will see below, this misclassification will introduce bias into measures such as odds ratios and relative risks.

Table 7.4 The 'true' results of a hypothetical case–control study with no measurement error.

	Cases	Controls	Total
Exposed	300	250	550
Unexposed	100	150	250
Total	400	400	800

$$OR = \frac{300 \times 150}{100 \times 250}$$
$$= 1.80$$

When assessing the likely effects of measurement error, the most important consideration is whether the errors and any subsequent misclassification are likely to be *the same* or *different* in the various study groups. In a case–control study we are usually concerned about whether errors in *exposure* measurement are the same for cases and controls. In a cohort study or a clinical trial we are often more concerned about whether the *outcome* measurement may have differed between the exposed and unexposed groups, although exposure measurement can also be an issue.

Non-differential misclassification

When measurement error and any resulting misclassification occur equally in all groups being compared, they are described as being *non-differential* (because they are the same or 'not different' in the various groups). For example, **non-differential error** occurs when the amount and type of error in exposure measurement is the same for cases and controls in a case–control study; or error in measurement of outcome is the same for the exposed and unexposed groups in a cohort study.

Imagine a case–control study in which everything is measured perfectly, with no error. The results of this hypothetical study are shown in Table 7.4 and the true odds ratio for the association between exposure and outcome is 1.80.

Now in practice the instrument used to measure exposure (this could be a biological test of some sort, a measuring device or a questionnaire) will rarely be perfect and, as a result, there will almost always be some degree of random error that results in non-differential misclassification. Imagine that 10% of all people who are exposed are misclassified as unexposed and 10% of all unexposed people are misclassified as exposed. (Note that this is the same as saying that the instrument has 90% **sensitivity** and **specificity**; it correctly identifies 90% of those who are exposed (sensitivity) and 90% of those who are unexposed (specificity). We will discuss sensitivity and specificity in more detail in Chapter 15.) The key point here is that the misclassification is *non-differential*, namely it affects everyone in the study. In this situation 10% or 30 of the 300 exposed cases and 25 of the 250 exposed controls will be misclassified as unexposed. In addition, 10% or 10

Table 7.5 The effect of non-differential random measurement error: 10% of all cases and controls are misclassified with regard to their exposure status.

	Cases	Controls	Total
Exposed	$300 - 30 + 10 = 280$	$250 - 25 + 15 = 240$	520
Unexposed	$100 - 10 + 30 = 120$	$150 - 15 + 25 = 160$	280
Total	400	400	800

$$OR = \frac{280 \times 160}{120 \times 240}$$
$$= 1.56$$

of the 100 unexposed cases and 15 of the 150 unexposed controls will be misclassified as exposed. This means that, instead of obtaining the true picture shown in Table 7.4, we would find results that looked like Table 7.5.

Because we have randomly misclassified some of the cases and controls, we have obtained an odds ratio of only 1.56 instead of the true odds ratio of 1.80. This makes the association seem weaker than it really is; i.e. the effect estimate, in this case an odds ratio, is biased towards the null. Note that some complex exposures, particularly things like diet, are particularly hard to measure and levels of misclassification are likely to be much greater than 10%. In this situation any measures of relative risk would be biased even closer towards 1.0 and real effects can disappear completely. For example, if the level of misclassification in the above example had been 20% instead of 10%, the odds ratio would have been 1.37 ((260×170) ÷ (140×230)); with 30% misclassification it would have been only 1.23 ((240×180) ÷ (160×220)).

As we discussed above, non-differential misclassification due to random measurement error is a fact of life but it is also possible to have non-differential misclassification due to systematic measurement error if the systematic error occurs equally in all study groups. For example, 'food frequency questionnaires' ask people to report how often, on average, they eat each of a list of individual food items. When confronted with a list of ten or twenty different vegetables people will often overestimate the total number of servings of vegetables they eat each day. If we then classify them according to whether or not they ate the recommended number of servings of vegetables per day, we would systematically misclassify some people with low vegetable intake into the high-intake group and this might happen equally for cases and controls. If, for example, in the study shown in Table 7.4, 20% of all unexposed people, both cases and controls, were systematically misclassified as exposed then we would obtain an odds ratio of 1.71, which would again underestimate the true value of 1.80. Note that while these examples have all considered the effects of non-differential misclassification on a case–control study, exactly the same effects occur in a cohort study (see question 5 at the end of the chapter for an example of this).

In the presence of non-differential misclassification, either random or systematic, estimates of the association between exposure and outcome will usually be underestimates of the true effect. In other words, the odds ratio or relative risk

Box 7.6 When non-differential misclassification does not bias towards the null

If an exposure has more than one level then misclassification between two of the groups will make those two groups look more similar than they really are. In a case–control study of smoking and respiratory disease, for example, participants might be classified as non-smokers, light smokers and heavy smokers. The distinction between smoker and non-smoker is likely to be fairly clear (and for simplicity we will assume that it is perfect), but there will inevitably be some misclassification between the light and heavy smoking groups. If the non-smokers form the reference group, the misclassification will make the odds ratios for light and heavy smokers more similar than they should be. The effect of this will be to bias the odds ratios for the highest group (heavy smokers) towards the null again but the odds ratio for the *middle group* (light smokers) will now be biased away from the null (Table 7.6). Overall, however, the net result is that the association is weakened.

Table 7.6 Non-differential misclassification can bias away from the null when there are more than two exposure groups.

	Cases	Controls	Odds ratio
Truth			
Non-smokers	150	200	1.0
Light smokers	120	125	1.3
Heavy smokers	130	75	2.3
20% of light smokers misclassified as heavy smokers and vice versa			
Non-smokers	150	200	1.0
Light smokers	122	115	1.4
Heavy smokers	128	85	2.0

will almost always be biased towards the null and the true effect will therefore be further from the null than the observed effect. This means that if a study gives a relative risk of 2.0 but there is likely to be non-differential misclassification, then the true association is likely to be even stronger than that observed (i.e. >2.0). Similarly, if a study gives a relative risk of 0.8 in the presence of non-differential misclassification, then the true relative risk is likely to be lower than this (i.e <0.8), again making the real association stronger than that observed. Although this is the norm, it is important to note that in some situations non-differential misclassification can bias estimates away from the null. This can happen simply by chance but is more common when we classify exposure into more than two groups (see Box 7.6 for an example).

Differential misclassification

When the measurement error and resulting misclassification occur to a greater extent in one group than another they are described as being **differential**. The effects of differential misclassification are generally harder to predict than those of non-differential misclassification.

In contrast to random error, which, as discussed above, is commonly non-differential because it is usually an inherent property of the exposure being measured or the measuring device and thus affects everyone in the study, systematic error is often differential. It is a particular problem in standard case–control studies in which cases already have the disease of interest when the exposure information is collected or measured and so might recall their exposure differently from controls; this type of error is known as **recall bias**. For example, the cases in a case–control study of respiratory disease might systematically overestimate the amount of passive smoking they had been exposed to because they thought that this might have caused their disease. The controls, however, would have no such reason to overestimate their exposure. This might make it look as if passive smoking was associated with respiratory disease even if there was really no difference between the cases and controls.

Imagine that, in the hypothetical study shown in Table 7.4, cases overestimated their exposure and, as a result, 20% of unexposed cases were systematically misclassified as exposed, but controls were not affected.

How many of (a) the 100 unexposed cases and (b) the 150 unexposed controls would have been misclassified as exposed?

So, in total, how many (a) cases and (b) controls would have been classified as exposed and how many as unexposed?

What would the odds ratio have been?

Would it have been an underestimate or an overestimate of the true odds ratio?

In this situation, 20% or 20 of the 100 unexposed cases but none of the unexposed controls would be misclassified as exposed and, instead of the true picture shown in Table 7.4, we would obtain results that looked like Table 7.7, giving an odds ratio of 2.4.

We have now overestimated the true odds ratio of 1.80, making the association seem much stronger than it really is. If the systematic misclassification had gone the other way and exposed cases had been misclassified as unexposed, or unexposed controls had been misclassified as exposed, then the bias would have gone in the opposite direction and we would have underestimated the effect.

Random error is less likely to be differential unless, for example, we use different measuring devices with differing levels of precision in the different study groups; however, if present, it too can make an association look either weaker or

Table 7.7 The effects of differential systematic misclassification: 20% of unexposed cases, but *not* controls, are misclassified as exposed.

	Cases	Controls	Total
Exposed	$300 + 20 = 320$	250	570
Unexposed	$100 - 20 = 80$	150	230
Total	400	400	800

$$OR = \frac{320 \times 150}{80 \times 250}$$
$$= 2.40$$

stronger than it really is (see question 6 at the end of the chapter for an example). *The best way to avoid differential random error and any consequential misclassification is thus to ensure that exactly the same instruments and methods are used in all of the different study groups.*

To summarise, if there is misclassification, either systematic or random, in a study and this occurs *to a different extent in the two study groups* (cases and controls or exposed and unexposed) then the study results can be biased either up or down, i.e. towards or away from the null value, and it is often impossible to know which way the bias would have gone or how large the effect might be. This type of misclassification can be very difficult to deal with because, unless you have some idea of how much misclassification is occurring and where it is occurring, you cannot work out what the true results should have been.

Sources of measurement error

As you will have gathered, almost every study will be subject to some degree of measurement error. One common but easily avoidable source of bias is the use of different instruments or measuring systems for different study groups or parts of groups. Examples of this include the use of different laboratories to analyse biological specimens, different locations for interviews of cases and controls (e.g. hospital versus home) and different interview methods (face-to-face versus telephone interview or postal questionnaire). Other particularly troublesome sources of error are the possibilities of recall bias and interviewer or observer bias.

Recall bias

Some degree of recall error is inevitable in any epidemiological study that requires participants to remember their past exposures. If this error is random and if, in a case–control study, it occurs in both cases and controls (i.e. it is non-differential) then the effects will usually be to bias the effect estimates towards the null. What can be more problematic is **recall bias**, which, as we noted above, can occur in case–control studies and cross-sectional studies if cases (or those with disease in a cross-sectional study) are systematically more likely to over- or underestimate their exposure than controls. For example, if an exposure is thought to cause disease, then cases might be more likely to recall or to exaggerate their past exposure than controls, leading to overestimation of the effect of that exposure on disease (as in the passive smoking example above). The opposite effect would occur if cases tended to underestimate their exposure because they feel guilty about it. This could occur, for example, in a study of the effects of sunburn in childhood on the occurrence of childhood skin cancer. If mothers are asked whether their children have ever been sunburnt, the mothers of children with cancer might tend to underestimate (or under-report) the occurrence of sunburn in their children because they feel guilty about admitting they allowed their children to become burned when they were young. This could lead to falsely low estimates of the frequency of sunburn in cases and consequently a weakened association between sunburn and skin cancer.

It is obviously difficult to know, even qualitatively, the extent to which such bias may operate in any given study, so a great deal of effort is put into designing information collection systems to limit the likelihood of it occurring; for example, through the use of highly structured questionnaires, standard prompts and so forth. One situation where it is sometimes possible to assess the extent of recall bias is in a nested case–control study when information collected from cases and controls *after* diagnosis of disease in the cases could be compared to information collected earlier in the follow-up period *before* the cases were diagnosed. Few such empirical studies have actually been done, but the limited evidence is somewhat reassuring. For example, recall bias has been a major concern in the field of melanoma epidemiology because of the growing public awareness of the risks of sun exposure and use of sunbeds. However, analysis of data from nested case–control studies does not give any consistent evidence of substantive recall bias being present for these exposures (Gefeller, 2009). Nonetheless this does not mean that we can ignore the need to capture data as objectively as possible to minimise this potentially important measurement flaw.

An equivalent bias has occasionally been seen in cohort studies when information about outcomes has been obtained from the participants themselves. In this situation the problem arises when members of the exposed group are more (or less) likely to recall having had the outcome of interest than are those in the unexposed group. For example, in a telephone follow-up ascertaining self-reported medical conditions in American veterans, those who had served in Vietnam (the *exposure* of interest) reported higher rates of a variety of conditions than did non-Vietnam veterans; but when a sub-set of the veterans was examined more thoroughly, there was little real difference between those who had and had not served in Vietnam (CDC, 1988). Note that the analysis presented in Box 7.3 above was based on routine statistics and not on self-report by the veterans themselves so it is not subject to the same types of error.

Interviewer or observer bias

Differential error may also occur if data collectors ask questions or record information in a different way for cases and controls (or for exposed and unexposed groups in a cohort study). For instance, an interviewer who knows the case/control status of a subject may probe more deeply with the cases than with the controls, resulting in differences in the quality of exposure data obtained for the two groups. Similarly, if in a cohort study or trial the observers know whether or not a person is exposed or unexposed (or treated/untreated), they may be more or less likely to diagnose the outcome of interest. A logical way to avoid these possibilities is to blind the interviewers/observers to the subject's status, although this is often not possible. Again, the use of objective criteria for outcome assessment, structured questionnaires and interview schedules, training and tape-recording interviews for quality control all help minimise interviewer bias.

Control of measurement error

It is difficult to get rid of measurement error once it has occurred and so it is important to minimise the potential for error at the design stage of the study. Whether you are conducting your own research or reading the reports of others, some important things to consider include the following.

Definitions

Everything that is measured in a study needs to be carefully defined. If the exposure is smoking, what makes someone a smoker? Anyone who has ever smoked a cigarette? 10 cigarettes? 100 cigarettes? A cigarette a day for six months? In practice most people probably try a cigarette at one time or another, so to classify them all as smokers would not be sensible. Common definitions that have been used are that someone should have smoked at least 100 cigarettes in their lifetime or that they should have smoked at least one cigarette a day for a defined period, usually a few months.

In addition to the important distinctions of exposed/unexposed (and of case/non-case in a cohort study or trial), it is also essential to have clear definitions and good measurements of the co-factors being measured. These are other factors that may influence (or 'confound' – see Chapter 8) the results of a study, e.g. age, socioeconomic status and smoking.

Choice of instrument

Instruments in epidemiological studies can include sophisticated laboratory tests, detailed questionnaires, or even simple observations. Inevitably the method of measurement used will influence the degree of error in the data. A set of scales that weigh to the nearest 100 g would be more accurate than scales that weigh to the nearest kilogram. Ideally the instrument used should be that which minimises both *random* and *systematic* error. Consideration should also be given to the circumstances of time and place of use of the instrument, since these may also affect the results obtained. For example, a face-to-face interview with a trained interviewer might elicit more reliable information than a questionnaire completed by the study participants themselves, but it would also be more expensive. And there are always exceptions – use of self-completed computer-based questionnaires may well capture more reliable data on use of illicit or socially stigmatised behaviours than in-person interviews.

Quality control

Whatever measuring devices are used, they need to be standardised. Instruments need regular calibration against a standard value and interviewers need training in a standard approach to obtaining data. Structured questionnaires help here, too. If the study continues for some time, consistency should also be monitored and maintained.

Assessment of measurement error

The two main issues in measurement are (i) is the instrument accurate (i.e. no systematic error)?, and (ii) is it precise (minimal random error)? The accuracy and precision of an instrument can be assessed by conducting validation and repeatability studies.

Assessing accuracy

In some situations accurate measuring devices or tests are available but too complex or costly to use on everyone in the study, so the investigators have to use a simpler or cheaper and less accurate tool. In this situation it is good practice to conduct a *validation study* in which both the accurate expensive ('gold standard') test and the simpler, potentially less accurate test are used on a sub-set of people in the study and the results are compared. In this situation it may then be possible to 'correct' the results of the study for any inaccuracies in the cheaper test (we will not consider the mechanics of this here).

Assessing precision

Another desirable way to test how well a measuring device performs is to measure its 'repeatability' or precision. If the same thing is measured on two different

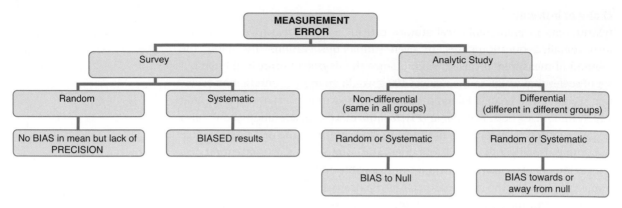

Figure 7.3 Overview of the types and consequences of measurement error.

occasions or by two different people, how well do the two measurements compare? This might simply be a case of repeating laboratory tests on some samples or it might involve asking some study participants to complete a study questionnaire twice on two different occasions to see how well their answers agree. In a cohort study that has repeated measures over time (such as the Nurses' Health Study) it is sometimes appropriate to average the values to give better precision.

Assessment of the likely effects of measurement error on the results of a study

By now it will be clear that there will always be some random measurement error in any data and thus if subjects have been classified into different exposure groups, there will always be some misclassification, the extent of which will depend on the variable being studied and the tool used to measure it. Things like age and height do not change (or change predictably) and can be measured fairly easily. In contrast we have alluded to the fact that complex factors like diet and physical activity are very hard to measure and so will be associated with a lot more misclassification. On top of this there may also be systematic error such as recall bias, particularly when we use case–control and cross-sectional designs.

The important thing is to assess the likely impact of any such error on the results of the study. Is it possible that an observed association is entirely due to error, or would the association still exist (and perhaps be even stronger) if the error could be eliminated? As shown in Figure 7.3, the key question in a survey is whether the error is random or systematic. Random errors should not lead to biased estimates of descriptive statistics such as means but systematic errors will. In contrast, when looking for associations between exposure and outcome in analytic studies, the central issue is whether any error and resulting misclassification is likely to be differential or non-differential; i.e. is it likely to have

Table 7.8 The likely effects of misclassification on the results of a case–control study.

Type of error / misclassification	True odds ratio (OR)	Study results	Type of bias
Non-differential	2.0	≥1.0 but <2.0	Result biased towards null but not below
	1.0	1.0	No effect if there is no association
	0.5	0.5 but ≤1.0	Result biased towards null but not above
Differential – cases overestimate (or controls underestimate) exposure	2.0	>2.0	Result biased upwards with no upper limit. An inverse association (OR < 1.0) could appear to be a positive association (OR > 1.0)
	1.0	>1.0	
	0.5	>0.5	
Differential – cases underestimate (or controls overestimate) exposure	2.0	<2.0	Result biased downwards with no lower limit. A positive association (OR > 1.0) could appear to be an inverse association (OR < 1.0)
	1.0	<1.0	
	0.5	<0.5	

occurred to the same extent in all study groups or to a differing extent in different groups? As you have seen, the likely effects of **non-differential misclassification** (either random or systematic) are to bias the estimates of effect (RR or OR) towards the null, making associations look weaker than they really are or, in some situations, masking them altogether. However, **differential misclassification** can bias estimates upwards or downwards, towards or away from the null. If information from a validation study is available, it may be possible to 'correct' the results of a study to allow for the fact that the measurements were not perfect, although any such correction will also be imperfect. **Sensitivity analysis** involves repeating the data analysis using different assumptions in the same way as we did to assess the effects of loss to follow-up above (look back to Box 7.5): if a proportion of subjects were misclassified, what effect would this have had on the results?

At the very least, it is essential to assess the likely degree of measurement error and/or misclassification and then make some judgements as to how this might have affected the results. Table 7.8 summarises the likely effects of misclassification on the estimates of an odds ratio under different scenarios.

- If the error or misclassification is non-differential, how bad is it likely to be? If the study found an association, e.g. an odds ratio of 1.8, then, in all probability, the real association is even stronger, i.e. >1.8. If the study did not find an association, is it possible that there was so much error that a real association could have been missed? (Note that non-differential misclassification is very unlikely to make it appear that an association exists when in reality there is none, although this can happen.)

- If the error or misclassification is likely to be differential, is it possible to predict what the differences might have been? For example, are cases more or less likely to have over-reported exposure? If cases overestimate their exposure then the OR is likely to be biased upwards, conversely if they underestimate their exposure (or controls overestimate theirs) then the bias is likely to be downwards. Could the observed association be due to misclassification? Or might the real association be stronger than that observed? (Note that, as well as making associations look weaker or stronger than they really are, differential misclassification can make an association appear where there is none, it can make it seem that there is no association when in reality there is one and it can even make a positive association look like an inverse association and vice versa.)

Summary

No epidemiological study will be perfect. The important thing, therefore, is to minimise errors and then evaluate the likely effect of any remaining error and we will come back to this again when we look at how to read (or write) and interpret epidemiological papers in Chapter 9. For now we can summarise the problem of error as follows: errors can be *random* or *systematic* and can relate to *subject selection* or to *measurement* of exposure and/or outcome. *Random sampling error* can be assessed from a confidence interval, but *systematic selection bias* is not so easily assessed, and is therefore a major problem in surveys. It can also be a problem in case–control studies, particularly with regard to selection of the control group. In cohort studies or clinical trials, selection bias is more likely to occur if people are lost to follow-up. In a survey, *systematic measurement error* is a bigger problem than random error. In analytic studies, the important distinction is between *non-differential error* (it occurs equally in all study groups), which will usually bias the study results towards the null, and *differential error* (it occurs to a different extent in the different study groups), which can bias the study results either towards or away from the null.

We have now considered two of the three possible 'alternative explanations' for an observed association, namely chance and bias. In the next chapter we will discuss the third major threat to the internal validity of epidemiological and other health research: confounding.

Questions

1. Imagine that a research team wanted to estimate the prevalence of vegetarianism in the community by means of a short questionnaire distributed with a women's health magazine. Would this give an accurate picture of the percentage of people who were vegetarians?

2. In a case–control study of liver disease and alcohol consumption, all patients in a community who had newly been diagnosed with liver disease were recruited as cases and people without liver disease were selected at random from the community to act as controls. All of the cases and controls were then asked about their alcohol intake. Only 25% of the controls selected from the community agreed to take part in the study.

   (a) Do you think that people with a high alcohol intake would be more or less likely to agree to take part in the study than average?

   (b) Is alcohol consumption in the controls likely to be higher, the same as or lower than in the whole community?

   (c) What effect would this have on the estimate of the association between alcohol and liver disease?

3. Look back at the hypothetical study shown in Table 7.4 and imagine that the measurement instrument *systematically* overestimated people's exposure and, as a result, 15% of all unexposed people, both cases and controls, were misclassified as exposed.

   (a) Is this misclassification differential or non-differential? Why?

   (b) In the presence of this misclassification is the observed odds ratio likely to be an overestimate or an underestimate of the true odds ratio?

   (c) How many of (i) the 100 unexposed cases and (ii) the 150 unexposed controls would have been wrongly misclassified as exposed?

   (d) So, in total, how many (i) cases and (ii) controls would have been classified as exposed and how many as unexposed using the flawed measuring tool?

   (e) What would the odds ratio have been?

4. Now imagine that cases underestimated their exposure and, as a result, 20% of exposed cases were falsely classified as unexposed, but that the classification of controls was not affected.

   (a) Is this type of misclassification random or systematic? Is it differential or non-differential? Why?

   (b) What effect would it have had on the results of the study?

   (c) Compare your answer to (b) with that in Table 7.7, where cases systematically *overestimated* their exposure.

5. The hypothetical results of a cohort study in which everything is measured correctly are shown in Table 7.9. Imagine that at the start of the study 30% of *all exposed people* were misclassified as unexposed.

   (a) Is this misclassification random or systematic? Non-differential or differential? And why?

   (b) What effect would the misclassification have on the incidence of disease in (i) the unexposed cohort and (ii) the exposed cohort?

   (c) What effect would this have on the observed relative risk?

6. Imagine that all of the cases in a case–control study had their blood pressure measured by a single doctor at the local hospital but, for practical reasons,

Table 7.9 The 'true' results of a hypothetical cohort study with no measurement error.

	Total	Cases	Cumulative incidence (%)
Exposed	10,000	200	2.0
Unexposed	10,000	100	1.0
Total	20,000	300	1.5

$$RR = 2.0 \div 1.0$$
$$= 2.00$$

the controls had their blood pressure measured by their local doctor. In this situation it is likely that there would be less random error in the blood pressure readings for cases that came from a single doctor than in those for controls that came from a number of different doctors.

(a) Re-calculate the results of the hypothetical case–control study shown in Table 7.4 assuming that the measurement of exposure among cases was perfect but 20% of exposed controls were randomly misclassified as unexposed and vice versa.

(b) Is this misclassification differential or non-differential and why?

(c) What effect has it had on the odds ratio and why?

(d) What would the effect have been if we had misclassified cases instead of controls?

REFERENCES

CDC (Centers for Disease Control). (1988). Health status of Vietnam veterans. II. Physical health. *Journal of the American Medical Association*, **259**: 2708–2714.

Dobson, A. J., Alexander, H. M., Heller, R. F. and Lloyd, D. M. (1991). Passive smoking and the risk of heart attack or coronary death. *Medical Journal of Australia*, **154**: 793–797.

Gefeller, O. (2009). Invited commentary: recall bias in melanoma – much ado about almost nothing? *American Journal of Epidemiology*, **169**: 267–270.

Kinsey, A. C. (1948). *Sexual Behavior in the Adult Male*. Philadephia: W. B. Saunders.

Maslow, A. H. and Sakoda, J. M. (1952). Volunteer error in the Kinsey study. *Journal of Abnormal Psychology*, **47**: 259–262.

Pandeya, N., Williams, G. M., Green, A. C. *et al.* (2009). Do low control response rates always affect the findings? Assessments of smoking and obesity in two Australian case-control studies of cancer. *Australian and New Zealand Journal of Public Health*, **33**: 312–319.

Wilson, E. J., Horsley, K. W. and Van Der Hoek, R. (2005). *Australian Vietnam Veterans Mortality Study 2005*. Canberra: Department of Veterans' Affairs.

8

Muddied waters: the challenge of confounding

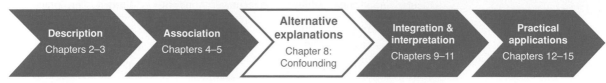

Box 8.1 Are university admissions biased towards men?

Table 8.1 shows that in one year a prestigious university admitted 52% of male applicants compared with only 45% of female applicants, suggesting that there was a bias in favour of men. When quizzed about this, the two main faculty heads said that it couldn't be true, they had both admitted a higher proportion of women than men: the success rate in arts was 38% for women and only 32% for men and that in science was 66% for women compared with only 62% for men. How can this be?

(continued)

Box 8.1 *(continued)*

Table 8.1 University admissions.

| | Men | | | Women | | |
Faculty	Applicants	Admitted	Percentage	Applicants	Admitted	Percentage
Arts	4,100	1,300	32	8,250	3,150	38
Science	8,200	5,100	62	2,900	1,900	66
Total	12,300	6,400	52	11,150	5,050	45

This is an example of *Simpson's paradox*, an extreme form of confounding where an apparent association observed in a study is in the opposite direction to the true association. In this example it arose because women were much more likely to apply to arts courses, for which applicants had a lower overall success rate.

(Based on an analysis of graduate admissions data conducted at the University of California, Berkeley (Bickel *et al.*, 1975).)

In Chapters 6 and 7 we considered two reasons why the results of a study might not be the truth, namely chance and error or bias. In this chapter we will consider a third possible 'alternative explanation' – confounding.

Confounding refers to a mixing or muddling of effects that can occur when the relationship we are interested in is confused by the effect of something else, just as we see in the striking example in Box 8.1. Here the true relation between sex and university admission – admission rates were higher for women – was 'confounded by faculty', such that a crude comparison actually suggested that admission rates were lower for women. Confounding is a major problem that has to be addressed in all non-randomised research and in some randomised trials as well, especially if they are small. As in previous chapters, we will mainly discuss confounding in the context of studies of the causes of a disease but, as with all epidemiological methods, everything that we say will apply equally to any study looking at associations in human (or animal) populations.

The following hypothetical case–control study of alcohol and lung cancer illustrates how easily confounding can arise and how it can be diagnosed. It also suggests how confounding can be dealt with and we will discuss this in more detail later in the chapter.

An example of confounding: is alcohol a risk factor for lung cancer?

Imagine a (very small) case–control study with 20 cases (people with lung cancer ☹) and 20 controls who do not have lung cancer (☺). Is drinking alcohol

Cases	Controls
☹ ☹ ☹ ☹ ☹	☺ ☺ ☺ ☺ ☺
☹ ☹ ☹ ☹ ☹	☺ ☺ ☺ ☺ ☺
☹ ☹ ☹ ☹ ☹	☺ ☺ ☺ ☺ ☺
☹ ☹ ☹ ☹ ☹	☺ ☺ ☺ ☺ ☺

Figure 8.1 A hypothetical case–control study of alcohol and lung cancer (blue = drinkers, black = non-drinkers).

Table 8.2 Calculation of the odds ratio for the association between alcohol and lung cancer.

	Cases	Controls
Alcohol drinkers	10	5
Non-drinkers	10	15

$$\text{Odds Ratio} = \frac{a \times d}{b \times c}$$
$$= \frac{10 \times 15}{5 \times 10} = 30$$

associated with the risk of lung cancer? If all the cases and controls were asked about their alcohol consumption we could classify people as 'drinkers' (☹,☺) or 'non-drinkers' (☹,☺) (Figure 8.1) and calculate an odds ratio to estimate the strength of the association between alcohol and lung cancer.

What is the odds ratio for the association between alcohol and lung cancer?

Can we conclude that alcohol consumption is associated with lung cancer?

As Table 8.2 shows, the odds ratio for the association between alcohol and lung cancer is 3.0, suggesting that the risk of developing lung cancer is three times higher in people who drink alcohol compared to non-drinkers.

However, we know that smokers are much more likely to develop lung cancer than non-smokers, and it is possible that they are also more likely to drink alcohol than non-smokers. Could smoking have affected the association we saw between alcohol and lung cancer? To investigate this we need to separate the smokers from the non-smokers and look at the association between alcohol and lung cancer – the 'alcohol effect' – in each group. Figure 8.2 shows that 12 of the 16 smokers were also alcohol drinkers compared with only three of the 24 non-smokers.

Calculate the odds ratio for alcohol and lung cancer separately for (i) smokers and (ii) non-smokers. (Hint: first draw up the appropriate 2 × 2 tables.)

Is alcohol associated with lung cancer among smokers? Among non-smokers?

How do you explain the change in the pattern of the alcohol–lung cancer relationship?

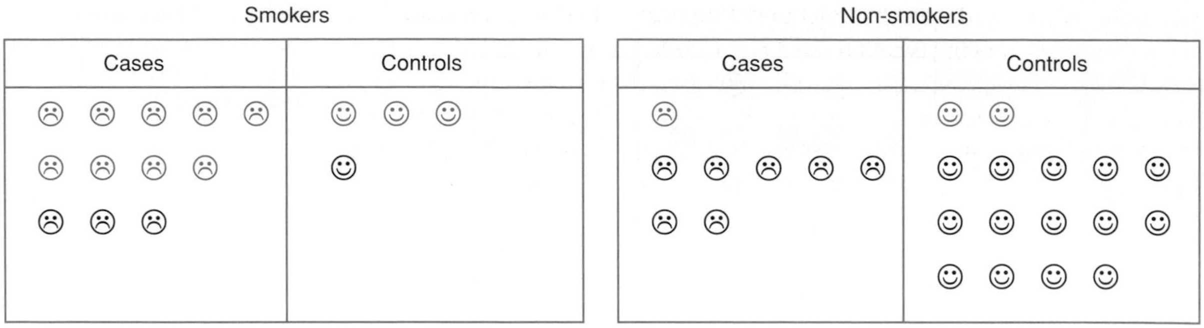

Figure 8.2 Separating smokers and non-smokers (blue = drinkers, black = non-drinkers).

Table 8.3 Calculation of the odds ratio for the association between alcohol and lung cancer, stratified by smoking status.

		Cases	Controls
Smokers	Alcohol drinkers	9	3
	Non-drinkers	3	1
Non-smokers	Alcohol drinkers	1	2
	Non-drinkers	7	14

$$\text{Odds Ratio} = \frac{9 \times 1}{3 \times 3} = 1.0$$

$$\text{Odds Ratio} = \frac{1 \times 14}{2 \times 7} = 1.0$$

The odds ratio for the association between alcohol and lung cancer among smokers is 1.0. Fewer of the non-smokers drink alcohol but again the odds ratio is 1.0 (see Table 8.3). This process in which we divide or *stratify* the study participants into two or more separate groups (*strata*) is known as **stratification**.

So, although there appears to be an association between alcohol and lung cancer in the whole study population, it disappears when we consider smokers and non-smokers separately. We could then go on to combine the odds ratios in smokers and non-smokers to calculate a *pooled* odds ratio that is *adjusted* for the effects of smoking. In this example the adjusted odds ratio is also 1.0. (We will not discuss the methods for calculating an adjusted odds ratio here, but a common method, developed by Mantel and Haenszel (1959), is shown in Appendix 6.)

The apparent (*crude*) overall relationship we saw between alcohol and lung cancer arose because while those with lung cancer were indeed more likely to drink alcohol than those without lung cancer, alcohol and smoking go together so they were also more likely to be smokers than those without lung cancer. The increased risk of lung cancer among alcohol drinkers was in fact due entirely to their smoking.

This situation, in which an apparent relationship between an exposure and an outcome is really due, in whole or in part, to a third factor that is associated both with the exposure and with the outcome of interest, is known as **confounding**. In the example, smoking is said to be a **confounder** of the alcohol–lung cancer link. Confounding is a *mixing of effects* because the effect of the exposure we are interested in (e.g. alcohol) is mixed up with the effect of some other factor (e.g. smoking). To look at the real effect of the exposure we have to first deal with the effect of the confounder.

Criteria for a confounder

For something to be a confounder it must
- be a risk factor for disease among those who are not exposed to the factor of interest
- be associated with the exposure of interest (in the source population or among the controls in a case–control study) and
- not be an intermediate between exposure and the outcome (i.e. it must not lie on the causal pathway).

Look back to Figure 8.2 and check that smoking fulfils the criteria for a confounder in the alcohol and lung cancer example.
- *Among non-drinkers* what proportion of (i) cases and (ii) controls smoked?
- *Among the controls* what proportion of (i) smokers and (ii) non-smokers drank alcohol?
- Is alcohol likely to *cause* smoking? (That is, could smoking lie on a causal pathway between alcohol and lung cancer?)

In the alcohol example, smoking was a confounder for the following reasons.
(1) *It was associated with lung cancer*: among people who did not drink alcohol, 3 out of 10 cases were smokers (30%) compared with only 1 of 15 controls (7%). That is, among non-drinkers, the cases were more likely to smoke than were the controls.
(2) *It was associated with alcohol among the controls*: 3 out of 4 controls who smoked also drank alcohol (75%), compared with only 2 out of 16 controls who did not smoke (12.5%). That is, among the controls, smokers were more likely to drink alcohol than were non-smokers.
(3) *It is not on a causal pathway between alcohol and lung cancer*: although alcohol and smoking often go together, drinking alcohol does not 'cause' someone to be a smoker.
An example of the third criterion is seen in the association between obesity and heart disease. High blood pressure is related both to obesity (the exposure) and to heart disease (outcome) and could, therefore, be a potential confounder of this association. However, since raising blood pressure is part of the causal

Figure 8.3 Confounding (e.g. alcohol, smoking and lung cancer).

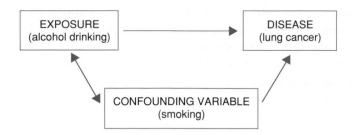

path through which obesity acts to increase the risk of heart disease (obesity → increased blood pressure → heart disease), it would be misleading to adjust for this, since it would remove part of a real causal effect of being heavy.

Figure 8.3 illustrates these criteria, showing how a confounder is related both to the exposure and to the outcome of interest. If an exposure is related to a confounding variable and this is, in turn, related to disease, the exposure itself may appear to be related to the disease even when it is not.

The effects of confounding

In the example above, the apparent effect of alcohol on lung cancer was entirely due to the effect of smoking, but confounding does not necessarily create an apparent effect where really there is none. Confounding can lead to either overestimation or underestimation of the size of a real effect, it can completely hide a real association that exists and in very extreme situations it can even reverse the direction of an effect, making it appear that a cause of a disease actually protects against it. (This is known as *Simpson's paradox* and it explains the apparent contradiction in the university admissions data in Box 8.1 at the start of the chapter.)

Age, sex and socioeconomic status (SES) are common confounders. As an example, many diseases occur more frequently in older people. If the exposure of interest also occurs more commonly in the elderly, e.g. a poor diet, then the confounding effects of age would have to be considered.

Confounding in a case–control study

Authors of early studies that looked at the relation between diet and heart disease found that the more a person ate the lower their risk of heart disease. This apparent association was all the more surprising because we know that obesity is a risk factor for heart disease. However, one factor that the studies did not take into account was physical activity and, on average, people who are physically active eat more than those who are inactive. Could this have affected the results

Table 8.4 Results of a hypothetical case–control study of high energy intake and heart disease, stratified by level of physical activity.

Energy intake	Total		High physical activity		Low physical activity	
	Heart disease	Controls	Heart disease	Controls	Heart disease	Controls
High	730	600	520	510	210	90
Low	700	540	100	150	600	390

of the studies? The results of a hypothetical case–control study evaluating the association between energy intake and heart disease are shown in Table 8.4.

What is the odds ratio for the *crude* association between high energy intake and heart disease?

What is the odds ratio for the association between high energy intake and heart disease in people with (i) high and (ii) low levels of physical activity?

Is the association between high energy intake and heart disease confounded by the level of physical activity?

The crude odds ratio for the association between high energy intake and heart disease in this study is (730 × 540) ÷ (700 × 600) = 0.9, i.e. those with high energy intake appear to have a 10% *lower* risk of coronary heart disease (CHD). When we stratify by physical activity the odds ratio is (520 × 150) ÷ (100 × 510) = 1.5 among the physically active and (210 × 390) ÷ (600 × 90) = 1.5 among the inactive. Thus, when we remove the confounding effects of physical activity by stratification, high energy intake is associated with a 50% *higher* risk of CHD (OR = 1.5).[1] In this example the confounding meant that the observed odds ratio (OR = 0.9) was an underestimate of the true association between obesity and CHD (OR = 1.5).

Confounding in a cohort study

Now imagine that, instead of a case–control study, we had conducted a cohort study to look at the effects of high energy intake on heart disease. The results of this study are shown in Table 8.5.

---

[1] In this example, the effect was exactly the same (OR = 1.5) among both the inactive and the active groups. In practice the *stratum-specific* estimates are unlikely to be identical and we will discuss this further under **Stratification** on page 213.

Table 8.5 Results of a hypothetical cohort study of high energy intake and heart disease, stratified by level of physical activity.

Energy intake	Total		High physical activity		Low physical activity	
	Person-years	Developed heart disease	Person-years	Developed heart disease	Person-years	Developed heart disease
High	60,000	720	50,000	500	10,000	220
Low	55,000	700	15,000	100	40,000	600

What is the crude rate ratio for the association between high energy intake and heart disease?

What is the rate ratio for the association between high energy intake and heart disease in people with (i) high and (ii) low levels of physical activity?

Is the association between high energy intake and heart disease confounded by the level of physical activity?

The overall incidence rate of heart disease among those with a high energy intake is $720 \div 60,000 = 12.0/1,000$ person-years (py) and the incidence rate among those with a low energy intake is $700 \div 55,000 = 12.7/1,000$ py, giving a *crude* rate ratio of 0.9 ($12.0 \div 12.7$). However, when we stratify by level of physical activity we see a different picture:

- in the active group, the incidence rate of heart disease among those with a high energy intake is $500 \div 50,000 = 10.0/1,000$ py, whereas that among those with a low energy intake is $100 \div 15,000 = 6.7/1,000$ py, giving a rate ratio of 1.5;
- in the inactive group, the incidence rate of heart disease among those with a high energy intake is $220 \div 10,000 = 22.0/1,000$ py, whereas that among those with a low energy intake is $600 \div 40,000 = 15.0/1,000$ py, again giving a rate ratio of 1.5.

As in the case–control example above, when we remove the effects of physical activity the true association between a high energy intake and heart disease is stronger ($RR = 1.5$) than when we did not allow for the effects of physical activity. Confounding is just as much a problem in cohort studies (or any other non-randomised follow-up studies, including non-randomised trials) as it is in case–control studies.

So how can we tell if an association is confounded?

If when you stratify or adjust for a potential confounder the effect estimate changes then confounding is present. In the lung cancer example at the start of

Table 8.6 Characteristics of women at time of recruitment into a study of oral contraceptive use and coronary heart disease.

	Oral contraceptive use	
	Yes	No
Percentage aged less than 30 years	60%	30%
Percentage of low SES	50%	40%
Percentage smoking >15 cig/day	17%	12%
Mean body mass index (weight (kg) / height (m)^2)	26.5	27.0
Percentage with a history of:		
Hypertension	1%	1%
Stroke	0.03%	0.3%
Venous thromboembolism	1%	8%

(Figures adapted from Vessey and Lawless, 1984.)

the chapter the odds ratio dropped from 3.0 to 1.0 when we adjusted for smoking, indicating that smoking was a strong confounder. In the heart disease example the estimate increased from 0.9 to 1.5 when we adjusted for physical activity, so again this was confounding the association. A general rule of thumb is that, if when you adjust for a potential confounder the crude and adjusted effect estimates differ by 10% or more, then the crude estimate is confounded to some degree and it is more appropriate to present the adjusted value.

When will a possible confounder actually be a confounder in practice?

There are many things that could confound an association between exposure and outcome but in practice they might not actually do so.

Table 8.6 shows the characteristics of a group of women at the time of recruitment into a cohort study of oral contraceptives (OCs) and coronary heart disease (CHD).

Assume that all the factors are known risk factors for CHD. Which of them might be confounders of the OC–CHD relationship? Why?

For something to be a confounder it has to be associated both with the exposure of interest (OC use) and with the outcome of interest (CHD). All of the factors listed are known risk factors for CHD, so they are all associated with CHD. Some are also associated with OC use – we can see from Table 8.6 that, compared with non-users, OC users are

- twice as likely to be under the age of 30 as non-users (60% versus 30%)
- slightly more likely to be of low SES (50% versus 40%)
- slightly more likely to be current smokers (17% versus 12%)

Table 8.7 Likely effects of potential confounders in a study of oral contraceptive use and coronary heart disease when the true RR = 3.0.

| | Oral contraceptive use | | Likely observed RR[a] |
	Yes	No	
Percentage aged less than 30 years	60%	30%	2.5
Percentage of low SES	50%	40%	3.2
Percentage smoking >15 cig/day	17%	12%	3.3
Mean body mass index (weight (kg) / height (m)^2)	26.5	27.0	2.9
Percentage with a history of:			
Hypertension	1%	1%	3.0
Stroke	0.03%	0.3%	2.9
Venous thromboembolism	1%	8%	2.4

[a] Estimated RR for OC use and CHD, assuming that the RRs for the associations between the potential confounders and CHD are: 2.0 for age, 2.0 for SES, 4.0 for smoking, 4.0 for BMI, 10.0 for stroke and 5.0 for venous thromboembolism.

- 10 times less likely to have had a stroke (0.03% versus 0.3%) and
- 8 times less likely to have had a venous thromboembolism (1% versus 8%).

So will these factors confound the association between OC use and CHD?

In practice, it turns out that only age, history of thromboembolism and, to a lesser extent, smoking are likely to affect the results appreciably. Since CHD rates increase with age, the rate in the OC users will be lower than in the non-users simply because they are younger. If OC use truly increased the risk of CHD, say the true RR = 3.0, then the effect of confounding by age might reduce the observed RR (unadjusted for age) to about 2.5 (Table 8.7) thus reducing the (real) difference between the groups. Similarly, the eight-fold difference between the OC users and non-users in terms of their history of thromboembolism, a strong risk factor for CHD, will also bias the observed RR downwards to about 2.4. Conversely, CHD rates are higher in smokers and OC users are slightly more likely to be smokers than non-users, thus the effect of confounding by smoking would be to increase the apparent RR, making the effect look stronger than it really is.

This contrasts strikingly with the confounding influence of a history of stroke. Theoretically this looks sure to be an important confounder, given the 10-fold difference between OC users and non-users in terms of their past stroke experience, i.e. a very strong association between OC use and stroke (note that this occurs because women who have had a stroke would not normally be prescribed the OC pill), and the very strong known link between stroke and heart disease

Table 8.8 Results of a hypothetical case–control study of high energy intake and heart disease, stratified by level of physical activity (present in only 6% of the population).

Energy intake	Total		High physical activity		Low physical activity	
	Heart disease	Controls	Heart disease	Controls	Heart disease	Controls
High	472	231	52	51	420	180
Low	1210	795	10	15	1200	780
OR	1.3		1.5		1.5	

(due to their common set of risk factors). However, because stroke is so rare in young women this imbalance affects only a tiny proportion of the total study group, and so has a trivial effect on the crude RR, biasing it downwards by <5%, from 3.0 to 2.9. Even if a history of stroke had been five times more common in the study groups (0.015% and 1.5%), the RR would have been biased downwards by only about 10%, from 3.0 to 2.7.

More predictably, strong independent risk factors for CHD such as low SES and body-mass index also fail to confound when their distributions in the groups being compared are reasonably similar. So for something to be a confounder in practice it must not only be associated quite strongly *with the exposure and the outcome*, it must also be quite prevalent in the population.

As another example, consider the case–control study of energy intake and heart disease shown in Table 8.4. In this study the prevalence of the confounder (physical activity) in the population was very high – 660 of the 1,140 controls or 58% were physically active. What would have happened to our analysis if the population had been much less active? Table 8.8 shows results from a similar study for a population in which only 6% of controls were physically active. (To obtain these numbers we have just divided the numbers in the physically active group by 10 and multiplied the numbers in the inactive group by 2.) The stratum-specific odds ratios, and thus the *adjusted* odds ratio, are unaffected but the crude odds ratio is now 1.3 instead of 0.9; i.e. it is much closer to the unconfounded value of 1.5 and there is much less confounding by physical activity because this is now much less common.

We can summarise this by saying the following.
• If the association between a potential confounder and *either* the exposure *or* the outcome is weak then the confounder is unlikely to have much effect on the results of a study.
• If a potential confounder is either *rare* or almost *ubiquitous* then it is unlikely to have much effect on the results of a study because these will be driven by

the large number of people who are not exposed to the rare confounder or by the many who are exposed to the very common confounder.

The most important confounders are therefore those that are both *relatively* common and strongly related to the exposures and health outcomes of interest. The typical confounders that we mentioned above – sex, age and SES – fulfil all of these criteria. Another common confounder is smoking as this is strongly associated with many lifestyle factors, including high alcohol and coffee consumption, a less healthy diet (less fresh fruit and vegetables) and low levels of physical activity, and is also a major risk factor for many diseases. There are also many other disease-specific confounders: sun-exposure is a major confounder in studies of other risk factors for skin cancer, obesity may be a confounder in studies looking for causes of type-2 diabetes and so on. Although note that, in this latter example, it is also possible that obesity may lie on the casual pathway for diabetes, for example in studies of physical activity where it is likely that lower physical activity → obesity → heart disease. In this situation we have to think carefully about whether obesity is simply a confounder or whether it might explain some of the effects of physical activity on diabetes risk.

Control of confounding

There are two strategies for dealing with confounding. The first is to try to prevent it from occurring in the first place and this can be done at the study design stage by *randomisation, restriction* or *matching*. The alternative is to deal with it when it occurs by using analytic techniques such as stratification and statistical modelling. The effectiveness of all of these strategies except randomisation depends on the ability to identify and measure any confounders accurately.

Control of confounding through study design

Confounding occurs when a confounding variable is distributed unevenly across our study groups (e.g. in the lung cancer example at the start of the chapter, cases were more likely to be smokers than controls). One way to avoid confounding is therefore to design a study so that all groups are similar with respect to any potential confounders.

Randomisation

The most effective way to prevent confounding is to allocate people to the different study groups *at random*. Clearly, this is possible only in an intervention study and it is for this reason that randomised trials are usually considered to provide the strongest evidence of any of the epidemiological study designs (note that non-randomised trials are particularly prone to a type of confounding called

Box 8.2 Confounding by indication

If in a trial the participants are *not* randomly allocated to the various treatment groups then confounding is still a major problem, particularly what is often called ***confounding by indication*** (Miettinen, 1983). This arises because, even among a group of people who all have the same medical condition, those who choose to take or who are prescribed a particular medication may well differ from those who do not take it or who are not prescribed it. Those who take the drug might tend to have more (or less) severe disease than those who do not take it and, conversely, anyone who has a medical condition or exposure that is contra-indicated for the drug should certainly not be taking it. As a result, the outcomes of those who take the drug may well differ from the outcomes of those who do not in a way that has nothing to do with the treatment itself, i.e. they might differ simply because those taking the group are less sick or do not have other major health conditions (co-morbidities). The obvious solution to this problem is a randomised trial in which people are allocated to the various treatment groups at random.

confounding by indication – see Box 8.2). When a trial is large enough, random allocation will generally ensure a balanced distribution of all characteristics between the intervention (exposed) and control (unexposed) groups. *However, even randomisation cannot guarantee the absence of confounding, especially in smaller studies*, so it must always be looked for. The analysis of a randomised study must then include all participants in the groups to which they were originally randomised (regardless of whether they actually received the intervention). This is known as '*intention to treat*' analysis and we will discuss the importance of this further in Chapter 15 when we consider randomised evaluations of screening programmes.

A major advantage of randomisation over other forms of control of confounding is that it deals not only with confounders that we know and can measure, but also with other unrecognised and unmeasured (or unmeasurable) confounders. These too will, on balance, be evenly distributed by the randomisation process. Such *unknown confounders* (e.g. aspects of personality that affect complex lifestyle patterns) cannot be dealt with by any other method.

Restriction

Since randomisation is not possible in the majority of epidemiological studies, are there any alternatives? One option is to *restrict* the study sample to people with or without the confounding characteristic. This can be done by restricting a study to a particular age or socioeconomic group, thereby removing confounding by age or SES, or by restricting a study to non-smokers if smoking is a potential confounder. For example, we know that infection with human papillomavirus (HPV) is a major factor (potentially a **necessary cause**, see Chapter 10) in the development of cervical cancer and we also know that HPV infection is strongly associated with a number of other lifestyle factors such as smoking and use of oral contraceptives. This makes it very difficult to evaluate the association between smoking and cervical cancer because it is hard to be sure that any association observed is not simply due to confounding by HPV infection. (Smokers are more likely to be HPV-positive than non-smokers, so this could explain why they are more likely to develop cervical cancer.) By restricting a study to include only HPV-positive women, any confounding by HPV status would be removed, making it possible to evaluate the effects of other co-factors, such as smoking. Restriction is, however, of limited practical value when it is necessary to control for more than one or two likely confounders.

Matching

The third possibility is to select study subjects so that major known confounders are evenly distributed across the study groups. This is achieved by matching subjects on the presence or absence of the confounding variable(s). This is most often done in case–control studies in which controls are selected to match the cases in some predetermined way, e.g. by age and sex. Matching can be done on an individual basis, with one or more controls matched to each case so that, for instance, each control is matched by sex and year of birth to a specific case. Alternatively, **frequency matching** aims to select controls to match the general distribution of the confounding variable in cases. For example, adenocarcinoma of the oesophagus is about seven times more common in men than women so in a study of this cancer, controls might be selected to give a similar ratio of males to females (i.e. 7:1). If, in this situation, controls were simply selected as a random sample of the population, it is likely that about half would be female and half male. There would therefore be many more female controls than female cases but many fewer male controls than male cases. Sex would be a potential confounder in the analysis (because it is associated with the disease and many of the potential risk factors), but any adjustment for sex would be statistically inefficient because of the large sex imbalance between cases and controls.

Matching can also be used in the same way in cohort studies. This has historically been much less common but, with the increasing use of record linkage to conduct historical cohort studies, it is likely to become more common in the future. For example a group used records from blood donation centres in the USA to identify a cohort of 10,259 adults whose blood samples tested positive for hepatitis C virus (HCV) antibodies between 1991 and 2002 and another 10,259 blood donors who tested negative. The HCV-negative group were frequency-matched to the HCV-positive group by age, sex, year of blood donation and post code (as a surrogate marker for ethnicity and socioeconomic status). They then used record linkage to the National Death Index to identify the dates and causes of death of people in the two groups. They found that after an average of 7.7 years follow-up, the risk of dying was three times higher in the HCV-positive group than in the HCV-negative group (hazard ratio[2] = 3.1, 95% CI 2.6–3.8) (Guiltinan *et al.*, 2008).

While it may seem tempting to match cases and controls (or the exposed and unexposed groups in a cohort study) on as many factors as possible in the hope of removing all possible confounders, this can lead to *over-matching*, which greatly decreases the efficiency and increases the cost of a study. It is much harder to find a suitable control who matches a long list of criteria than it is to find someone who is only the same age and sex as the case (and even that is not always as easy as it sounds).

Finally, *it is essential that any matching factors are accounted for in the analysis*. The process of matching does not itself remove confounding – it can actually introduce different confounding, which must then be allowed for. If the matching factor is associated with the exposure of interest then, even if it is *not* associated with disease and so is not a true confounder (see criteria for a confounder above), the fact that cases and controls have been matched for that factor *will make it a confounder in the study*. In general, if a matching factor is positively associated with the exposure, the matching process will make cases and controls look more similar than they should. This means that, if the matching is not taken into account in the analysis, the calculated odds ratios will underestimate the true association between exposure and disease (they will be closer to 1.0) as shown in the example in Box 8.3. If frequency matching has been used it is sufficient to treat the matching factors as normal confounders (see 'Control of confounding' below), but there are special techniques for analysing individually matched data (see Box 8.3). The only exception to this rule is if, in practice, it turns out that a matching factor is *not* associated with exposure in a case–control study. In this situation matching cases to controls on that factor will not have introduced any additional confounding and the factor need not be allowed for in the analysis.

Matching was a primary technique for control of confounding in the early decades of the modern case–control study (from the mid twentieth century until the 1980s). The ready availability now of flexible and reasonably straightforward computing packages that allow effective control for confounding at the stage of data analysis (either by stratified or multivariable analysis) has somewhat lessened its importance, although it continues to be used to increase efficiency in a variety of situations.

---

[2] The hazard ratio is a measure of relative risk. It is essentially the same as an incidence rate ratio and is often calculated in cohort studies.

Box 8.3 Analysis of individually matched data

To analyse the data from a simple matched case–control study you have to compare each case with their matched control (or controls if more than one control is selected for each case). In Table 8.9 the numbers no longer represent individual people but 155 matched pairs of cases and controls so there are 40 pairs for which both the case and the control are exposed, 25 pairs for which only the case was exposed and so on.

Table 8.9 Analysing data from an individually matched case–control study.

Cases	Controls	
	Exposed	Unexposed
Exposed	40	25
Unexposed	10	80

Matched odds ratio = $25 \div 10 = 2.5$

If a case and their matched control are both exposed (or both unexposed) that pair (or set) cannot tell us anything about the association between exposure and disease. The interesting case–control pairs are those for which one member is exposed and the other is unexposed. The matched odds ratio is calculated by simply dividing the number of pairs for which the case was exposed and the control unexposed by the number of pairs for which the control was exposed and the case unexposed:

$$\text{Matched OR} = \frac{\text{\# of pairs where the case was exposed and the control unexposed}}{\text{\# of pairs where the control was exposed and the case unexposed}} \quad (8.1)$$

Note that, if we had not taken the matching into account in the analysis, we would have said that 65 (40 + 25) out of the 155 cases were exposed and 90 (10 + 80) were unexposed compared with 50 (40 + 10) exposed and 105 (25 + 80) unexposed controls, giving an unmatched odds ratio of (65 × 105) ÷ (90 × 50) = 1.5, which is considerably less than the matched value of 2.5.

Does increasing the size of a study help?

In any observational epidemiological study increasing the size of the study will not make any difference to the amount of confounding. (To convince yourself of this, go back to one of the earlier examples and try doubling the numbers of people in each group. This will not alter the odds ratios or rate ratios and will not get rid of the confounding.) The only time study size does matter is in the context of a randomised controlled trial. The bigger a randomised trial is, the more likely it is that any confounders (known and unknown) will be balanced across the study groups and the less likely it is that there will be any confounding.

Control of confounding in data analysis

If you have designed a study using restriction or matching to reduce the effects of confounding, it is no longer possible to study the effects of the confounding variables. For example, if you have restricted your study to people aged between 60 and 70 years, or have matched cases and controls for age, it would no longer be possible to look at the direct effects of age on disease. This means that it is often preferable to collect information on potential confounders and then to control for these in the analysis. The aim of the analysis is exactly the same as the design options mentioned above, namely to ensure that the confounders are balanced across the groups, and in practice this is achieved by comparing exposure–disease patterns within narrow ranges of one or more confounders. These approaches apply equally to case–control and cohort studies and also to intervention studies if they are not randomised or if, in a randomised study, the randomisation did not lead to an equal balance of important confounders across the study groups.

Stratification

This is the method that we used in the alcohol and lung cancer example where we stratified by smoking status, and the steps are shown in Figure 8.4 (where RR stands for relative risk and may be a rate, risk or odds ratio). Study subjects are split into groups, or strata, based on levels of the confounding variable. The association between the exposure and outcome of interest is then measured separately in each stratum because if the people in each stratum are homogeneous (the same or similar) with respect to the confounding variable, there can no longer be any confounding by that factor. An analysis could be done separately for men and women to remove confounding by sex, for different age groups, for smokers and non-smokers (as in the example of alcohol and lung cancer) and so on.

In the examples we have looked at so far, the stratum-specific odds ratios were exactly or almost exactly the same, but this is rarely the case in practice. If the stratum-specific estimates are similar then it is reasonable to assume that the small differences between them are simply due to chance. In this situation it is possible to combine the estimates from each separate stratum to summarise the overall effect in the whole group. There are several ways to do this and the effect is then said to be 'adjusted' for the confounder (see Appendix 6). This process is

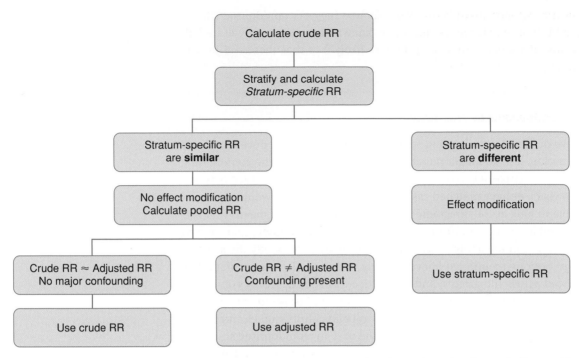

Figure 8.4 A scheme for identifying and dealing with confounding and effect modification.

analogous to the standardisation that you met in Chapter 2. If the adjusted measure of association is *different* from the original crude measure, then we know that the crude association was confounded. In the alcohol and lung cancer example the crude OR was 3.0 and the adjusted OR was 1.0, showing that the crude OR was heavily confounded by smoking.

If, however, the stratum-specific estimates are quite different then there may be *effect modification* or in other words the 'effect' (the association between exposure and outcome) may be truly different in the different strata. For example, regular physical activity might reduce the risk of a particular disease among people who are overweight but it might confer no benefit for those of normal weight. In this situation obesity *modifies* the effect of physical activity on disease and it would be inappropriate to treat obesity as a confounder (see Figure 8.4). In practice, however, there is always some variation in the odds ratios across the different strata and it can be very difficult to know whether this indicates a meaningful difference or just random variation. There are statistical tests (tests for heterogeneity) that can be used to help decide whether the variation could just be due to chance. However, these are not very powerful and are unlikely to detect variation unless the difference is very great (in which case it would be apparent without a statistical test) or the study is very large. In this situation it is still possible to use statistical packages to 'adjust' for the effect modifier but it is important to consider whether this is appropriate. If the effects in different groups really are different then combining them will just average out the differences and give a measure that may not reflect the true association in any of the groups.

Finally, it is important to note that although stratification can also be used for studies in which cases and controls have been frequency matched, it is generally not appropriate for individually matched studies. These should be analysed using a special 'matched' analysis (See Box 8.3) or modelling techniques (see below).

Multivariable modelling

Stratification may be impractical when a study is small or you need to control for several confounders simultaneously, because you are likely to end up with small numbers in any one stratum. If, for example, you wanted to control for sex, age with five 10-year age groups (20–29, 30–39, 40–49, 50–59 and 60–69) and smoking (non-smoker versus smoker), you would end up with 20 different strata (five age groups for smokers and five for non-smokers for each sex). On average, each stratum will contain only 5% of your study population and, with small numbers, it can be difficult to obtain precise estimates of the stratum-specific associations. An alternative is to use statistical modelling techniques to estimate the strength of the relationship of interest while controlling for all of the potential confounders. The most commonly used multivariable approach for unmatched (or frequency-matched) case–control studies is *multiple logistic regression*. Individually matched case–control data can be analysed by a variation of this called *conditional logistic regression*, which takes the individual matching between cases and controls into account. A common technique used to analyse person-time data from a cohort study is *Cox proportional hazards regression*. (Note that this generates *hazard ratios* which, as you saw on page 211, are essentially the same as incidence rate ratios.) We will not discuss the details of these procedures here – they can be found in any standard medical statistics text. See also Box 8.4 for examples of some other newer and more complex approaches to controlling for confounding.

A word of caution, however: multivariable modelling can be performed very easily with modern statistics software but it is important to know what you are doing. The models can be complex and they are based on a number of underlying assumptions. If you are not familiar with the techniques it is wise to seek advice from a statistician before diving in. Furthermore, it is important to be familiar with your data before starting any modelling and nothing can replace simple stratified analyses, as outlined above, for this.

Box 8.4 More advanced ways to identify and control for confounding

Directed acyclic graphs (DAGs) or causal diagrams are gaining popularity as a graphical way to aid causal analysis (Greenland *et al.*, 1999). Explicitly considering the relation between different components of a potential causal pathway can help to identify possible confounding (and/or selection bias) that might otherwise go unmissed. For example, Figure 8.5 shows the relation between neighbourhood violence and cardiovascular disease (CVD). The arrows show that even if there is no direct relation between violence and CVD, these variables are linked via ethnicity/race and income so these will be potential confounders of the violence–CVD association.

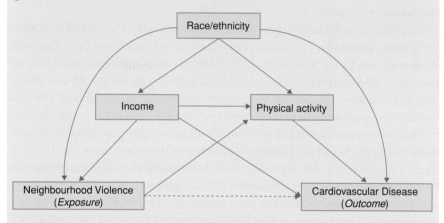

Figure 8.5 A directed acyclic graph showing that race/ethnicity and income will confound the association between neighbourhood violence and cardiovascular disease. (Drawn from: Fleischer and Diez Roux, *Journal of Epidemiology and Community Health*, 2008; 62: 842–846, with permission from BMJ Publishing Group Ltd.)

Propensity scores are mainly used in non-randomised trials when the probability that an individual receives a particular treatment may depend on multiple characteristics of the individual, such as other co-morbidities, that might themselves affect the outcome. The first step is to calculate how individual characteristics (potential confounders of the relation between treatment and outcome) affect the probability that someone receives the treatment of interest. It is then possible to calculate, for each individual, their probability of receiving treatment based on their particular characteristics. If we then match or stratify study participants on the basis of this '*propensity score*', the net effect is to balance the *measured* confounders between the study groups and thus reduce the effects of confounding (Joffe and Rosenbaum, 1999).

(continued)

Box 8.4 (continued)

Instrumental variables are also used for non-randomised treatment studies and for other observational studies. In this case the aim is to find a variable that is associated with treatment selection but not with outcome. This instrumental variable must be associated with the exposure (treatment) and must affect the outcome only via this exposure, i.e. it must not have any independent effect on outcome. It must also not share any common cause with the outcome. This variable can then be used in the analysis instead of the treatment variable. The strength of this approach over propensity scores is that it controls for both *measured* and *unmeasured* confounders; the major challenge is to find an appropriate variable that meets all of the criteria for an instrumental variable. For example, observational treatment data from the US Surveillance Epidemiology and End Results (SEER) program were used to assess whether chemotherapy improved survival from advanced lung cancer in the elderly. The authors did not look at whether the individual themselves received chemotherapy or not but instead used the probability that the healthcare centre the patient attended would offer chemotherapy. This fitted the criteria of an instrumental variable because, by definition, it would affect whether someone received chemotherapy but should not otherwise be related to outcome. The results suggested that chemotherapy did increase one-year survival by approximately 9% (Earle *et al.*, 2001).

In some situations a genetic marker is used as an instrumental variable and this is known as *Mendelian randomisation*. For example, studies looking at the relation between serum cholesterol levels and cancer could be confounded by a multitude of lifestyle factors such as diet that could affect both cholesterol levels and cancer risk. However, there are genetic variants that affect cholesterol levels but are unlikely to be related to diet or lifestyle (nobody would know which variant of the gene they carried). These provide an instrumental variable that can be used to estimate the unconfounded relation between low serum cholesterol and cancer (Davey Smith and Ebrahim, 2004).

Residual confounding

In practice it is rarely possible to remove all confounding so we will be left with some **residual confounding**. For example, in a study of US health professionals the crude RR (0.56; 95% CI 0.38–0.84) suggested that men who consumed high levels of fruit and vegetables had almost half the risk of lung cancer of those who ate little fruit and vegetables (Feskanich *et al.*, 2000). When the authors adjusted their analysis for a simple measure of smoking status (never, past, current smoker) the RR increased to 0.86 (95% CI 0.58–1.29), suggesting that the crude RR was confounded by smoking. When they also adjusted for more detailed measures of smoking, including time since stopping and current amount smoked, the RR increased still further to 1.07 (95% CI 0.71–1.61). This shows convincingly that the simple adjustment for smoking status was not sufficient to remove all of the confounding by smoking and there was considerable residual confounding. If they had not adjusted for the additional smoking variables the results would have left some room for optimism that improving diet might confer some benefit, whereas the fully adjusted result suggests that unfortunately this is not the case. In general, if adjustment changes an observed odds ratio quite markedly, e.g. it reduces it from 5.4 to 2.6, then it is likely that, if we could have controlled for the confounding perfectly, the true odds ratio would have been even less than 2.6. We then have to decide whether we think that there is a *true* association between the exposure and disease or whether all the *observed* association could be due to confounding. However, if the control for confounding only changed the odds ratio from 5.4 to 5.1 then it is likely that, even if we could have controlled completely for confounding, the true odds ratio would still have been close to 5.0, suggesting that this is more likely to be a real association.

Confounding: the bottom line

Confounding is almost ubiquitous in practice and almost any paper that reports associations between two factors will say that the authors have 'adjusted' for this, that and the other to control for confounding. If a paper does *not* mention adjustment for confounding then it is important to consider whether this is a possibility; we will discuss this further in the next chapter.

As we discussed in the previous chapter, it can be hard to know what effects bias might have on the results of a study; in contrast, *known* confounders can be identified and addressed *if information about the confounders has been collected.*

Even if an analysis has 'adjusted for confounders' there is likely to be *residual confounding* either by measured confounders or by unmeasured/unknown confounders. For *known confounders*, a big difference between the unadjusted and adjusted measures suggests that there may be considerable residual confounding; a small difference implies that residual confounding is not a big problem. Unless we are talking about a randomised trial we will not know anything about the likely effects of any *unknown or unmeasured confounders*, but if we see a strong association between exposure and outcome then the confounding would have to be enormous (very strong associations between the confounder and both the exposure and the outcome) to explain the whole association. In practice we might hope that we would know about such strong confounders!

Table 8.10 Results of a study of head injury and helmet use.

	Driver		Passenger		Total	
	Head injury	Other injury	Head injury	Other injury	Head injury	Other injury
No helmet	17,869	51,900	3,052	12,522	20,921	64,422
Helmet	7,342	86,212	485	7,971	7,827	94,183
Total	25,211	138,112	3,537	20,493	28,748	158,605

(Lardelli-Claret *et al.*, 2003.)

We have now covered the three main issues that we have to consider before we conclude that the results of a study are real: namely chance, bias and confounding. In the next chapter we will bring these all together to look at how we can make sense of the epidemiological literature.

Questions

Table 8.10 shows some data from a study of injuries involving moped riders in Spain. The authors obtained information from the Spanish Registry of Traffic Crashes regarding 187,353 moped riders injured in traffic accidents between 1990 and 1999. They then compared the group with head injuries (cases) with those with other types of injury (controls).

1. What is the crude odds ratio for the association between not wearing a helmet (exposed) and head injury?
2. What is the odds ratio for the association between not wearing a helmet and head injury among (i) moped drivers and (ii) moped passengers?
3. Was the crude association between not wearing a helmet and head injury confounded by position on the moped?
4. Does the position of the rider (driver or passenger) on the moped affect their chances of sustaining a head injury? (Hint – first calculate the crude odds ratio for the association between moped position and head injury and then consider whether this could be confounded by helmet use.)
5. If we are interested in the association between drinking coffee and incidence of heart disease, which of the following factors are likely to be confounders and why:
   a. age and sex
   b. smoking
   c. physical activity
   d. fruit and vegetable intake.

6. Go back to Table 8.8 and re-calculate the crude (overall) and stratum-specific odds ratios assuming that the study had (i) half as many people (i.e. divide all the numbers of cases and controls by 2) and (ii) twice as many people. What effect does changing the size of a study have on the confounding effect of physical activity?

REFERENCES

Bickel, P. J., Hammel, E. A. and O'Connell, J. W. (1975). Sex bias in graduate admissions: data from Berkeley. *Science*, **187**: 398–404.

Davey, Smith G. and Ebrahim, S. (2004). Mendelian randomization: prospects, potentials, and limitations. *International Journal of Epidemiology*, **33**: 30–42.

Earle, C.C., Tsai, J. S., Gelber, R. D. *et al.* (2001). Effectiveness of chemotherapy for advanced lung cancer in the elderly: instrumental variable and propensity analysis. *Journal of Clinical Oncology*, **19**: 1064–1070.

Feskanich, D., Ziegler, R. G., Michaud, D. S. *et al.* (2000). Prospective study of fruit and vegetable consumption and risk of lung cancer among men and women. *Journal of the National Cancer Institute*, **92**: 1812–1823.

Fleischer, N. L. and Diez Roux, A. V. (2008). Using directed accylic graphs to guide analyses of neighbourhood health effects: an introduction. *Journal of Epidemiology and Community Health*, **62**: 842–846.

Greenland, S., Pearl, J. and Robins, J. M. (1999). Causal diagrams for epidemiologic research. *Epidemiology*, **10**: 37–48.

Guiltinan, A. M., Kaidarova, Z., Custer, B. *et al.* (2008). Increased all-cause, liver, and cardiac mortality among hepatitis C virus-seropositive blood donors. *American Journal of Epidemiology*, **167**: 743–750.

Joffe, M. M. and Rosenbaum, P. R. (1999). Invited commentary: propensity scores. *American Journal of Epidemiology*, **150**: 327–333.

Lardelli-Claret, P., Luna-del-Castillo, J. D. D. and Jimenez-Moleon, J. J. (2003). Position on the moped, risk of head injury and helmet use: an example of confounding effect. *International Journal of Epidemiology*, **32**: 162–164.

Mantel, N. and Haenszel, W. (1959). Statistical aspects of the analysis of data from retrospective studies of disease. *Journal of the National Cancer Institute*, **22**: 719–748.

Miettinen, O. S. (1983). The need for randomization in the study of intended effects. *Statistics in Medicine*, **2**: 267–271.

Vessey, M. P. and Lawless, M. (1984). The Oxford Family Planning Association contraceptive study. *Clinical Obstetrics and Gynaecology*, **11**: 743–757.

Reading between the lines: reading and writing epidemiological papers

Description	Association	Alternative explanations	Integration & interpretation	Practical applications
Chapters 2–3	Chapters 4–5	Chapters 6–8	Chapter 9: Reading papers	Chapters 12–15

In Chapters 4, 6, 7 and 8 we looked at the different epidemiological study designs and examined the various misfortunes that can befall them. Good studies are difficult to design and implement, and interpretation of their results and conclusions is not always as straightforward as we might hope. How, then, can we make the best use of this information? The central question we have to answer when we read a study report is '*Are the results of the study valid?*' If the authors report an association between exposure and outcome, is it real? If they find nothing, do we accept this? Or could there be an alternative explanation for the results, namely chance, bias and/or confounding?

Frank and Ernest

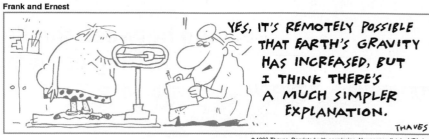

© 1990 Thaves. Reprinted with permission. Newspaper dist. by NEA, Inc.

Much of the following discussion will pick up and integrate the core epidemiological issues covered in the previous chapters. We will concentrate mainly on analytic studies looking for associations between 'cause' and 'effect', the study designs that you met in Chapter 4, but the same general principles apply equally to descriptive epidemiology. To extract the maximum information from a paper we need a systematic approach to identifying its strengths and weaknesses. Some quite detailed sets of guidelines for 'critical appraisal' of the health literature exist already and we do not intend to add to this list (although we do offer a flowchart for more general guidance). Instead we will focus on the essence of the challenge: what are the practical effects of the ways in which subjects were selected and information collected, and the likely influence of confounding and chance on the results we see? While the elements of the general strategy we propose are universal, the approach can (and should) be tailored to suit your own personal style. In practice you will almost certainly have to read individual papers and reports and, if you are involved in research, you may write some of your own. Both activities demand a very practical approach and this is what we will focus on here. We will emphasise the perspective of the reader, but the writer should be thinking about exactly the same things, since good writing demands that the readers' needs and perspectives are kept firmly in mind.

The research question and study design

When reading a paper, the first step is to identify the *research question* that the authors set out to answer and then the strategy they used to attempt to answer that question. Was the *study design* appropriate to answer the question posed? This involves consideration of what the *ideal* type of study would be and also what would be *practical* in that particular situation.

As you have seen, the *ideal* study to answer a question of cause and effect would often be some sort of randomised trial, but in many situations this will be impossible for numerous ethical and/or practical reasons. Next best would generally be a cohort study in which exposure is measured prior to the development of disease, but again the resources, time and money required to conduct a large enough study often make it unfeasible. So, from a practical viewpoint the key question should be 'Was the research design the best that could have been done in the circumstances to answer that particular question?' If it was not the best, can it still provide useful information? Are there existing studies addressing the same issue that were of better design against which the findings of the current study can be compared?

Many studies are conducted not because they will provide the strongest possible evidence for a causal association between exposure and outcome, but because they can answer a range of other more indirect questions of interest. For example, the results from the ecological study of *Helicobacter pylori* infection and stomach cancer rates in China shown in Figure 3.7 cannot directly answer the question 'Does *H. pylori* infection cause stomach cancer?' We can, however, answer the question 'Are stomach cancer rates higher in areas where *H. pylori* infection is more common?' Trials, and to a lesser extent cohort studies and case–control studies, can address issues of causality more directly, whereas other types of study provide more circumstantial evidence, but if the results are valid each can increase our understanding of the relation between an exposure and outcome. As an example, ecological and migrant studies conducted across countries with widely differing levels of solar ultraviolet (UV) radiation have consistently revealed an association between sun exposure in childhood and melanoma rates. In contrast, case–control studies, which have generally been conducted within a single country or region with a narrow range of UV exposures, have not given consistent results (Whiteman *et al.*, 2001). In this particular situation ecological studies with their wide variety of exposure levels provide a valuable additional perspective to the case–control studies.

So how do we decide whether the results of a study are valid? We have to consider the three main alternative explanations that we discussed in the preceding chapters: bias (both the *selection of participants* for the study and the *information* that was *measured* or collected from or about them), confounding and chance.

The study sample: selection bias

Who was included in the study, how were they selected and are there possible sources of selection bias? Specific questions to ask when reading a paper include those below.

- Is the comparison group appropriate?
  In a case–control study are the controls really representative of the population from which the cases arose? In a cohort study where the comparison cohort

was recruited separately from the exposed cohort, are the two groups really comparable?

- What proportion of eligible participants actually took part in the study and, if appropriate, what proportion was lost to follow-up?

  Participation or follow-up rates less than 90% (some would say 80%) may be cause for some concern. If the rates are lower than this, could participation (or loss to follow-up) be related to either the exposure or the outcome of interest? That is, could those who refused to take part (or who were lost to follow-up) have differed in some way from those who did take part? If so, might this have led to an overestimation or underestimation of the level of exposure and/or outcome? Most importantly, could this have differed between study groups?

- Finally, what is the likely effect of any selection bias on the results of the study? Ideally the authors of the paper will have considered all of these issues in their discussion, but if they have not then it is up to the reader to decide whether bias might be present and, if so, what effect it may have had on the results. In practice there will almost certainly be some potential for selection bias. Participation rates are never 100% and in many developed countries it is becoming increasingly hard to persuade people to take part in research, especially when they see no benefit to themselves. This is a major issue in case–control studies when the motivation for a 'case' to take part may be much greater than that of an unaffected 'control'. Also, people are becoming increasingly mobile, so follow-up in a cohort study that runs for more than a few years is never likely to be 100%.

If we were to reject all studies with less than 100% participation or follow-up rates, we would be left with nothing to review. In practice, participation or follow-up rates greater than 80% or 90% are generally considered to be good, but rates lower than this do not necessarily invalidate the findings (see Example 2 below). The challenge for both investigator and reader is to think practically and to decide whether any potential biases related to selection might have compromised the study results (the **internal validity**) and, if so, how and to what degree the results might be biased. It is often impossible to quantify this, but **sensitivity analyses** making various assumptions about the size and direction of possible bias can be informative (see Chapter 7).

Example 1: case–control studies of blood transfusion and Creutzfeldt–Jakob disease

In five case–control studies of Creutzfeldt–Jakob disease (CJD) the controls were more likely to report having had a blood transfusion than cases (Riggs *et al.*, 2001). Does this tell us that blood transfusions might protect against CJD (a finding contrary to the causal hypothesis)? If we consider the control groups, we find that in three of the five studies they were selected from among hospitalised patients and in another study more than 12,000 telephone calls were made in order to recruit just 784 controls.

The use of hospital controls and the very low participation rate among controls should ring alarm bells. Why?

People who are in hospital are more likely to have had a blood transfusion than those who are not; and in addition, given the publicity surrounding 'mad cow disease', people who have had a blood transfusion may well be more likely to agree to take part in a study of CJD. Indeed, in these four studies approximately 20% of controls reported having had a blood transfusion – an improbably high proportion, probably due at least in part to these selection pressures. So what can we conclude about the association between transfusion and CJD from these studies? Not much. The high transfusion rate in controls almost certainly overestimates the base rate in the population from which the cases came. We have no idea whether the true background rate is similar to that in cases (i.e. there is no association) or lower than in cases (i.e. there is a positive association). Our next example shows how external information can help resolve such dilemmas.

Example 2: a case–control study of oesophageal cancer and smoking in Australia

In an Australian case–control study of oesophageal cancer, the authors considered the relation with smoking. In this study approximately 70% of eligible cases but only 49% of the controls who were contacted agreed to participate – this is a fairly typical response rate in many countries these days, but is far from ideal. The authors found that current smoking rates were higher among cases with oesophageal adenocarcinoma than controls (OR compared to never smokers = 2.7; 95% CI 1.9–3.9), but could this be due to selection bias?

In general, smokers are less likely to agree to take part in a study than non-smokers. What effect might this have had on the odds ratio?

If smokers were less likely to take part the prevalence of smoking in the control group would be *lower* than that in the general population. This would exaggerate the difference between cases and controls and so increase the odds ratio, making it look as if smoking is associated with oesophageal adenocarcinoma when in reality it might not be. To address this issue the authors used data from a National Health Survey conducted at about the same time to estimate the likely prevalence of smoking in the controls who did *not* agree to take part in the study. If they assumed that the whole control population had a smoking rate equal to that seen in the national survey, they found that the odds ratio for the association between smoking and oesophageal adenocarcinoma was slightly weaker but still significantly greater than 1.0 (imputed OR = 2.4; 95% CI 1.7–3.4). This suggested that even though only about half of the controls invited to take part in the study actually agreed to participate, the overall results for the association with smoking were not seriously biased (Pandeya *et al.*, 2009).

Measuring disease and exposure: measurement bias

We also have to consider the information collected from or about the people in the study – particularly the measurement of 'outcome' and 'exposure' but also measurement of other factors that might be important confounders. Attention to unbiased measurement of *outcome* is crucial for cross-sectional, cohort and intervention studies. It is of relatively less importance in a case–control study, in which cases are selected because they have already experienced the outcome of interest (although a clear definition of what constitutes a case is still essential). Accurate measurement of *exposure* is important in every study, and in a case–control study it is critical to ensure that there are no systematic differences in measurement between cases and controls. Good measurement of *confounders* is often overlooked, but this is also essential to enable optimal control of confounding in the analysis (see comments on residual confounding in Chapter 8).

Some questions to ask when reading a paper are the following.
- Were the outcome/exposures/confounders clearly defined, and how were they measured?
- Have all relevant outcomes and/or exposures and/or confounders been included and, if not, how important are those omitted?
- Were the same definitions and methods of measurement used in all of the study groups?
- Is measurement error likely to be a problem and, if so, could there be **non-differential misclassification** (look back to Chapter 7 if you are unsure about this)?

No measurement is perfect and some measurements are very poor. The effect of the ubiquitous random error and consequent non-differential misclassification must always be considered. The practical implication of this is that effects (OR, RR) estimated in the face of equal measurement error in the compared groups will usually appear *weaker* than they truly are. Thus a finding of a positive association, despite poor measurement, should not be dismissed because of this – the true association is likely to be more impressive. On the other hand, a null finding or a very weak effect in the presence of non-differential misclassification is uninformative since it may reflect the imprecise measurement (thereby masking a true association) or there may truly be no effect.
- Is the extent of any measurement error likely to differ between groups (e.g. could there be **recall** or **interviewer bias** in exposure measurement in a case–control study) and so could there be **differential misclassification**?

Differential misclassification can bias results in either direction. It is particularly important to consider this possibility in cross-sectional and case–control studies when exposure is measured after the outcome has occurred. In analytic research it is generally easier to distinguish clearly between outcome states (diseased versus non-diseased) than it is to measure exposures precisely, but the avoidance of differential outcome assessment is central to the integrity of cohort studies and trials, and again for cross-sectional studies.

- Finally, what practical effects might any measurement bias (outcome or exposure) have had on the results of the study?

Example 3: a case–control study of body-mass index (BMI) and asthma in Mexico

A significant association between asthma and obesity (defined as BMI > 30 kg/m^2 based on self-reported weight and height) was observed among women (adjusted OR = 1.7; 95% CI 1.1–2.7), with a weaker non-significant association (adjusted OR = 1.3; 95% CI 0.6–2.9) seen among men (Santillan and Camargo, 2003); but how reliable are self-reported data on body size and could measurement error have affected the results? The authors specifically addressed this question by weighing and measuring all of the participants. They found that, on average, people tended to report that they were taller and lighter than they really were, particularly the men. As a result, the *true* prevalence of obesity based on measured BMI was higher than that based on self-reported BMI and the difference was somewhat greater for cases (40% versus 24% for men and 44% versus 38% for women) than for controls (28% versus 22% for men; 24% versus 23% for women).

Is the error in the self-reported information on body-size differential or non-differential?

Assuming that the measured BMI values are correct, is the *true* association between obesity and asthma likely to be stronger or weaker than that seen for self-reported obesity?

In this example there is *differential* error since cases, particularly men, were more likely to underestimate their weight and overestimate their height than controls. The effect of these errors would be to reduce the association seen and this is what happened. When the authors calculated the association between asthma and *measured* obesity, the OR was 2.3 (95% CI 1.5–3.8) for women and 2.5 (95% CI 1.1–5.9) for men, i.e. the associations were much stronger than those based on self-reported BMI above. (Note that although the OR based on measured BMI is likely to give a more accurate estimate than that based on self-reporting, even this may be an underestimate of the 'true' effect since there is still likely to be some *non-differential* random misclassification.) Validation studies such as this

Box 9.1 Sensitivity analysis: kangaroos and Ross River virus (RRV) infection

Authors of a case–control study found an odds ratio of 4.3 (95% CI 0.9–21) for the association between seeing kangaroos in the backyard and risk of RRV infection, possibly because kangaroos provide a host for the mosquitoes that spread RRV. However, information was missing for a number of cases and controls, so the authors performed a sensitivity analysis.

If they assumed that all cases and controls for whom exposure data were missing had seen kangaroos, the OR was 1.9 (95% CI 0.7–5.1); if they assumed that none had seen kangaroos the OR was 3.5 (0.9–14.1). If they assumed that cases were more likely to remember exposure than controls (i.e. there is recall bias) and, therefore, that cases with data missing had not seen kangaroos whereas controls had seen them, then the association disappeared completely (OR = 1.0, 95% CI 0.4–2.8). This analysis raised questions about the validity of the observed association between sighting of kangaroos and RRV infection.

(Harley *et al.*, 2005)

can provide valuable insights into the accuracy of study results, as can sensitivity analyses such as that described in Box 9.1.

Confounding

The next major issue to consider is that of confounding.
- Have the authors considered all important confounders and controlled for them in their analysis?
- Could there be residual confounding by variables that have not been considered or because of incomplete adjustment for factors that have?
- If so, what effect might this have had on the study results?

Again, the important thing is to think practically: in which direction is any residual confounding likely to operate? If when the authors adjusted for confounding the association became *stronger* (i.e. the confounding had originally biased the effect towards the null) then, if there is residual confounding, the real effect is likely to be even more extreme than that observed. Conversely, if the adjustment brought the estimate *closer* to 1.0 (i.e. the confounding had biased the estimate away from the null) then the true result may be even closer to the null than that reported. In the latter situation our confidence in the value of a positive effect estimate would decrease, unless it was very large. A large effect is less likely to be wholly due to confounding because, to explain away a very strong RR (e.g. 10.0), the confounder itself would have to be an even stronger risk factor for the disease. If this is the case then it is likely to be known already, and hence should have been measured and controlled for.

Example 4: a cross-sectional study of risk factors for depression in the UK

Among 14,217 adults aged over 75 years, the risk of depression appeared to be somewhat higher among women than among men (crude OR = 1.3, 95% CI 1.1–1.5) (Osborn *et al.*, 2003). After adjustment for potential confounding factors including age, marital status, living alone, smoking and alcohol consumption, the adjusted OR was 1.1 (95% CI 1.0–1.3).

What do these results suggest about the association between sex and risk of depression?

The adjustment has reduced the OR, bringing it closer to 1.0. It is also likely that there is further residual confounding, which might bring the true OR even closer to 1.0, suggesting that sex is not associated with depression (at least in this study). This example also highlights the need to consider the clinical or practical significance of the results of a study. A very large study can show what appears to be a very small effect with great precision (a narrow confidence interval); even though the result might be statistically significant ($p < 0.05$) the key question is whether such a small difference is meaningful.

Example 5: a cohort study of statin use and atrial fibrillation in the USA

A cohort of patients with coronary artery disease was followed for a minimum of 12 months to document the incidence of atrial fibrillation (AF, an abnormal heart rhythm); 263 of the patients were using statins (cholesterol-lowering drugs) and 186 had never used them (Young-Xu *et al.*, 2003). (Note that this was an observational study, not a randomised trial.) Overall, the rate of AF was lower among the group taking statins, giving a crude relative risk of 0.5 (95% CI 0.3–0.8). When the authors adjusted for potential confounding factors including age, systolic blood pressure, alcohol consumption, history of heart failure and total serum cholesterol level, the RR was 0.4 (95% CI 0.2–0.8).

Assuming that there are no important selection or measurement errors, what conclusions can we draw about the association between statin use and AF?

It appears that there was some confounding by the other factors such as age since the RR dropped from 0.5 to 0.4 after adjustment, indicating that the real effect of statin use was even stronger than the crude RR suggested. However, doctors prescribe treatment partly on the basis of prognostic judgements, which are difficult to measure. There may thus be other unknown and unmeasured confounders that have not been controlled for, so we would still need to be cautious about this particular result which, as you saw in Chapter 8, could be due to **confounding by indication**. Large, well-conducted RCTs remove this potential problem.

Chance

Finally, it is important to consider the role of chance. Have the authors included confidence intervals for their estimates? How narrow (good precision) or wide (poor precision) are they? If an association is seen, how likely is it that there is really no effect (i.e. the association arose by chance)? If there is no clear association (e.g. if the confidence limits are very wide and include 1.0), is it possible that there is a real effect but the study was simply too small to detect it? Is the study useful or are the results inconclusive? As well as *statistical significance* it is also important to consider whether the results are *socially* or *clinically* significant (see *Statistical versus clinical significance* in Chapter 6). A large study may give an association that is statistically significant, for example the odds ratio of 1.1 (95% CI 1.0–1.3) seen for the association between sex and depression in Example 4 above, but we would then have to ask whether a 10% higher risk of depression in women than men was a meaningful difference.

Study validity

Once we have considered all of these aspects (summarised in Figure 9.1) we can make an overall judgement of the validity of the study results. There are two separate issues here. The first and most important, often called **internal validity**, is the extent to which the results of a study reflect the true situation *in the study sample* in the absence of any alternative explanations. These alternative explanations, namely chance, bias and confounding, have been the focus of this and the previous chapters. *The prime objective of study design, implementation, analysis and interpretation is to maximise the internal validity of a study*. The second issue is one of **generalisability** or **external validity**. Are the results of a study applicable to populations other than the study population?

Internal validity

Have the authors discussed the limitations of their study? What conclusions do they draw with respect to the research question? Are these conclusions justified? Does the study appear to be internally valid or could the results be due to chance, bias or confounding? It is important to remember that in public health we are dealing with real people and complex exposures that are often difficult to measure and/or impossible to control adequately and we are, quite rightly, constrained as to what we can do by codes of ethics. Any study is thus likely to fall short of perfection and it is important to realise this. Research should be appraised in the light of what it has been able to achieve – there will be

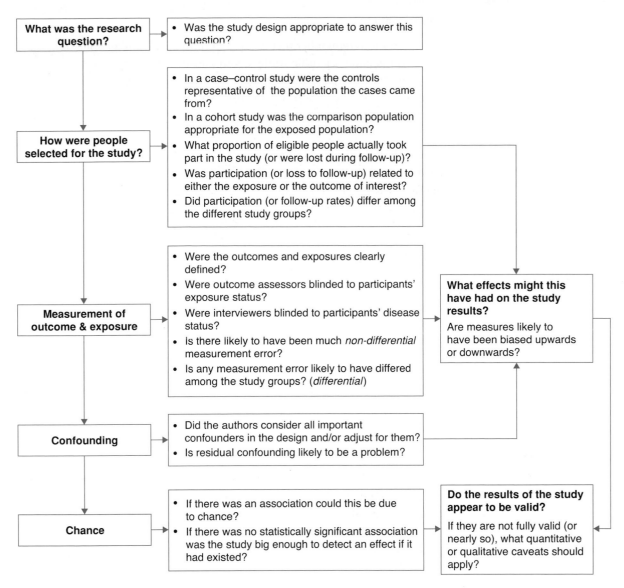

Figure 9.1 Issues to consider when reading epidemiological papers.

deficiencies but, given the particular circumstances, could things realistically have been improved? The evidence reported in a research paper might not always be strong but, if it is the best that is likely to be available, we should not discount it because of the flaws. Rather we should draw from it what information we can that bears on the question in hand.

External validity

It is important to remember that the aim of the 'causal arm' of epidemiology is to discover general scientific truths about cause and effect. Can the results of a study of, for example, American men aged 50–65 be generalised to older or younger men? Women? Non-Americans? (Note that such a question presumes the internal validity of a study: *if a study is not internally valid, then the results should not be applied to anyone.*)

There are no firm rules to help with generalising from a study to the wider population. In case–control comparisons, population-based studies are the ideal in order to reduce the possibilities of selection bias and, as a result, it might not require such a leap of faith to extrapolate the results from one population to another. However, the process is not simply a matter of statistical representativeness, but is more fundamentally one of biological insight. The question then is 'How relevant (biologically) is a result for a given population?' Can a study in a very select population (e.g. urban-living Japanese, Czech women, Brazilian men) inform us about disease causation more generally? Well, we certainly hope so. As an example, careful follow-up of the survivors of the atomic bomb blasts in Hiroshima and Nagasaki, Japan, has yielded volumes of information regarding the relation between exposure to ionising radiation and subsequent risks of mortality, cancers and other rare diseases. While this information comes only from the Japanese, no one would argue that radiation would not have similar effects in other nationalities, and we certainly do not want to see this 'unnatural experiment' repeated. While this generalisation is perhaps easier than many because of the magnitude and timing of the effects and the well-understood physical and biological properties of ionising radiation, the principle is identical for other abstract causal speculation.

Generalising from clinical and other trials raises additional issues. For practical reasons, many clinical trials are conducted on highly selected groups of people who are almost certainly not representative of the general population. This can make the results of the specific trials easier to interpret (internal validity), but means that they can be harder to generalise to other groups (see Chapter 11).

Descriptive studies

The discussion above has focused on papers evaluating associations between exposure and outcome and that, therefore, address the 'Why?' of epidemiology. It is equally important to evaluate the results of descriptive studies that provide the 'Who?', 'Where?' and 'When?' information that is essential to make a community diagnosis and, as you will see in Chapter 14, also play an important role in evaluating the effects of public health interventions. In practice this requires us to consider exactly the same issues: selection and measurement error, confounding and chance.

- How was the survey sample selected? Is it representative of the wider population?
- How was the factor of interest measured? Is it likely to be over- or under-reported?
- If we are making comparisons, are we comparing like with like or is there a need for standardisation (to remove confounding by, e.g., differences in the age structure of populations)?
- Could any observed excesses (or deficits) of disease in different populations, in different places or at different times be due to chance? For example, it is unlikely that several cases of a rare disease would occur in the same small community (what is known as a 'cluster' – see Chapter 12), but it is not impossible for this to occur by chance. Similarly, rates of disease (particularly rare diseases) will naturally vary from year to year, so could an apparent increase or decline just be due to chance?

It is also important to note that, although *representativeness* is not the primary issue in studies of aetiology, it is crucial for applying the results of a descriptive study to a wider population. If a sample of people is surveyed to identify the health needs of an area then, if those participating do not represent the whole population, the results could be very misleading. If, for example, they were unusually healthy then the needs of the population might be greatly underestimated, and vice versa.

Writing papers

We have focused on the information that you need to look for when reading a paper and, as we suggested at the start of this chapter, it goes without saying that this is also the information that you need to provide when writing a paper. To improve the reporting of experimental research, some journals now require that authors follow the checklist of points contained in the Consolidated Standards of Reporting Trials or CONSORT statement (Moher *et al.*, 2001). This document has since been modified to give the TREND (Transparent Reporting of Non-randomised Designs) checklist for reporting results of studies of behavioural and public health interventions with non-randomised designs (Des Jarlais *et al.*, 2004). Similar guidelines have been developed for observational studies including the STROBE (STrengthening the Reporting of OBservational studies in Epidemiology) statement (von Elm *et al.*, 2007), and the STREGA (STrengthening the REporting of Genetic Association Studies) statement, a modification of STROBE for genetic studies (Little *et al.*, 2009), as well as a guide specific to longitudinal studies (Tooth *et al.*, 2005).

Box 9.2 The problem of multiple testing

The more hypotheses that we test, the more likely it is that some apparently statistically significant results will arise by chance. For this reason statisticians often recommend 'correcting' for this problem of multiple testing. A simple form of this is to reduce the α-level at which a result is considered to be statistically significant based on the number of tests performed. For example, if 20 separate tests are conducted within a single study then the p-value at which a result is considered statistically significant would be reduced from 0.05 to $0.05 \div 20 = 0.0025$. The net result is that fewer results, those with the strongest associations, will be deemed statistically significant and, hopefully, these are also the results that are less likely to be due to chance. However many epidemiologists have pointed out the illogicality of such an arbitrary rule (for example, should an epidemiologist adjust their results based on the number of statistical tests performed that day or for the number of tests they have ever done? (Rothman, 1990)) and prefer to take a more common-sense approach. One notable exception is in the context of modern genetic studies which may evaluate tens or hundreds of thousands of genetic markers at the same time. In this situation, increased stringency is essential to minimise the thousands of spurious results that will arise simply by chance if we accept a significance level of 5% (5% of 100,000 genes is ~5000 significant results by chance!). Results from the new 'genome-wide association studies' (GWAS) which may look at 1 million or more genetic variants in relation to disease are usually not considered statistically significant unless p is less than about 0.0000001.

Summary: one swallow doesn't make a summer

We will end with a note of caution. The ultimate aim of much public health research is to change practice or policy to improve health outcomes, but even if a well-written paper that is (largely) free from major sources of bias and confounding finds what appears to be a statistically and practically significant association between an exposure and health outcome, we cannot rush out to act on this. Despite our best efforts and those of the investigators it is still possible that statistically significant results can arise by chance. As you saw in Chapter 6 the probability of this happening is usually defined as <5%; however, in many modern studies the investigators study multiple associations so the probability that one will arise by chance is greatly increased. Some authors recommend correcting results for this problem which is known as 'multiple testing' (see Box 9.2); however, we and many others prefer to rely more on a common-sense approach that places less emphasis on the question of statistical significance and more on the overall strength, coherence and plausibility of an observed association. We will discuss some of these issues further in Chapter 10. With the possible exception of a large randomised trial, no practical or policy decision should be made on the basis of the results of a single study, however good. As you have seen, individual studies can never be perfect so it is important to consider all of the evidence on a given subject before attempting to make policy or practical decisions. We will come back to the ways in which you can do this in Chapter 11.

Questions

We have not included any questions for this chapter, but the Epidemic Intelligence Service of the US Centers for Disease Control and Prevention has developed an excellent exercise, 'Cigarette smoking and lung cancer', that draws on many of the issues covered in this and the previous chapters. This and other similar exercises are freely available from http://www.cdc.gov/eis/casestudies/casestudies.htm.

REFERENCES

Des Jarlais, D. C., Lyles, C., Crepaz, N. and the TREND Group. (2004). Improving the reporting quality of non-randomized evaluations of behavioral and public health interventions: the TREND statement. *American Journal of Public Health*, **94**: 361–366.

Harley, D., Ritchie, S., Bain, C. and Sleigh, A. C. (2005). Risks for Ross River virus disease in tropical Australia. *International Journal of Epidemiology*, **34**: 548–555.

Little, J., Higgins, J. P. Y., Ioannidis, J. P. A. *et al.* (2009). Strengthening the Reporting of Genetic Association Studies (STREGA) – an extension of the STROBE statement. *PLoS Medicine*, **6**(2): e1000022.

Moher, D., Schultz, K. F. and Altman, D. G. for the CONSORT Group. (2001). The CONSORT statement: revised recommendations for improving the quality of reports of parallel-group randomised trials. *Lancet*, **357**: 1191–1194.

Osborn, D. P. J., Fletcher, A. E., Smeeth, L. *et al.* (2003). Factors associated with depression in a representative sample of 14,217 people aged 75 and over in the United Kingdom: results from the MRC trial of assessment and management of older people in the community. *International Journal of Geriatric Psychiatry*, **18**: 623–630.

Pandeya, N., Williams, G. M., Green, A. C. *et al.* (2009). Do low control response rates always affect the findings? Assessments of smoking and obesity in two Australian case-control studies of cancer. *Australian and New Zealand Journal of Public Health*, **33**: 312–319.

Riggs, J. E., Moudgil, S. S. and Hobbs, G. R. (2001). Creutzfeld–Jakob disease and blood transfusions: a meta-analysis of case–control studies. *Military Medicine*, **166**: 1057–1058.

Rothman, K. J. (1990). No adjustments are needed for multiple testing. *Epidemiology*, **1**: 43–46.

Santillan, A. A. and Camargo Jr, C. A. (2003). Body mass index and asthma among Mexican adults: the effect of using self-reported versus measured weight and height. *International Journal of Obesity*, **27**: 1430–1433.

Tooth, L., Ware, R., Dobson, A., Purdie, D. and Bain, C. (2005). Quality of reporting of observational longitudinal research. *American Journal of Epidemiology*, **161**: 280–288.

von Elm, E., Altman, D. G., Egger, M. *et al.* (2007). The Strengthening the Reporting of Observational Studies in Epidemiology (STROBE) Statement: guidelines for reporting observational studies. *PLoS Medicine*, **4**(10): e296.

Whiteman, D. C., Whiteman, C. A. and Green, A. C. (2001). Childhood sun exposure as a risk factor for melanoma: a systematic review of epidemiologic studies. *Cancer Causes and Control*, **12**: 69–82.

Young-Xu, Y., Jabbour, S., Goldberg, R. *et al.* (2003). Usefulness of statin drugs in protecting against atrial fibrillation in patients with coronary artery disease. *American Journal of Cardiology*, **92**: 1379–1383.

Who sank the boat? Association and causation

Description	Association	Alternative explanations	Integration & interpretation	Practical applications
Chapters 2–3	Chapters 4–5	Chapters 6–8	Chapter 10: Causality	Chapters 12–15

Box 10.1 Who sank the boat?

As the story goes, there were five animals living by the sea, a cow, a donkey, a sheep, a pig and a mouse. One fine day they decided to go rowing on the bay.

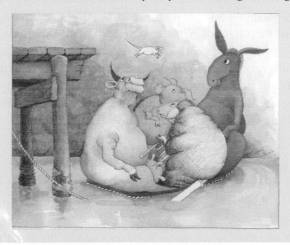

(*continued*)

Box 10.1 *(continued)*

First the cow got into the boat, it rocked a bit but she settled herself down comfortably at the back. Then the donkey got in carefully and sat down at the front to balance the boat. Next the pig climbed in, clutching her umbrella – the boat is low in the water by now. Then the sheep climbed in carrying her knitting and she sat down opposite the pig.

   The boat is still afloat, but only just. Finally the little mouse jumped aboard and – disaster! The boat capsized and the animals had to swim to the shore.

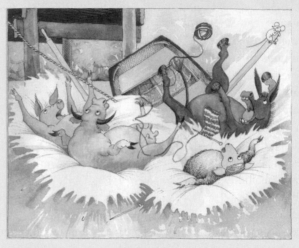

So who sank the boat?

(Storyline (adapted) and pictures from '*Who Sank the Boat?*' (Allen, 1983), reproduced with permission from Penguin Books Australia Ltd.)

The search for the causes of disease is an obvious central step in the pursuit of better health through disease prevention and Box 10.1, abstracted from a wonderful children's picture book, illustrates perfectly the complexity of assigning causality. In the previous chapters we have looked at how we measure health (or disease) and how we look for associations between exposure and disease. Being able to identify a *relation* between a potential cause of disease and the disease itself is not enough, though. We need to go one step further and decide whether this relation is causal.

What do we mean by a cause?

It is tempting to think that a cause is a single condition or event that inevitably leads to a particular effect or outcome; i.e. that there is a one-to-one relationship such that wherever or whenever the cause occurs the effect will follow. If we consider this more closely, it quickly becomes apparent that things are not so simple and that everyday causal phenomena are rather more complicated than they might seem at first. For example, while it might appear that all we need to do to turn on a computer is press the 'on' button, we know better: what if the wiring is faulty, there is no power supply or the hard drive has died an untimely death? To 'cause' the computer to come on we need power, good wiring, a functioning hard drive and relevant software in addition to the pressure of our finger on the button. We could describe each of these separate requirements as **component causes**, since they are all part of the one **sufficient cause** that will inevitably lead to the effect – in this case the computer turning on. In this situation they are also **necessary causes** because in the absence of just one of these things the computer will not work.

In the same way, disease rarely occurs as the result of a single event or exposure. Even though it might seem that an infectious agent would be a sufficient cause in its own right, not everyone develops disease following exposure to a particular bug. The real-life food-poisoning example in Chapter 1 made this clear – although people who ate the cold chicken were 3.8 times more likely to suffer from food poisoning than those who did not, almost one-quarter (23%) of those who ate the cold chicken suffered no ill effects. Whether someone does become ill depends both on their susceptibility to the agent and on the dose they receive. For tuberculosis (TB), for example, a person's susceptibility is determined by whether they have been infected before and are now immune, and also their overall level of health at the time. The infectious agent, the tubercle bacillus, is only a component of the total or sufficient cause that will lead to TB. It is, however, a **necessary cause** in that, by definition, TB cannot occur without it. We will look at causation and infectious diseases in more detail in Chapter 12.

Some definitions

There are many definitions of a cause but the following, from Rothman (1986; p. 11), is appealing because of the brevity with which it captures the concept:

a cause is *'an event, condition or characteristic* [or a combination of these factors] *that plays an essential role in producing an occurrence of the disease'.*

There are also many ways in which such entities (causes) can be classified, but the following subdivision serves well.

- A **sufficient** cause is a factor (or more usually a combination of several factors) that will inevitably produce disease.
- A **component** cause is a factor that contributes towards disease causation but is not sufficient to cause disease on its own.
- A **necessary** cause is any agent (or component cause) that is required for the development of a given disease (for example the specific infectious agent).

Figure 10.1 A conceptual scheme for the causes of a hypothetical disease. (From: Rothman, Causes. *Am. J. Epidemiol.*, 1976; 104: 589, by permission of the Society for Epidemiological Research.)

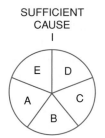

SUFFICIENT CAUSE I

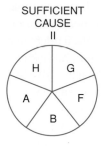

SUFFICIENT CAUSE II

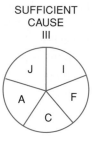

SUFFICIENT CAUSE III

In terms of working out 'who sank the boat' we can say that each one of the animals was a **component** cause and that together they created the **sufficient** cause that caused the disaster. Probably none was actually **necessary** to sink the boat – any group of similarly sized animals would have had a similar effect. The ordering of the events, i.e. whether the mouse got in first or last, also did not matter; it was the sum of the weights that caused the boat to sink. This may also be true in much disease causation, but sometimes the component causes will have to occur in a specific order or they will have to be present at the same time. For example, TB infection will occur only if the individual is susceptible at the time they are exposed to the infection; and thrombosis (blood clotting) in an artery leading to a heart attack or stroke rarely occurs unless the blood vessel is already damaged or partly blocked.

A useful model for considering causal mechanisms is the 'pie' diagrams used by Rothman (1976) and shown in Figure 10.1. In this scheme

- I, II and III are three different **sufficient causes** for a disease;
- A is a **necessary cause** for the disease because it is present in all three sufficient causes; and
- A, B, C, D, E, F, G, H, I and J are component causes.

So, for example, if 'A' were the cow, 'B' the donkey, 'C' the pig, 'D' the sheep and 'E' the mouse, we would have sufficient cause I, while the other 'pies' show that different combinations of animals or other objects would also have led to the boat overturning.

In practice, when considering causes of disease we mostly find ourselves dealing with component causes. Aside from something like a major disaster such as an earthquake or nuclear explosion, it is hard to imagine identifying a single factor that is truly necessary and sufficient to cause disease. We also have to accept that, other than for something like an injury, we are unlikely to know either the precise nature of any sufficient cause or many of the possible component causes of disease. This need not matter – we do not have to eliminate all components of a particular cause in order to prevent disease due to that cause. If any one of them is identified and removed (e.g. B in the example above), then we will prevent cases of disease due to sufficient causes that contain component

Table 10.1 The percentage of DALYs due to ischaemic heart disease which can be attributed to various risk factors, shown separately for low- and middle-income and high-income countries.

	Percentage of DALYs attributable to various risk factors		
	Low- and middle-income countries	High-income countries	World
High blood pressure	44%	48%	45%
High cholesterol	46%	57%	48%
Low fruit and vegetable intake	30%	19%	28%
Physical inactivity	21%	21%	21%
Overweight and obesity	16%	27%	18%
Smoking	15%	23%	17%

(Lopez *et al.*, 2006.)

B (i.e. I and II). Some disease will still occur, however, as a result of sufficient cause III.

The causes of many diseases, and especially those like cancer that develop over many years, are going to be complex and we may never identify all their components. It is thus encouraging to know that by just identifying one or two we may still prevent a large proportion of the disease. If we could have stopped any one of the animals, even the mouse, from getting into the boat then it would not have turned over at that point in time. However, if the wind blew up or a wave came along once they had pushed off then they may have sunk later: a different sufficient cause leading to a similar outcome. Searching for modifiable causes that are associated with a large population attributable risk, i.e. ones which cause a large number of cases of disease, will give the greatest benefit in terms of public health. (We will take this up again in Chapter 14.)

Look at Table 10.1. The population attributable risks for ischaemic heart disease sum to more than 100%. Why is this so? Is it a problem?

If we assume that each of the causes of ischaemic heart disease shown can be represented by one of the letters in Figure 10.1 (for example, if low fruit and vegetable intake were cause 'A', overweight and obesity were cause 'B' and smoking were cause 'C'), we can immediately see that the total amount of disease attributable to each component cause will be much greater than 100%. Ensuring that everyone had adequate fruit and vegetable intake (i.e. removing cause 'A') would prevent all disease due to sufficient causes I, II and III. However, if we have already removed the problem of obesity and overweight (cause 'B') and so prevented disease due to sufficient causes I and II, then the extra benefit of improving fruit and vegetable intake could only prevent the extra disease due to sufficient cause III. Similarly, although stopping everyone smoking would prevent some disease on its own, once we have removed the problems of diet and obesity it would have little extra benefit.

In thinking about how component causes might act together, we need to keep in mind that in no sense need they be similar: one component might be the absence of a protective factor and another the presence of a quite different harmful factor. For instance, if we consider the underlying causes of lung cancer we would probably find that cigarette smoke is a component in most sufficient causes. However, since not all smokers develop lung cancer we can surmise that smoking is not a sufficient cause on its own but also requires other factors (for example weakened DNA-repair capacity) to complete a sufficient cause. Similarly, since lung cancer can develop in the absence of smoking, we can presume that there is at least one sufficient cause that does not have personal smoking as a component cause.

Association versus causation

In preceding chapters we have considered how we can determine whether a particular exposure is *associated* with the outcome of interest. The next stage is to determine whether such an association may be causal. Just because a particular exposure is associated with the development of a disease does not automatically imply cause and effect. We must attempt to draw appropriate causal inferences explicitly from our data, in the light of other evidence.

In London during the cholera epidemics of the nineteenth century one common belief, the 'miasma' theory, was that cholera was caused by noxious vapours in the air. While John Snow was conducting his pioneering work implicating contaminated water, William Farr, director of the Office of the Registrar General, was also interested in the transmission of cholera. He had noticed that cholera mortality seemed to be higher in lower-lying areas and so collected mortality data for a number of districts in London at different elevations. This revealed a dramatic inverse relation between elevation and mortality and Farr was able to calculate a formula that could accurately predict the mortality rate for any given elevation. Figure 10.2 shows a graph of actual cholera death rates for various levels of elevation above the River Thames as well as the death rates predicted by Farr's theory. These data were taken as strong evidence in favour of the miasma theory, under which it was felt that the vapours would be most concentrated and, therefore, most dangerous at lower elevations.

However, as you saw in Chapter 3, like most ecological research (the graph compares rates of cholera in areas at various elevations, not individual data), these observations provide weak evidence for a true causal association, and we

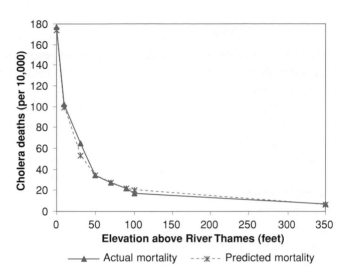

Figure 10.2 Actual (——) and predicted (- - - -) cholera death rates at various levels of elevation above the River Thames in London, England, 1849. (Data source: Farr, 1852.)

must consider whether other differences between people living at different elevations could explain them. As it happened, people living closest to the river were also more likely to be exposed to contaminated water than their neighbours in the higher areas. This confounding factor could explain the apparent association between elevation and cholera mortality entirely, and today it is John Snow, not William Farr, whom we recognise as having solved the mystery of cholera. Ironically, in trying to prove his own 'airborne' theory, Farr also provided much of the crucial evidence that ultimately supported Snow's theory of contaminated water.

This example highlights the necessity of not accepting the results of any study, however exciting, at face value. There are two substantial steps to be taken before we can reasonably promote an exposure–disease relation as warranting serious attention with respect to disease control. We must first thoroughly consider alternative non-causal explanations for an association: could it be an artefact due to chance, bias or confounding? We need to apply the approach outlined in Chapter 9 to decide whether the results we are looking at (our own or those reported by someone else) are believable. In the cholera example we have postulated that confounding by water supply is the most likely explanation for the close association seen in Figure 10.2, and that the relation with elevation is an artefact. If, however, the answer to the question 'Is it real?' is at least a qualified 'yes' then we can move on to the next step – a formal evaluation of whether the observed relation could be causal.

Evaluating causation

How should we do this? The nature of causation has been a central theme of philosophy for centuries (see Box 10.2) and in recent times has been given a fair

Box 10.2 Some potted philosophy

Do we learn about the world from observation and experience or by reason? This was the major tension in Western causal thinking for many centuries. Broadly speaking, observation or learning from our own experience (*induction*) gradually replaced more abstract reasoning about how the world worked (*deduction*). The practical inductive approach fits pretty well with public health and epidemiology – we collect facts, decide what they mean and then act accordingly – but, of course, it is not perfect. Starting with David Hume in eighteenth-century Scotland, many philosophers have demonstrated that induction can never *prove* a cause-and-effect relationship (this became known as Hume's problem). Just because we observe that the computer turns on the first 99 times we press the button does not mean that it will turn on again the 100th time (we are all familiar with this phenomenon). Final proof is thus unobtainable by this process. In Europe in the middle decades of the twentieth century, Karl Popper in a sense turned Hume's problem around and said that, although induction based on supportive observations could never finally *confirm* a hypothesis, contrary data could be used to *refute* one. Consider the statement 'all swans are white'. We may see only white swans but can never prove that this statement is true – it just takes one black swan to disprove it. The hypothesis can stand only until we see that one black swan.

We will never know anything with absolute certainty and this is something we must learn to live with comfortably. You will note that the subsequent guidelines to causal reasoning incorporate both judgement and probabilistic elements – implying that we do not demand certainty. If we did we would

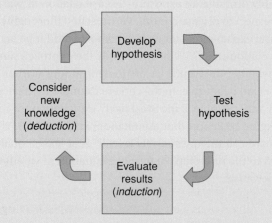

Figure 10.3 An integrated cycle of causal reasoning.

(continued)

Box 10.2 (*continued*)

never act, the antithesis of the remit of public health. In pursuit of making good judgements on how and when to act, epidemiologists have long sought to bring good evidence to bear on a question. In the past decade or so this has come into sharper focus with research increasingly aiming to test critical elements of causal belief or hypothesis along the lines proposed by Popper and his followers last century. This has led to an integrated cycle of causal reasoning that essentially combines both induction and deduction (Figure 10.3).

bit of attention by epidemiologists. This has given a useful perspective on thinking about how we operate, but epidemiologists are fundamentally pragmatic and seek practical tools. Unfortunately, in the causal realm our tools are not as precise as we might like and views on how to apply them differ somewhat.

Various sets of guidelines have been proposed to assist our causal evaluations. There are many similarities among them, and arguably the best known – certainly the best written – were set forth by a British statistician, Sir Austin Bradford Hill, in an after-dinner speech. He put forward a list of nine aspects of an association to be considered when assessing whether it was likely to be causal (Hill, 1965). He was adamant that these should serve only as '*aids to thought*' and were not absolute requirements to be met before an exposure could be considered to cause a disease. Various modifications of this list have been suggested, and many of the elements remain cornerstones of judgement on whether an exposure really does cause a disease, or whether an intervention is effective in preventing or treating disease. These elements are discussed below.

Temporality

For an exposure to cause a disease it must precede the development of the disease. This might seem obvious, but in some instances, say for a condition like cancer that is often present for many years before diagnosis, it can be difficult to decide whether an exposure really did occur before the true origin of disease. If we find that people with stomach cancer have lower levels of vitamin C in their blood than those without stomach cancer, can we be sure that the low levels of vitamin C really preceded the growth of the cancer? Or might the lower vitamin C levels be a result of the disease process? As you will recall from Chapter 4, these questions can frequently be answered only by performing cohort studies and, even then, it may be difficult to establish the order of exposure and effect with certainty. *Of all Bradford Hill's factors this is the only one that is an absolute requirement.*

Figure 10.4 The relation
between higher egg
consumption and ovarian cancer
risk in five population-based
studies. The squares represent
the relative risk, with the size
of the square being proportional
to the size of the study, and the
horizontal lines represent the
95% confidence intervals. The
open diamond represents the
relative risk and 95% confidence
interval from all five studies
combined.

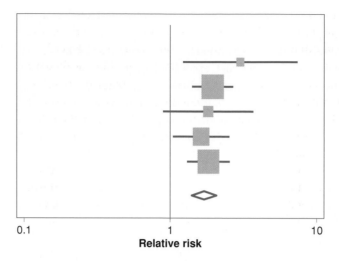

Strength of association

The stronger an association is (usually as described by the relative effect, OR or RR), the less likely it is to be due solely to either bias or confounding. A strong association is thus more suggestive that the effect is real. However, just because a relation is weak does not mean that it cannot be causal: only that it is harder to eliminate study error as a possible explanation for the apparent effect.

What constitutes a 'weak' or a 'strong' effect? There is no universal agreement on this but we would generally consider an effect (OR, RR) greater than 2.0 to be moderately strong and an effect greater than 5.0 to be strong. Note, however, that a small effect observed consistently in many studies, especially if these are of different designs and performed in different settings, may well give stronger evidence of causality than an effect that is strong in one or two studies but not found in others (see 'Consistency' below, and Chapter 11). It is important not to be too dismissive of 'weak' effects, since these can be of great public health importance when the exposure is common and the consequences severe.

Consistency

An effect found consistently across a range of studies of different types and/or in different populations gives some reassurance that it is not an artefact. An Australian ovarian cancer case–control study found an association between higher egg consumption and ovarian cancer (Pirozzo *et al.*, 2002). This seemed unlikely to be a real effect, but a literature search showed that all four population-based studies that had previously looked at this had also reported an increase in risk of ovarian cancer among women who ate more eggs (Figure 10.4).

Figure 10.4 summarises the data neatly and accurately. If we look first at the square boxes that represent the relative risks, we see that, while there is some variability, all are greater than 1.0 and in four the association is statistically significant (i.e. their 95% confidence intervals do not cross 1.0). When the data from all five studies were combined the overall 'pooled' RR was 1.9 (95% confidence interval 1.5–2.3), suggesting that there was an almost two-fold increase in risk among women who ate the most eggs. The results are, therefore, quite consistent and so increase belief that the association between eggs (or some component of, or contaminant in, eggs) and ovarian cancer might be causal. (Note: more recent studies have not seen an association between egg consumption and ovarian cancer, suggesting that these earlier results could have been due to chance, despite the consistency across several studies. It is also possible that eggs nowadays are less likely to be contaminated by, for example, pesticide residues than they were in the past and this could potentially explain the different results.)

However, lack of consistency need not in itself rule out causality. Differing results could reflect variation in study design or quality, or an exposure could have a different effect in people with a different genetic make-up or with different exposures to other factors that might modify (interact with) the possible cause of interest. In any review of a topic it is important to give thoughtful consideration to why studies might give different results (heterogeneity); we will discuss reviews further in Chapter 11.

Dose–response relationships

If a factor does cause a disease, then the risk of developing the disease is likely to be related to the amount or 'dose' of exposure. This is often a function of both *level* and *duration of exposure*. Figure 10.5 shows some data from the first eight years of follow-up of the US Nurses' Health Study. The investigators calculated the age-adjusted relative risk that a woman would develop type-2 diabetes on the basis of her body-mass index (BMI; weight/height^2) and found that the risk of diabetes increased dramatically with increasing body size, particularly for women with a BMI greater than 25 kg/m^2 (the upper limit of what is usually considered to be 'normal'). Among the heaviest women, those with BMI of 35 kg/m^2 or greater, the risk of diabetes was almost 60 times that of women with BMI less than 22 kg/m^2. Similarly, we saw that the risk of lung cancer increases sharply with increasing numbers of cigarettes smoked (Figure 1.1). Patterns of relative risk like these add credence to the idea that an association is causal. Note, however, that measurement of dose is not always straightforward. In the British Doctors Study discussed in previous chapters, Doll and Hill used a simple measure of dose of smoking, namely 'average number of cigarettes smoked per day'. This clearly worked very well, but does not capture other important information such as the number of years that someone has smoked. These days this additional information would almost always be included in any assessment of effects of

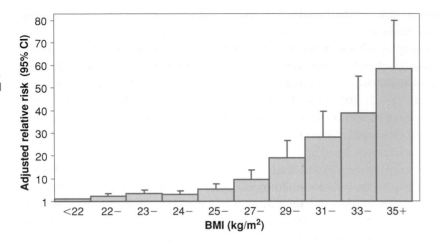

Figure 10.5 Age-adjusted relative risks and 95% confidence intervals for type-2 diabetes in relation to body-mass index. (From: Colditz *et al.*, Weight as a risk factor for clinical diabetes in women. *Am. J. Epidemiol.*, 1990; 132: 505, reprinted by permission of the Society for Epidemiological Research.)

smoking, often in a combined variable called 'pack-years', where one pack-year is equivalent to smoking 20 cigarettes a day for 1 year (or 10 cigarettes a day for 2 years, etc.).

Of course, some genuine cause-and-effect relationships will not give such a regular pattern. For instance, there may be a 'threshold' effect, whereby any exposure above a certain level will lead to disease. A dose–response relationship can therefore add weight to an evaluation of causality but its absence need not count against making a causal link.

Biological plausibility

A causal hypothesis should obviously be viewed in the light of its plausibility. If there is a likely biological mechanism through which an exposure might cause the disease, this can add substantial weight to a causal argument. Lack of plausibility does not necessarily rule out causality, because increasing knowledge of disease mechanisms may make an association appear more credible in time. The characteristic of plausibility is also tempered by the realisation that scientists are ingenious by nature and can probably come up with a plausible-sounding hypothesis in most situations if they believe an association to be causal!

Specificity

Bradford Hill presented this concept somewhat less clearly than the others on his list – he suggested that, if an association were limited to a specific outcome, then this would argue in favour of causation. He went on to say that this characteristic should not be over-emphasised because factors could cause more than one disease and diseases might have more than one cause. This concept was crudely interpreted as 'one cause – one disease' in attempts to argue that cigarette smoking did not cause lung cancer: cigarettes were linked to many different diseases, therefore their effects were not specific, therefore they caused none of them.

When we recall that many diseases are based on similar underlying patholo-gies (e.g. vascular diseases of the brain, heart and other organs frequently stem from atherosclerosis) it is hardly surprising that a single exposure (e.g. a high-fat diet) can be linked to a variety of different conditions. Nonetheless, we would still not expect an exposure to be linked to *all* outcomes; thus there must be some degree of specificity that we can use to inform an evaluation of causality (Weiss, 2002). For example, bicycle helmets would be expected to reduce the risk of head injury but not of other types of injury (specificity of outcome). If results of stud-ies suggested that helmet use did indeed reduce the risk of injuries to the head only, then this would strengthen belief that it was a causal (or in this case pro-tective) association. An association seen only for one particular type of analgesic (as in the Phenacetin study described in Box 4.4) could again strengthen belief in causality (specificity of exposure). Similarly, individuals might be susceptible to an exposure only if they have a particular genetic make-up, so, if the relation is seen only for those with the specific genotype (specificity of susceptibility), then belief in causality is again strengthened.

Pulling it all together

Bradford Hill also suggested that consideration should be given to any **exper-imental data** – these could come from studies in animals or other organisms or from intervention studies in humans. Such evidence in humans is crucial to assessing the benefits of interventions. The final two characteristics that he put forward are sensible but of less direct help than the others: **coherence** – a cause-and-effect interpretation should not conflict with the known facts; and **analogy** to existing known causal associations. An additional aspect to consider is that, if a relation is causal, then removal of the exposure should lead to a reduction in the effect – as was seen in the time trends of cigarette sales and lung cancer mortality in Figure 3.6.

Consideration of these issues can help us decide whether an association is likely to be causal. Sometimes the decision may be clear cut, but it is equally likely to be controversial, and in this situation there can be no 'right' answer. It is important to remember that these elements do not provide an infallible check-list that will lead to the correct decision. Rather, they provide a framework for an evaluation of causality.

Bradford Hill (Hill, 1965) summarised the questions that should guide a con-sideration of causality as follows:

Is there any other way of explaining the set of facts before us, is there any other answer equally, or more likely than cause and effect?

Evaluating causality in practice: does *H. pylori* cause stomach cancer?

You have seen in earlier chapters that there appears to be a link between infection with *H. pylori* (a bacterium that infects the stomach) and stomach cancer rates. Now let us consider whether this relation might be causal. Many case–control studies have been conducted to evaluate this, but these are fraught with problems, in particular because people with stomach cancer may test negative for *H. pylori* even if they have been infected in the past. As a result there is the potential for differential misclassification of cases as *H. pylori*-negative, thereby biasing the odds ratio towards the null. Cohort studies are impractical because of the logistics of testing thousands of cohort members for *H. pylori*. The best evidence therefore comes from well-designed *nested case–control studies* (see Chapter 4) in which blood samples were collected prior to the diagnosis of cancer. In 2001, a group pooled the data from all 12 such studies to evaluate this association (*Helicobacter* and Cancer Collaborative Group, 2001). (We will discuss *pooled* studies further in Chapter 11.) In all of the studies the cases and controls were matched for age and sex and there were no other major confounders; there were also no obvious sources of selection or measurement bias. Authors of all 12 studies reported an increased risk of stomach cancer associated with infection, which was statistically significant (i.e. unlikely to be due to chance) in nine. The odds ratio from all 12 studies combined was 2.4 (95% CI 2.0–2.8).

So could the relation be causal? The association is quite *strong* and also *consistent* across these better studies. In all of them the blood samples used for testing for *H. pylori* were collected before diagnosis of cancer, suggesting that infection does indeed *precede* cancer. Since, by and large, someone is either infected or not infected, it is not possible to look for a *dose–response* relationship, but the association appears to be fairly *specific* for stomach cancer and laboratory studies have shown that some types of *H. pylori* may be more carcinogenic than others. Further *experimental evidence* comes from studies that have shown that *H. pylori* infection induces cancer in some animal models. A relation is also biologically *plausible* because the bacterial infection directly affects the stomach, which is where the cancer occurs. Taken together, there is thus good evidence for the conclusion, now widely accepted, that *H. pylori* infection is indeed a cause of stomach cancer.

And then what?

Once a cause-and-effect association has been established beyond any reasonable doubt, action can be taken to change public policy, legislation, health education, clinical practice or the direction of research. Thalidomide is no longer given to women during pregnancy because it causes birth defects;

diethylstilboestrol is no longer prescribed to prevent miscarriage because it can cause vaginal cancer in the women's daughters; dietary advice and drugs are used to lower cholesterol levels to prevent heart disease; the hazards of smoking are publicised, and legislation restricting smoking in public has been enacted in many countries; seat-belt wearing is becoming ubiquitous internationally – the list goes on.

It is worth noting that it has taken a long time, decades even, to establish causality for some of these associations. Although wholly reliable criteria for truly establishing causality do not exist, modern society often demands rapid 'proof', increasingly for legal rather than social or health reasons. This tension between the desire for full knowledge and the social need for action is a given in public health. The clearer our insight into the evidence the better our judgements will be. Remember, however, that we are all fallible and absolute proof is impossible.

So, to conclude, if we had stopped the mouse from jumping into the boat (i.e. removed one component cause) it would not have overturned at that precise point in time (we would have prevented that particular outcome). But who is to say what would have happened if the other animals had ventured out into the rougher water in the middle of the lake ...

REFERENCES

Allen, P. (1983). *Who Sank the Boat?* Thomas Nelson Australia. Republished by Penguin Books Australia Ltd., 1998.

Farr, W. (1852). Influence of elevation on the fatality of cholera. *Journal of the Statistical Society London*, **15**: 155–183.

Helicobacter and Cancer Collaborative Group. (2001). Gastric cancer and *Helicobacter pylori*: a combined analysis of 12 case–control studies nested within prospective cohorts. *Gut*, **49**: 347–353.

Hill, A. B. (1965). The environment and disease: association or causation? *Proceedings of the Royal Society for Medicine*, **58**: 295–300.

Lopez, A. D., Mathers, C. D., Ezzati, M. *et al.* (Eds) (2006). *Global Burden of Disease and Risk Factors*. World Bank and Oxford University Press.

Pirozzo, S., Purdie, D., Kuiper-Linley, M. *et al.* (2002). Ovarian cancer, cholesterol and eggs: a case–control analysis. *Cancer Epidemiology Biomarkers and Prevention*, **11**: 1112–1114.

Rothman, K. J. (1976). Causes. *American Journal of Epidemiology*, **104**: 587–592.

Rothman, K. J. (1986). *Modern Epidemiology*. Boston: Little Brown & Co.

Weiss, N. S. (2002). Can the "specificity" of an association be rehabilitated as a basis for supporting a causal hypothesis? *Epidemiology*, **13**: 6–8.

11

Assembling the building blocks: reviews and their uses

Description	Association	Alternative explanations	Integration & interpretation	Practical applications
Chapters 2–3	Chapters 4–5	Chapters 6–8	Chapter 11: Reviews	Chapters 12–15

While it is important to be able to read and interpret individual papers, the results of a single study are never going to provide the complete answer to a question. To move towards this we need to review the literature more widely. There can be a number of reasons for doing this, some of which require a more comprehensive approach than others. If the aim is simply to increase our personal understanding of a new area then a few papers might provide adequate background material. Traditional *narrative reviews*, which give less emphasis to complete coverage of the literature and tend to be more qualitative, have value for exploring areas of uncertainty or novelty, but it is harder to scrutinise them for flaws. In contrast, a major policy decision might require a *systematic review* of all the relevant literature. We will focus on the systematic approach here, but this can of course be tailored according to need.

What is a systematic review?

Like a primary research paper, an epidemiological review should aim to produce a helpful synthesis of primary data – looking for patterns but not hiding differences – and it should normally offer a formal causal interpretation. Although its primary data units are whole studies rather than individuals, the review process should have the same rigour as its component studies. A **systematic review** should be a response to a clearly formulated question and involve the identification of *all* relevant primary research studies that address that question. Each study found should be included or excluded according to predetermined selection criteria, and critically appraised. The findings should then be summarised and appropriate conclusions drawn. In some situations this process can be taken one step further by combining the results of the component studies in a **meta-analysis**. An even more rigorous approach, known as a **pooled analysis** or re-analysis, is to obtain the original data from all relevant studies and re-analyse them as a single large study.

It follows from this that such a review should be structured in the same way as a primary paper: an *introduction* to show why the research question is of interest; a *methods* section to explain how studies were identified, included/excluded and appraised, and how the data were abstracted; the *results*, where patterns are highlighted and differences assessed; and, finally, a *discussion*, where the results are interpreted, threats to validity considered and conclusions drawn.

So how should we go about conducting a systematic review? Box 11.1 shows a condensed excerpt from the methods section of a review of the benefits of a low-fat diet for weight loss (Pirozzo *et al.*, 2003), and gives a sense of the detailed approach required. The following summary focuses on the various stages of the review process as a guide to both reading and writing a systematic review, but we stress that this is an overview of the main principles and methods; more detailed 'how to' manuals are fairly widely available (e.g. Glasziou *et al.*, 2001).

Identifying the literature

The first challenge when conducting a systematic review is to identify all of the relevant literature. The potential sources of data are numerous. MEDLINE

Box 11.1 Should we recommend low-fat diets for obesity?

Research question

To determine the effectiveness of low-fat diets in achieving sustained weight loss in obese or overweight people.

Search strategy

The following sources were included in the literature-searching process: The Cochrane Library (Issue 2, 2001), MEDLINE, EMBASE, the Science Citation Index, bibliographies and handsearching. The original searches of MEDLINE and EMBASE were conducted from the beginning of each database until January 2001. The search was updated in February 2002. The references of all relevant studies were searched in the Science Citation Index to identify any additional trials.

Trial selection

The titles and abstracts of the records identified were independently screened by two investigators. Articles were rejected if the reviewers determined from the title and abstract that the study (a) was not a report of a randomised controlled trial, (b) did not address a low-fat diet, (c) did not have a follow-up period that was at least 6 months in duration, or (d) concerned persons less than 18 years old. When a title/abstract could not be rejected with certainty, the full text of the article was obtained for further evaluation. The full text of all selected articles was examined independently by two investigators to identify all relevant trials. Differences in opinion were resolved by consensus.

Quality assessment of trials

The trials were assessed independently by two investigators using specific quality criteria related to the following aspects of study methodology:
(1) randomisation and concealment of allocation;
(2) blinding of caregivers, participants and, in particular, outcome assessors; and
(3) follow-up and intention-to-treat analysis.
Trials were categorised according to the extent to which they met the quality criteria:
  A = all criteria met,
  B = one or more criteria only partially met and
  C = one or more criteria not met.

Data extraction

Three reviewers independently extracted data from the studies, with any differences resolved by the fourth reviewer. A specially developed data-extraction form was used. This form incorporated general trial information, trial characteristics, details of the intervention, patient-selection procedures and characteristics of sample, study outcomes and results.

(Excerpted from Pirozzo *et al.*, 2003.)

is probably the most commonly used source for epidemiological papers, but only about one-third of the approximately 10 million medical articles on library shelves are indexed in the MEDLINE database (which is freely accessible through the US National Library of Medicine search engine PubMed at www.ncbi.nlm.nih.gov/pubmed/). EMBASE® is not so widely available but has some advantages over MEDLINE in that it includes many additional journals as well as conference abstracts. Another valuable database, particularly for systematic reviews of trials of the effects of healthcare interventions, is that of the Cochrane Collaboration (www.cochrane.org). There are also many other electronic databases that may be valuable sources of literature depending on the question you are researching (e.g. CANCERLIT® and PSYCHLIT each have an obvious specialised focus).

No electronic literature search is ever likely to be complete, so it is important to use multiple strategies. Once several relevant articles have been identified, it can help to check the papers that they cite, and also to look in the other direction, i.e. for papers that have cited them (e.g. using the Science Citation Index). Other sources include personal communication with experts in the field who may know of additional published articles (and unpublished material); theses, seminars, internal reports and non-peer-reviewed journals (sometimes described as the 'grey literature'); and other electronic information including topic-specific internet databases.

Publication and related biases

When searching the literature it is important to bear in mind that studies with positive and/or statistically significant findings may be more likely to be published than those without significant results. This *publication bias* is related not only to selective acceptance by journals but also to selective submission to journals by researchers who may decide not to submit reports from research that either finds no association at all (i.e. a null finding) or in which the results are not statistically significant.

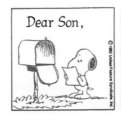 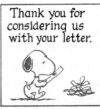 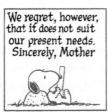 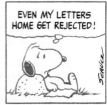

Closely related to publication bias are the problems of preferential detection of articles in English and studies with overlapping publications on the same topic. For an English speaker there are several barriers to the inclusion of non-English studies in a review, including the difficulties associated with translation and the

Table 11.1 System commonly used to classify levels of evidence.

Level	Evidence
I	Evidence from at least one properly randomised controlled trial
II-1	Evidence from well-designed controlled trials without randomisation
II-2	Evidence from well-designed cohort or case–control studies, preferably from more than one centre or research group
II-3	Evidence from comparisons over time or between places with or without the intervention; dramatic results in uncontrolled experiments could also be regarded as this level of evidence
III	Opinions of respected authorities, based on clinical experience, descriptive studies and case reports, or reports of expert committees

(Harris *et al.*, 2001.)

fact that non-English articles may be published in local journals that are not indexed by major bibliographic databases. This is also more likely to be the case for less exciting findings. A less-recognised problem is that of multiple but apparently unrelated publications from one study with (usually) positive results. Such a study is more likely to be identified than those published only once (or with all papers clearly from the one source) and, if included as separate studies in the review, could lead to overestimation of an association.

Different types of study

The amount and types of literature generated by a search will vary enormously depending on the subject area. For a review of a specific treatment the studies may all be clinical trials, whereas an aetiological review is likely to include observational studies of all types from case reports to cohort studies, with few or no trials. As you have seen, different types of study answer different types of questions, or may be subject to different biases when answering the same question, so it is sensible to group them separately, at least to start with. This grouping may then provide a logical framework to help organise the data within the review.

A common approach to grading the quality of individual studies has been to classify study designs according to a hierarchy such that those at the top are considered to provide stronger evidence of an effect than those further down the scale (Table 11.1). You will notice that this ranking puts randomised trials at the top of the pile. (Variations of this scheme include yet another layer at the top for systematic reviews of randomised controlled trials as the 'ultimate' evidence.) While a classification of this type may be appropriate in the clinical context where RCTs are the norm, a ranking based largely on evidence from trials is often not much help for an aetiological review. In 2003, the British Medical

Journal published an entertaining systematic review of randomised controlled trials of 'parachute use to prevent death and major trauma related to gravitational challenge' (Smith and Pell, 2003). Not surprisingly, the authors failed to find any randomised trials for this particular preventive intervention. The BMJ is well known for publishing more light-hearted articles in its Christmas issue but, despite the tongue-in-cheek nature of the report, the fact remains that not all interventions can be evaluated in RCTs and a lack of RCT evidence does not mean a lack of evidence. Even more important is the disregard for the quality of individual studies inherent in this approach. A well-designed and properly conducted cohort or case–control study could provide better evidence than a small or poorly conducted trial, but this rigid hierarchy would rate the evidence from the trial more highly. The need to move away from such a rigid approach has been well documented both for clinical research (Glasziou *et al.*, 2004) and for health services research in general (Black, 1996).

A preferable approach, adopted by decision-making bodies around the world such as the US Preventive Services Task Force (USPSTF) and the Canadian Task Force on Preventive Health Care (CTFPHC), is not to classify studies purely on the basis of their *design* but also according to the *quality of the evidence* they provide. As its name suggests, the USPSTF regularly reviews the evidence for and against a wide range of preventive interventions. They rate studies according to specific criteria for that design (based on the key questions of subject selection and measurement that we discussed earlier). A 'good' study would generally meet all of the specified criteria, a 'fair' study does not meet them all but is judged not to have a fatal flaw that would invalidate the results, and a fatally flawed study is classified as 'poor' (Harris *et al.*, 2001). We have examined specific quality issues for the various designs in earlier chapters (Chapters 4 and 7), and Box 11.2 considers the value of randomised and non-randomised designs in healthcare evaluation in more detail. (An additional marker of better study quality that appealed to us was the inclusion of an epidemiologist or statistician among the authors of a research paper (Delgado-Rodriguez *et al.*, 2001)!)

Study inclusion, appraisal and data abstraction

Studies should be selected for inclusion in the review on the basis of pre-defined criteria. Depending on the research question, it might be appropriate to restrict the review to specific research designs, for example only randomised trials, or to those with specific methodological features. Such features might include

- the study size (e.g. only those studies with more than a certain number of cases)
- the participants (e.g. a specific age range or sex)
- a specific outcome or the way in which outcome was measured (e.g. histological or serological confirmation)

Box 11.2 Randomisation versus observation

Most generic lists rank RCTs first in terms of study quality. For appropriate questions, i.e. about the effects of various interventions, this is reasonable, as you have seen. However, even for such questions caveats need to be applied. If a randomised trial is not competently conducted, or is too small, then its theoretical advantages disappear, and it can give misleading results (Schultz *et al.*, 1995). There are also many situations in which a trial would be unfeasible, unethical, undesirable or unnecessary (Black, 1996), and trials are generally irrelevant for questions related to frequency or measurement validation (e.g. of the performance of a screening or diagnostic test).

Estimates of the effects of treatment may differ between randomised and non-randomised studies, but when direct comparisons have been made neither method has consistently given a greater effect than the other (McKee *et al.*, 1999). Overall, it seems that dissimilarities between the participants in RCTs and non-randomised studies explain many of the differences; the two methods should therefore be compared only after patients not meeting the RCT eligibility criteria have also been excluded from the non-randomised study. Not surprisingly then, treatment effects measured in randomised and non-randomised studies are most similar when the exclusion criteria are the same and where potential prognostic factors are well understood and controlled for in the non-randomised setting. Taking this approach has helped reconcile some of the apparently major differences between the effects of hormone replacement therapy (HRT) as found in RCTs (evidence of harm) and cohort studies (evidence of health benefits). Closer consideration of the details of the different studies suggests that differences in the ages at which women started taking HRT – around menopause (average age 51 years in the USA) in the cohort studies but at a mean age of more than 60 years in the trials – could explain many of the differences (Manson and Bassuk, 2007). It is also important to consider the precision of the RCT effect estimates – some are based on so few events (especially when death is the outcome of interest) that chance differences from the true underlying effect are quite likely. (For an example of these issues from studies comparing the effectiveness of various interventions to unblock coronary arteries see Britton *et al.* (1998).)

The **generalisability** (see Chapter 7) of the results of RCTs can also be questionable, given the highly selected nature of the participants: patients excluded from randomised controlled trials tend to have a worse prognosis than those included (McKee *et al.*, 1999). When both randomised and non-randomised studies have been conducted and estimates of treatment effect are reasonably consistent for patients at similar risk, it allows more certain generalisation to the broader target populations of the non-randomised studies.

- the way in which exposure was measured or classified (e.g. a specific blood test to measure an infection, more than two levels of alcohol intake) and
- the duration of follow-up (e.g. more than 12 months).

The validity of studies that meet the criteria should then be evaluated as outlined in Chapter 9, and key information on design, conduct, potential for error and results abstracted onto purpose-designed forms. In an ideal world the appraisers should be blinded to the authors and the study results since this knowledge has been shown to influence judgements about validity. In practice this is not always possible, since the reviewers may already be too familiar with the literature. Rigorous systematic reviews of clinical interventions, such as those conducted through the Cochrane Collaboration, will often specify the need for multiple assessors to reduce the potential for bias, but this level of rigour is less common (and perhaps of limited added value) for aetiological reviews.

Summarising the data

The next step in any review is to draw the data together to simplify their interpretation and to assist in drawing valid conclusions. It is important to look both for consistency of effects across studies (homogeneity) and for differences between studies (heterogeneity). Could differences be due to chance variation or can they be explained by features of the studies or the populations they were conducted in? Graphs can be used to summarise the results of many studies in a simple format and in some situations the technique of **meta-analysis** can be used to combine the results from a number of different studies.

Graphical display of results

One way to display the results of a number of different studies is in a figure called a **forest plot**. Figure 11.1 shows a forest plot from a systematic review of the relation between weight/BMI and ovarian cancer risk (Purdie *et al.*, 2001). It shows the results of all 23 case–control studies whose authors had reported data on this association, ordered with the most recent study at the top and the oldest at the bottom. The odds ratio for each individual study is represented by the black square, with the size of the square indicating the size (or 'weight' – see *Meta-analysis* below) of that particular study. The horizontal bar through each box shows the 95% confidence interval for the odds ratio and the vertical line indicates the point where there is 'no effect', i.e. an odds ratio of 1.0. When the confidence interval crosses this line (i.e. it includes the null value) it indicates that the result is not statistically significant (i.e. $p \geq 0.05$). (Note the use of the logarithmic scale, which balances positive and inverse relative effects visually

Figure 11.1 Diagrammatic representation of the results of 23 case–control studies evaluating the relation between extremes of weight/BMI and ovarian cancer risk (Purdie *et al.*, 2001).

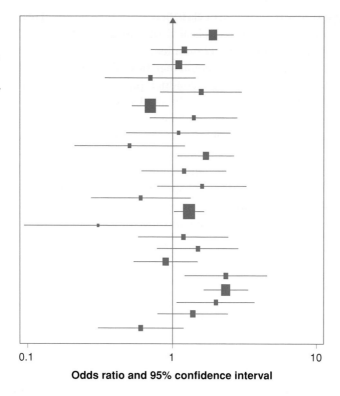

Odds ratio and 95% confidence interval

around the null; i.e. an OR of 2.0 would be the same distance from 1.0 as an OR of 0.5 in the opposite direction.)

Assessing heterogeneity

In this example the results of the 23 studies are scattered both sides of the line that marks an odds ratio of 1.0 (i.e. no effect), and they show no obvious pattern. The next step should be to evaluate this *heterogeneity* in more detail. Are there any differences between the studies that could explain some of the variation in their results?

One major methodological difference between the studies in this example is subject selection: some were population-based and others were hospital-based. We touched on some of the problems inherent in hospital-based studies in earlier chapters – could this difference explain any of the variation in the study results? Other possibilities to consider might include the geographical areas where the research was done – for example, separating high- and low-risk countries, and the ages of the participants. In this case, if we separate the hospital- and population-based studies (Figure 11.2) we start to see some regularity. In each of the 11 population-based studies at the bottom of Figure 11.2, the OR is

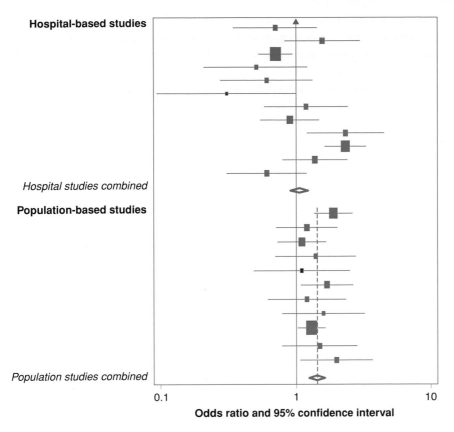

Figure 11.2 Diagrammatic representation of the results of 12 hospital-based and 11 population-based case–control studies evaluating the relation between extremes of weight/BMI and ovarian cancer risk (Purdie *et al.*, 2001).

greater than 1.0 (although many of the individual results are not statistically significant), suggesting that obesity/higher weight is associated with an increased risk of ovarian cancer. In contrast, the results of the hospital studies still vary widely. In this situation it was felt that using hospital-based controls might not be appropriate, since their use might well lead to overestimation of the prevalence of obesity in the population and thereby lead to underestimation of the obesity–cancer association.

Meta-analysis

Meta-analysis is a powerful technique that allows the results of a number of different studies to be combined. Each study is assigned a weight based on the amount of information it provides (e.g. the inverse of the standard error of the OR) and in general larger studies have greater weight. A weighted average of the individual study results can then be calculated. The assumption underlying this analysis is that all of the studies are estimating the same underlying effect and any variation between their results is due to chance. If their results are very different (i.e. they are *heterogeneous*), as in the hospital-based studies of BMI above, then this assumption may not be true and it might not be appropriate to combine the results.

The diamond at the bottom of Figure 11.2 represents the combined odds ratio for the 11 population-based studies; the centre indicates the point estimate and the ends show the 95% confidence interval. In this case, it indicates that being overweight increases the risk of ovarian cancer by 40% (pooled OR = 1.4; 95% CI 1.2–1.6). Notice that the diamond does not overlap the 'no-effect' line (i.e. the confidence interval does not include 1.0), so the pooled OR is statistically significant. If we draw a dotted line vertically through the combined odds ratio, it passes through the 95% confidence interval of each of the individual studies. This is an indication that the results of the studies are fairly *homogeneous*, but it is certainly not definitive. In this case a formal statistical test for heterogeneity gives a p-value of 0.63. If p were < 0.05, this would suggest that differences between the results of the individual studies were unlikely to be due to chance; however, the observed p-value is well away from this, suggesting there is no significant heterogeneity and thus supporting the 'eyeball' finding that the results are all fairly similar.

In contrast, if we combine the results of the 12 hospital-based studies, we find a combined OR of 0.9 (95% CI 0.9–1.2), but a line through this point would not pass through the confidence intervals of the individual studies. This suggests that the results of the hospital-based studies are heterogeneous, and this is confirmed by a statistical test for heterogeneity, which gives $p < 0.001$, which is highly statistically significant. In this situation it is inappropriate to combine the results into a single estimate of effect.

As we discussed in Chapter 5, absolute measures of effect such as the **attributable risk**, **absolute risk reduction** and **number needed to treat** can provide a better sense of the practical impact or clinical importance of an exposure–outcome relation than a relative measure. Combining these absolute measures from studies conducted in very different populations can, however, be problematic, since they will usually depend on the baseline risk in a population, and this may vary widely. For this reason, relative effect measures (OR or RR) are usually used to summarise the evidence, and then applied to the relevant baseline rate to show the predicted absolute difference.

Pooled analysis

A pooled analysis goes one step further than a meta-analysis. Instead of combining the summary results (OR or RR) from a number of different studies, the investigator obtains copies of the raw data from the original studies and re-analyses them. An excellent example is the Oxford-based Collaborative Group on Hormonal Factors in Breast Cancer which, since the mid 1990s, has been producing reports based on analyses of over 50,000 women with breast cancer and 100,000 without, from data provided by more than 50 separate studies. The collaboration's first paper showed with great precision the very low absolute risk of breast cancer conferred by the majority of patterns of oral contraceptive pill use (Collaborative Group on Hormonal Factors in Breast Cancer, 1996). This report removed a great deal of the uncertainty that remained about this relation, despite many prior publications from individual studies.

Until recently, such pooled analyses were relatively uncommon: the effort required to obtain the original data, clean, recode and re-shape each dataset to a common standard, conduct a new analysis and write the paper, all the while maintaining full approval of all contributing investigators, is monumental. However, the last few years have seen an explosion in the number of international consortia (and acronyms!) established specifically to bring together investigators from around the world to pool genetic and/or epidemiological data from different studies. This has been particularly true in the field of molecular cancer epidemiology where it seems likely that aside from a small number of 'high risk' genes, such as the *BRCA1* and *BRCA2* genes identified for breast and ovarian cancer, the effects of any individual genetic variant on cancer risk are likely to be small and, as a result, very large numbers of individuals are needed to show an association with any certainty. Examples of these consortia include BCAC (Breast Cancer Association Consortium), OCAC (Ovarian Cancer Association Consortium), PANC4 (Pancreatic Cancer Case Control Consortium), E2C2 (Epidemiology of Endometrial Cancer Consortium), BEACON (Barrett's and Esophageal Adenocarcinoma Consortium), ILCCO (International Lung Cancer Consortium)...the list is ever growing.

A word of caution

Finally, a few words of caution: the ability of meta-analysis to provide unbiased summary estimates has been seriously debated. Combining the results of a number of studies usually generates an estimate with narrow confidence limits, thereby giving a sense of precision and accuracy that may be illusory. The combined results of a meta-analysis will depend entirely on the studies selected for inclusion (or exclusion) and Box 11.3 gives an example of where two systematic reviews reached almost diametrically opposing conclusions due, at least in part, to the different sets of studies considered appropriate for inclusion. (Note, this is also another example of when simple descriptive data can be informative.)

Furthermore, as you saw in Chapters 7 and 8, there are numerous ways in which bias can occur and the old adage still holds true: 'rubbish in = rubbish out'. Combining results cannot get rid of bias or undetected confounding and, although a combined odds ratio from several poor studies may look good, it will not compensate for problems in the individual studies. Figure 11.3 shows

Box 11.3 Do mobile telephones cause brain cancer?

Given the unprecedented growth in the use of mobile telephones over the last 25 years such that usage is now almost ubiquitous in many countries, a major question is whether exposure to the radiofrequency fields they generate causes brain cancer. This is both a highly controversial and highly emotive area as brain cancers often occur at younger ages than many other cancers and, because of their location, are often fatal. In mid-2009, two meta-analyses attempted to address this question.

The first study focused on the long-term effects of mobile phone use and thus only included published studies where participants had used mobile phones for at least 10 years. Because the radiofrequency waves generated by mobile phones do not penetrate very far into the brain, they also restricted their review to studies with a 'laterality' analysis, i.e. that considered whether the cancer arose on the same side of the head preferred for phone use. A total of 11 studies met these criteria. They found that use of a mobile phone for 10 or more years approximately doubled the risk of being diagnosed with a brain tumour on the side of the head preferred for phone use, and that the association was statistically significant for two types of brain cancer: gliomas and acoustic neuromas. *They therefore concluded that there was adequate epidemiological evidence to suggest a link* (Khurana *et al.*, 2009).

The second group took a broader approach and included all published studies that had evaluated this association (>20 individual reports). They found that the current data did not show any increase in risk of brain cancer with up to 10 years of mobile phone use and concluded that the data *do not suggest a causal association between mobile phone use and fast-growing brain tumours such as gliomas* (Ahlbom *et al.*, 2009). The authors did, however, acknowledge that longer follow-up was needed before any conclusions could be drawn regarding longer-term use and the effects on slow-growing tumours.

So why did these two meta-analyses come to such different conclusions?

The individual studies included in the meta-analyses have given quite different results; some show a strong association and others see no effect. No one has, as yet, been able to adequately explain the reasons for this but it is likely that the different criteria used to determine which studies would be included/excluded from each of the reviews led to their differing conclusions. As to which is correct? It may be that only time and a longer follow-up period will tell although it is worth noting that, as yet, there have been no increases in reported incidence rates of brain cancer (Deltour *et al.*, 2009; Horner *et al.*, 2009).

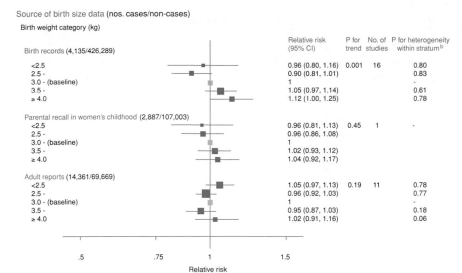

Source of birth size data (nos. cases/non-cases)
  Birth weight category (kg)

	Relative risk (95% CI)	P for trend	No. of studies	P for heterogeneity within stratum[b]
Birth records (4,135/426,289)				
<2.5	0.96 (0.80, 1.16)	0.001	16	0.80
2.5 -	0.90 (0.81, 1.01)			0.83
3.0 - (baseline)	1			-
3.5 -	1.05 (0.97, 1.14)			0.61
≥ 4.0	1.12 (1.00, 1.25)			0.78
Parental recall in women's childhood (2,887/107,003)				
<2.5	0.96 (0.81, 1.13)	0.45	1	-
2.5 -	0.96 (0.86, 1.08)			
3.0 - (baseline)	1			
3.5 -	1.02 (0.93, 1.12)			
≥ 4.0	1.04 (0.92, 1.17)			
Adult reports (14,361/69,669)				
<2.5	1.05 (0.97, 1.13)	0.19	11	0.78
2.5 -	0.96 (0.92, 1.03)			0.77
3.0 - (baseline)	1			-
3.5 -	0.95 (0.87, 1.03)			0.18
≥ 4.0	1.02 (0.91, 1.16)			0.06

.5   .75   1   1.5
Relative risk

Figure 11.3 Relative risk of breast cancer (and 95% confidence intervals) associated with increasing birth weight, stratified by source of birth weight data (From: dos Santos Silva *et al.*, 2008.)

the results of a pooled analysis of data from 32 studies looking at the relation between birth weight and subsequent risk of breast cancer (dos Santos Silva *et al.*, 2008). When the authors separated the studies according to the source of the birth weight information, they saw a clear trend towards increasing risk of breast cancer with increasing birth weight among the 16 studies where the information on birth weight came directly from birth records and was thus, presumably, most accurate. The association was much weaker in the one study where the information was provided by the women's mothers when the women themselves were children, and there was no association at all among the 11 studies that relied on the women reporting their own birth weight – almost certainly the least reliable source of information. (Note also that the results of the statistical tests for heterogeneity are all non-significant ($p > 0.05$, suggesting that the results of the various studies within each group are all quite consistent.) This is a striking example where error and subsequent non-differential misclassification (see Chapter 7) in the self-reported data have completely masked what appears to be quite a strong association based on the more accurate birth record information. If all of these studies had been pooled together, it is likely that this association would have been missed.

Assessment of causality

Systematic reviews, and particularly meta-analyses and pooled analyses, can contribute directly to an assessment of causality. Reviews that generate

Table 11.2 Guidelines for appraising the validity of a systematic review.

Criteria	What to look for	Comments
Focused research question	The main research question should be clear from either the title or the abstract. The exposure, such as a risk factor or therapy, and the outcome(s) of interest should be expressed in terms of a simple relationship.	If the review addresses multiple questions it is likely to be a general introduction to the area and may have limited sources of evidence for the conclusions drawn. Statements may be made with few citations and limited in-depth analysis of studies. Caution should be taken in accepting conclusions from this type of review.
Inclusion and exclusion criteria	The eligibility criteria used to select studies should be stated and should specify the participants, exposures and outcomes of interest and in some cases the study design.	If the eligibility criteria are not clearly stated you have no way of knowing whether studies were included (or excluded) solely on the basis of their results, which could bias the conclusions of the review.
Comprehensiveness of search strategy	Detailed search strategy indicating that the authors have searched all the relevant bibliographic databases with a variety of appropriate search terms. Other strategies such as hand searching and snowballing[a] may be used.	It is only possible to evaluate the thoroughness of the search strategies if the methods used by the authors are made explicit. If there is no methods section then you should be cautious in accepting any of the results.
Assessment of included studies	Statements that indicate whether individual included studies are scientifically sound as measured against established criteria.	The criteria for appraising the individual studies should reflect the study design. For example if the review was based on a therapy then the criteria should relate primarily to RCTs.
Reproducibility of assessments[b]	Statements that the appraisals were conducted independently by at least two reviewers and any differences resolved by consensus or by a third person.	Since appraisal of studies involves judgement calls, decisions based on these appraisals are subject to random errors or mistakes and systematic errors or bias. Having two independent reviewers should minimise these.
Similarity of results of included studies	Detailed reporting of the results of individual studies with some measure of the differences (heterogeneity) between them.	If the results are very different it may not be appropriate to combine them in a meta-analysis. Instead there should be some exploration of the reasons for the differences (e.g. different populations, different study methods, etc.)
Overall logic and insight	Discussion of how error and heterogeneity have been handled, also causality and practical importance.	These issues are central to making a comprehensive judgement.

(Adapted from Oxman *et al.*, 1994.)

[a] Snowballing refers to the iterative process of searching where the results of the initial search are used to identify missed papers through either a search of the reference list at the end of the identified paper or by using Science Citation Index to see who has cited the identified paper.

[b] Multiple assessors are used in rigorous systematic reviews of clinical interventions such as those conducted through the Cochrane Collaboration but this level of rigour is less commonly used for aetiologic reviews. This need not invalidate the results as long as the criteria used to include and exclude studies are clearly described.

combined effect estimates across studies provide more precise summary measures of the *strength* of an association and sometimes of the *dose–response* relationship. Our discussion above of the homogeneity (or otherwise) of study results addresses the concept of *consistency* in practice. We do not require that effect estimates be near-identical across studies to meet this criterion: simply showing that most are positive (or negative) and reasonably similar with respect to their confidence intervals (i.e. the 95% CIs are overlapping) may suffice. Also, if more extreme heterogeneity can be shown to be due to differing methodology or degrees of study error, and results among the better studies are reasonably consistent, then the review has again provided helpful causal information (Weed, 2000). The causal argument of the review should then be fully developed along the lines presented in Chapter 10.

Assessing the quality of a systematic review

A principal feature of a modern systematic review is that it must have a comprehensive methods section. As you saw in Box 11.1, the authors should have detailed their literature-searching strategy and the processes of study selection and appraisal and data extraction. Table 11.2 outlines a fairly comprehensive set of the key criteria for appraising the validity of a systematic review which summarises and extends the major points made above. Complementary sets of guidelines have been promoted to improve the reporting of meta-analyses. The 'Quality of Reporting of Meta-analyses' or QUOROM statement (Moher *et al.*, 1999) was developed specifically for reporting meta-analyses of randomised controlled trials and has recently been updated as the PRISMA statement (Preferred Reporting Items for Systematic reviews and Meta-Analyses; Liberati *et al.*, 2009). A parallel guide developed for reporting meta-analyses of observational studies is the 'Meta-analysis Of Observational Studies in Epidemiology' or MOOSE statement (Stroup *et al.*, 2000). Omitted from some such lists, however, but always central to making a comprehensive judgement, is a consideration of the logic and insight of the review, especially its treatment of error, heterogeneity, causality and practical importance.

Making judgements in practice

Primary epidemiological data (from individual studies) and secondary data (from reviews) are not ends in themselves. They aim to tell us about the healthiness of populations, what we might need to change to improve their condition, and how we might go about this. Judgements about need are primarily the remit of health departments and organisations (local, regional and global), using appropriate descriptive data. In contrast, identification of causes and preventive factors comes largely from academic research, and in addition a wide variety of professional, community and government groups have interests in specific topics. The aim of the whole enterprise is to take action to improve health. This is not a modern phenomenon and, as you have seen, many advances in public health pre-date epidemiology. The strong call to base all such actions on good evidence is, however, quite recent, and has spread rapidly from clinical medicine to public health. Much effort is spent these days on collating knowledge to answer practical questions as to what interventions might work, and a common starting point is a review. An existing review can be useful, but often one will need to be commissioned to address the precise question being asked. Newly emerging issues will sometimes not have been studied adequately, which leaves reviewers, planners and decision-makers in something of a quandary. This book is not primarily about how to make decisions under conditions of uncertainty, but the logic of epidemiology can certainly help. As one of the seminal figures in health services research said;

The absence of excellent evidence does not make evidence-based decision making impossible; what is required is the best evidence available not the best evidence possible. (Muir Gray, 1997)

A systematic epidemiological review, then, is often an early response to a question about the effects of an intervention, but it may also be used practically (as opposed to academically) to support broad overviews of causation aimed at informing and influencing health policy. Approaches vary depending on the specific purpose of the review, and we conclude this chapter with descriptions of how some influential national and international bodies engaged in disseminating helpful judgements and interpretations operate.

The US Preventive Services Task Force (USPSTF)

The USPSTF was convened by the US Public Health Service in the 1980s to assess the merits of preventive activities in clinical practice. It aims to provide simple practical guidelines for clinicians regarding the utility of preventive interventions that they might use in their practice (over 200 to date). Many of the interventions assessed relate to early detection of a wide range of conditions, counselling to change behaviour and primary chemoprevention (e.g. aspirin to prevent cardiovascular disease). Topic teams assigned by the task force prepare systematic reviews of the evidence according to a standard protocol. The *evidence* for a particular preventive service is classified as good, fair or poor and then combined with a judgement of the *net benefit* of the service (substantial, moderate, small or zero/negative). The USPSTF assesses the reviews centrally and then makes formal recommendations with specific ratings (AHRQ, 2004; Harris *et al.*, 2001), examples of which are given below. These recommendations translate into practice guidance for clinicians who are advised to offer or provide services with 'A' and 'B' recommendations to eligible patients; discourage the use of services with 'D' recommendations; offer or provide services with 'C' recommendations only if other considerations support this for an individual patient; and, for services with 'I' statements, carefully read the Clinical Considerations section for guidance, and help patients understand the uncertainty surrounding these services.

A The USPSTF *strongly recommends* screening for cervical cancer in women who have been sexually active and have a cervix. The USPSTF found *good evidence*... that screening with cervical cytology reduces incidence of and mortality from cervical cancer ... The USPSTF concludes that the *benefits of screening substantially outweigh potential harms* (January 2003).

B The USPSTF *recommends* structured breastfeeding education and behavioural counselling programmes to promote breastfeeding. The USPSTF found *fair evidence* that programmes combining breastfeeding education with counselling are associated with increased rates of initiation of breastfeeding ... (2003).

C The USPSTF makes *no recommendation* for or against routine osteoporosis screening in post-menopausal women younger than 60. The USPSTF found fair evidence that screening women at lower risk can identify women who may be eligible for treatment but it would prevent a small number of fractures. The USPSTF concludes that the *balance of benefits and harms of screening and treatment is too close* to make a general recommendation for this age group (September 2002).

D The USPSTF *recommends against* the use of beta-carotene supplements for the prevention of cancer or cardiovascular disease. The USPSTF found good evidence that beta-carotene supplementation provides no benefit in the prevention of cancer or cardiovascular disease in middle-aged and older adults ... The USPSTF concludes that beta-carotene supplements are *unlikely to provide important benefits and might cause harm* in some groups (June 2003).

I The USPSTF concludes that the *evidence is insufficient to recommend for or against* behavioural counselling in primary care settings to promote physical activity. The USPSTF could not determine the balance of benefits and harms ... (August 2002).

A parallel activity for community prevention, the Community Guide, was established by the US Department of Health and Human Services in 1996 and is conducted by the Task Force on Community Preventive Services (http://www.thecommunityguide.org/index.html). Some typical findings are summarised in Table 11.3.

Table 11.3 Some findings from the US Community Guide regarding community interventions.

Finding	Intervention	Date
Recommended (strong evidence)	Increasing alcohol taxes	June 2007
	Community water fluoridation	October 2000
	Worksite programs to control overweight and obesity	February 2007
Recommended (sufficient evidence)	Enhanced enforcement of laws prohibiting alcohol sales to minors	February 2006
	Vaccination programs in schools	June 2001
	Diabetes self-management education in the home – children and adolescents with Type 1 diabetes	March 2001
Insufficient evidence	Vaccination programs in childcare settings	June 1998
	Diabetes self-management education in school settings or the worksite	September 2000
	School-based programs to control overweight and obesity	October 2003

The International Agency for Research on Cancer (IARC): monographs programme

Three times a year the IARC convenes a working party of experts to review all of the literature relating a specific exposure or exposures to cancer. This process is one of the most comprehensive conducted anywhere; in addition to studies in humans, the working parties also include experts on the exposure itself (chemists, toxicologists, physicists, etc.), on animal studies and on molecular biology. The IARC secretariat performs comprehensive literature searches and sends the material to the individual scientists who are asked to summarise the literature in a particular area. During a week-long face-to-face meeting, subgroups of the working party (exposure data, human studies, animal studies and laboratory data) discuss and finalise the draft sections of the report and prepare a summary for their section. The full group then comes together to reach a final consensus. The human and animal data are first classified separately as providing *sufficient, limited* or *inadequate* evidence of carcinogenicity or, occasionally, evidence suggesting a lack of carcinogenicity. These data are then combined with the exposure data and molecular information to make a more formal assessment of causality, classifying agents as:

- carcinogenic to humans
- *probably* carcinogenic to humans
- *possibly* carcinogenic to humans
- *not classifiable* regarding carcinogenicity to humans or
- *probably not* carcinogenic to humans (http://monographs.iarc.fr).

As of December 2009 they had classified 108 agents or mixtures as clear carcinogens with another 63 classified as probable and 248 as possible carcinogens, reflecting the general lack of certainty when dealing with evidence of this type. (Only one compound has been classified as probably not carcinogenic!) A further 515 agents were found to be not classifiable because there was insufficient evidence to make any judgement.

The World Cancer Research Fund and American Institute of Cancer Research

The aim of the World Cancer Research Fund (WCRF) International is to 'lead and unify a global network of cancer charities dedicated to the prevention and control of cancer by means of healthy food and nutrition, physical activity and weight management'. (http://www.wcrf.org/index.php). In 1997, the WCRF joined forces with the American Institute for Cancer Research (AICR) to jointly publish a comprehensive review of the current state of knowledge regarding the relation between nutrition and cancer (WCRF and AICR, 1997). In 2007 the second edition of this report was published to incorporate new evidence that had accumulated since 1997 (WCRF and AICR, 2007). The reviews were contracted out to international teams of experts and their detailed methodological plans for the review were critiqued by others and refined before the reviews were conducted. These reviews (including a biological perspective) were themselves further evaluated and combined into a single report by a central scientific committee. While these reviews are not directly linked to policy, the aim is to provide good scientific evidence that can be used by policy makers, research scientists, health professionals and community groups around the world. To this end the final chapter of the review assesses policy implications directly.

Consensus conferences and working groups

Consensus conferences on many topics, often similar in format to the IARC working parties, are convened on an ad-hoc basis to evaluate the evidence in a specific area. Independent experts are usually invited to submit papers in advance and these are then discussed at a face-to-face meeting. These conferences may be conducted at an international level or on a smaller scale to provide specific information to inform local planning and practice. The outcomes are, however, necessarily dependent on the individual members and how strongly they advocate their own personal opinions. An alternative method that has been proposed to overcome this is the 'Cooke method', which weights the opinions of individual experts according to their individual proficiency, assessed perhaps by their responses to a set of relevant professional questions with widely accepted answers (Aspinall, 2010). It remains to be seen whether this approach will catch on.

Box 11.4 Should women under the age of 50 be offered routine mammographic screening?

The debate surrounding this question highlights the difficulties of interpreting evidence. In 1993, an expert panel at the US National Cancer Institute (NCI) concluded that there was no evidence for a benefit of mammographic screening for women aged 40–49 years and the NCI withdrew their recommendation for screening in this age group. In response, the American Cancer Society reaffirmed their recommendation *for* screening, which was based on the view of a separate expert panel. The publication of additional data in 1996 opened up the question again and the NCI responded by convening a consensus conference in 1997. The independent experts at the conference again concluded that there was insufficient evidence to recommend routine mammography for women under the age of 50 years. This conclusion led to such a public outcry that the NCI was forced to reconsider their position. The question went back to the National Cancer Advisory Board, a presidentially appointed committee, who voted 17 to 1 in favour of recommending mammographic screening for younger women. Since then the controversy has continued, with groups reaching opposing conclusions based on the same evidence.

As you will see in Chapter 15, the evaluation of screening programmes is not simple, and in this particular instance it appears that there is still no clear consensus. At the end of 2009, the USPSTF recommendation was against routine screening mammography in women aged 40 to 49 years (a Grade C recommendation), noting that 'The decision to start regular, biennial screening mammography before the age of 50 years should be an individual one and take into account patient context, including the patient's values regarding specific benefits and harms' (US Preventive Services Task Force, 2009). Or, as summarised by D. Petitti, Vice Chair of the US Preventive Services Task Force:

'So, what does this mean if you are a woman in your 40s? You should talk to your doctor and make an informed decision about whether mammography is right for you based on your family history, general health, and personal values' (19 November 2009; from http://www.ahrq.gov/clinic/uspstf/uspsbrca.htm, accessed 31 January 2010).

The end result

Policy makers invariably want a black-and-white answer to any question – does this cause/prevent/improve treatment of the condition in question? Unfortunately, as you will have gathered, this yearning for certainty can rarely be fulfilled. Nothing is absolute and, as we discussed in Chapter 10, it is impossible to prove something definitively. As a result you will find that the conclusions of many systematic reviews are couched in fairly cautious terms, but policy makers and planners have to act despite this and make the best of what is available. We will end with a question that still causes controversy: should we recommend widespread mammographic screening for women under the age of 50 years (Box 11.4)? (Or, some would argue, should we recommend it at all? (Various, 2004).)

Summary

In the previous chapters we have discussed the practical 'nuts and bolts' of epidemiology. In Chapters 2–4 we considered the ways in which we can measure health and quantify associations between 'exposures' and health 'outcomes'. We then looked critically at how we interpret the results of such studies in Chapters 5–9 so that we can start to make informed decisions as to whether reported associations might be real. In Chapter 10 we took this one step further to see how we can start to assess whether an association might be causal. In this chapter we have considered how we can bring together all of the information related to a particular association with a view to informing decision-making – whether this is to establish policy or to identify avenues for further research. However, as you have seen, this is not always as straightforward as we might wish. One of the big challenges in epidemiology, and indeed all health research, is to recognise when we have enough data to act or to plan with sufficient confidence that we are doing the right thing. We will return to this conundrum in the final chapter.

We will now move on to look at some practical applications of epidemiology that all aim to reduce the burden of disease in a community at some level: outbreak management, surveillance, prevention and screening. These will draw on the core concepts that you have learned so far and reinforce the epidemiological perspective – a mix of science and art that requires an open mind, attention to detail and the potential for error, a willingness to consider alternative explanations and, finally, the ability to be both constructively critical and pragmatic.

REFERENCES

Ahlbom, A., Feychting, M., Green, A. *et al.* (2009). Epidemiologic evidence on mobile phones and tumor risk. A review. *Epidemiology*, **20**: 639–652.

AHRQ. (2004). *Guide to Clinical Preventive Services, Third Edition: Periodic Updates. AHRQ Publication No.* 04-IP003, January 2004. Rockville, MD: Agency for Healthcare Research and Quality.

Aspinall, W. (2010). A route to more tractable expert advice. *Nature*, **463**: 294–295.

Black, N. (1996). Why we need observational studies to evaluate the effectiveness of health care. *British Medical Journal*, **312**: 1215–1218.

Britton, A., McKee, M., Black, N. *et al.* (1998). Choosing between randomised and non-randomised studies: a systematic review. *Health Technology Assessment*, **2** (No. 13): 1–124.

Collaborative Group on Hormonal Factors in Breast Cancer. (1996). Breast cancer and hormonal contraceptives: collaborative reanalysis of individual data on 53297 women with breast cancer and 100239 women without breast cancer from 54 epidemiological studies. *The Lancet*, **347**: 1713–1727.

Delgado-Rodriguez, M., Ruiz-Canela, M., De Irala-Estevez, J., Llorica, J. and Martinez-Gonzalez, A. (2001). Participation of epidemiologists and/or biostatisticians and methodological quality of published controlled clinical trials. *Journal of Epidemiology and Community Health*, **55**: 569–572.

Deltour, I., Johansen, C., Auvinen, A., Feychting, M., Klaeboe, L. and Schüz, J. (2009). Time trends in brain tumor incidence rates in Denmark, Finland, Norway, and Sweden, 1974–2003. *Journal of the National Cancer Institute*, **101**: 1621–1724.

dos Santos Silva, I., de Stavola, B., McCormack, V. and Collaborative Group on Pre-Natal Risk Factors and Subsequent Risk of Breast Cancer. (2008). Birth size and breast cancer risk: re-analysis of individual participant data from 32 studies. *PLoS Medicine*, **5**: e193.

Glasziou, P., Irwig, L., Bain, C. and Colditz, G. (2001). *Systematic Reviews in Health Care: A Practical Guide*. Cambridge: Cambridge University Press.

Glasziou, P., Vandenbroucke, J. and Chalmers, I. (2004). Assessing the quality of research. *British Medical Journal*, **328**: 39–41.

Harris, R. P., Helfand, M., Woolf, S. H. *et al.* for the Methods Work Group Third U.S. Preventive Services Task Force. (2001). Current methods of the U.S. Preventive Services Task Force: a review of the process. *American Journal of Preventive Medicine*, **20** (3S): 21–35.

Horner, M. J., Ries, L. A. G., Krapcho, M. *et al.* (Eds). (2009). SEER Cancer Statistics Review, 1975–2006, National Cancer Institute. Bethesda, MD, http://seer.cancer.gov/csr/1975_2006/, based on November 2008 SEER data submission, posted to the SEER web site, 2009.

Khurana, V. G., Teo, C., Kundi, M., Hardell, L. and Carlberg, M. (2009). Cell phones and brain tumors: a review including the long-term epidemiologic data. *Surgical Neurology*, **72**: 205–214.

Liberati, A., Altman, D.G., Tetzlaff, J. *et al.* (2009). The PRISMA statement for reporting systematic reviews and meta-analyses of studies that evaluate healthcare interventions: explanation and elaboration. *British Medical Journal*, **339**:b2700 doi: 10.1136/bmj.b2700.

Manson, J. E. and Bassuk, S. S. (2007). Invited commentary: hormone therapy and risk of coronary heart disease – why renew the focus on the early years of menopause? *American Journal of Epidemiology*, **166**: 511–517.

McKee, M., Britton, A., Black, N. *et al.* (1999). Interpreting the evidence: choosing between randomised and non-randomised studies. *British Medical Journal*, **319**: 312–315.

Moher, D., Cook, D. J., Eastwood, S. *et al.* (1999). Improving the quality of reports of meta-analyses of randomised controlled trials: the QUOROM statement. Quality of reporting of meta-analyses. *Lancet*, **354**: 1896–1900.

Muir Gray, J. A. (1997). *Evidence-Based Health Care – How to Make Health Policy and Management Decisions.* Edinburgh: Churchill Livingstone.

Oxman, A. D., Cook, D. J. and Guyatt, G. H. (1994). Users' guides to the medical literature VI. How to use an overview. *Journal of the American Medical Association*, **272**: 1367–1371.

Pirozzo, S., Summerbell, C., Cameron, C. and Glasziou, P. (2003). Should we recommend low-fat diets for obesity? *Obesity Reviews*, **4**: 83–90.

Purdie, D. M., Bain, C. J., Webb, P. M. *et al.* (2001). Body size and ovarian cancer: case–control study and systematic review (Australia). *Cancer Causes Control*, **12**: 855–863.

Schultz, K. F., Chalmers, I., Hayes, R. J. and Altman, D. G. (1995). Empirical evidence of bias. Dimensions of methodological quality associated with estimates of treatment effects in controlled trials. *Journal of the American Medical Association*, **273**: 408–412.

Smith, G. C. S. and Pell, J. P. (2003). Parachute use to prevent death and major trauma related to gravitational challenge: systematic review of randomised controlled trials. *British Medical Journal*, **327**: 1459–1461.

Stroup, D. F., Berlin, J. A., Morton, S. C. *et al.* (2000). Meta-analysis of observational studies in epidemiology. A proposal for reporting. *Journal of the American Medical Association*, **283**: 2008–2012.

US Preventive Services Task Force. (2009). Screening for breast cancer: U.S. Preventive Services Task Force recommendation statement. *Annals of Internal Medicine*, **151**: 716–726.

Various. (2004). Screening for breast cancer: point–counterpoint. *International Journal of Epidemiology*, **33**: 43–74.

WCRF (World Cancer Research Fund) and AICR (American Institute for Cancer Research). (1997). *Food, Nutrition and the Prevention of Cancer: A Global Perspective*. Washington DC: AICR.

WCRF (World Cancer Research Fund) and AICR (American Institute for Cancer Research). (2007). *Food, Nutrition, Physical Activity, and the Prevention of Cancer: A Global Perspective*. Washington DC: AICR.

Weed, D. L. (2000). Interpreting epidemiological evidence: how meta-analysis and causal inference methods are related. *International Journal of Epidemiology*, **29**: 387–390.

Outbreaks, epidemics and clusters

Description	Association	Alternative explanations	Integration & interpretation	Practical applications
Chapters 2–3	Chapters 4–5	Chapters 6–8	Chapters 9–11	Chapter 12: Outbreaks

Box 12.1 An unusual epidemic of pneumonia

On the 21st of February 2003, a doctor from southern China visited Hong Kong and stayed one night in a local hotel. Unwell for several days before the trip, he became seriously ill and the next day was admitted to a hospital with severe pneumonia; he died 10 days later. Before admission he had infected numerous people who came into contact with him, including his own family (wife, daughter, sister and brother-in-law) and 16 guests or visitors to the hotel. Some of the hotel guests left Hong Kong for Singapore, Hanoi and Toronto and outbreaks in those areas rapidly followed. Within a month large outbreaks arose in several Hong Kong hospitals, affecting staff, students, patients and visitors. As family members became infected they infected others and the disease began to spread in the community. On the 12th of March 2003, the World Health Organization issued a global alert on atypical pneumonia, called **severe acute respiratory syndrome** (SARS). By late March a huge outbreak in a Hong Kong housing estate was traced back to a patient discharged from one of the affected hospitals. In Hong Kong there were 1,755 cases and 300 deaths (case fatality rate, CFR = 17%), including 8 fatalities among the 386 health workers affected. The high-rise housing estate had 329 cases and 42 deaths. Hong Kong health authorities quarantined 493 households with 1,262 people, traced 26,520 contacts, and screened 36.3 million travellers. Globally, public health organisations collaborated to identify the organism, devise diagnostic tests, introduce control measures and stop the epidemic by August 2003 after 8,422 cases and 916 deaths worldwide (Chan-Yeung and Yu, 2003).

Investigation of disease outbreaks or epidemics such as that described above is part of the core business of epidemiology. An internet search yields more than a million scholarly references for 'outbreak' and, as you will see, the utility of epidemic investigations is obvious from the wide variety of applications. Many examples earlier in this book focused on 'chronic' disease. Now we will spotlight infectious diseases (although not exclusively) and use epidemiological principles to explain the occurrence of endemic, epidemic and pandemic infections. Historically, the study of epidemic infections helped develop methods for epidemiology, especially retrospective cohort analysis and case–control studies, and epidemic investigations still have a high profile in public health practice today. Emerging and re-emerging infections have become prominent over the last two to three decades and the threat of global epidemics (pandemics) mobilised resources to plan for, detect and combat such catastrophes. Over the same period, growing awareness of environmental pollution and community detection of clusters of rare diseases, especially cancer, increased demand for epidemiological investigation of 'outbreaks' of non-communicable disease. In response, statisticians are developing new methods for spatial analyses and epidemiologists are studying community risk perception and public communication of risk appraisals.

Infectious disease epidemiology is often presented as a different discipline from the epidemiology we have been describing, but in fact the fundamental principles are identical, as are the study designs used: cohort and case–control studies to investigate causality and experiments to evaluate preventive and therapeutic interventions. Causal reasoning is conceptually simpler but still has its own complexities, as we show below. The comparability of the two approaches has become more obvious as knowledge has expanded to include infectious agents as prime causes of a number of conditions generally considered to be 'chronic', a term often used as a synonym for non-infectious. For example, after decades of study, cervical cancer can now be characterised as a sexually transmitted infectious disease caused by strains of the human papillomavirus. The major difference for most infectious conditions, and other outbreaks we discuss here, is the urgency with which investigations take place. This is often extreme (as with SARS), and demands robust, practical methods for subject identification and selection, as well as for data collection.

Outbreaks, epidemics, endemics and clusters

What do we mean by an epidemic or **outbreak**? The two terms are often used interchangeably and generally they involve unexpected increases in incidence of a disease. Benenson (1990, p. 499) defines both as '*the occurrence in a community or region of cases of an illness clearly in excess of that expected*'. Others have defined them slightly differently; for example the 'Dictionary of Epidemiology' (Porta, 2008, p. 176) describes an outbreak as '*an epidemic limited to localised increase in the incidence of a disease. e.g., in a village, town or closed institution*'. Outbreak may also be used to refer to a small epidemic arising in an area that has had no cases for a long time – an epidemic with excess frequency compared with an expected frequency of zero. In such a setting a single case would not be considered an outbreak, but two or more cases could be.

You should also be clear on the distinction between epidemic and **endemic** disease. Endemic disease can be defined as '*the constant presence of a disease or infectious agent within a given geographic area or population group*' (Porta, 2008, p. 78). For example, malaria is endemic in much of Africa. Thus 'endemic' describes attributes of a disease, not an area; 'endemic area' is a frequent misuse of the term endemic. For some diseases, notably malaria, the word endemic has been further defined in reference to the degree of endemicity – with holoendemic the most extreme (children intensely infected, most adults immune), followed by hyperendemic (a disease constantly affecting a large proportion of all age groups in the population). Epidemics thus represent an unexpected increase in incidence of disease whereas endemic describes a constant presence of disease. Parallel terms referring to infections within animal populations are *epizootic* (an unexpected increase in incidence in an animal population) and *enzootic* (constant presence in an animal population). Sometimes an enzootic infection crosses to humans and causes an epidemic (the most likely explanation for SARS, hantavirus and many other infections). Other times an epizootic infection reaches humans and causes an epidemic (as periodically occurs with plague), or fizzles out after causing great alarm but without any epidemic human-to-human transmission (as has happened so far with H5N1 avian influenza).

When a disease affects a large number of people and crosses many international boundaries it is called a **pandemic**. Examples of pandemics last century include plague (around 1900), influenza (1918, 1957 and 1968) and cholera (since 1961). Certain pandemics in history caused great loss of human populations, notably plague in the late middle ages and 'Spanish' influenza at the end of World War I. The modern pandemics of HIV and multi-drug-resistant tuberculosis are of great concern. The organism causing the most recent pandemic – H1N1 influenza virus (often inappropriately described as 'swine flu') – first appeared in Mexico in 2009. It quickly spread and reached over 200 countries by the end of the year. So far the disease has been far less severe than anticipated for pandemic influenza. But it has tended to affect young adults and pregnant women more than the seasonal influenza it has replaced, and is likely to recur in several waves as did previous variants that caused pandemics.

One more term must be dealt with here – **cluster**. This can be defined as an *'aggregation of relatively uncommon events or diseases in space and/or time in amounts that are believed or perceived to be greater than could be expected by chance'* (Porta, 2008, p. 42). The word is usually used to describe a cluster of cases of a rare (usually non-infectious) disease, and putative clusters of disease are often suspected to have an environmental cause on the basis of anecdotal evidence. As a result, much effort is often expended in response to public outcry in attempts to determine whether a true cluster exists. Box 12.2 gives some idea of the range of outbreaks and clusters that can occur in practice.

Rare disease clusters

Clusters of rare diseases, especially cancer, are increasingly being reported by members of the community in many countries and public awareness of environmental hazards has increased demand for public health authorities to investigate them. Any apparently unusual frequency of any disease will now attract attention

Box 12.2 Some outbreak and cluster investigations

Re-emergence of fatal avian influenza in humans (China)

The first documented instance of avian influenza subtype H5N1 causing severe respiratory illness in humans was in Hong Kong in 1997 when it affected 18 patients, 6 of whom died. In January–February 2003 it re-emerged when a family from Hong Kong visited China. The seven-year-old daughter developed fever and respiratory symptoms two days after arriving and died of a pneumonia-like illness seven days later; her cause of death was not ascertained. The family returned to Hong Kong and the father was admitted on 11 February after four days of fever, sore throat and coughing. He died six days later and H5N1 was detected. On 12 February the eight-year-old son, who reported having close contact with live chickens in China, was also admitted with a flu-like illness. H5N1 was isolated and he recovered (Peiris *et al.*, 2004).

An outbreak of chromium ulcer in a manufacturing plant (Taiwan)

On 23 May 1989, managers of a manufacturing plant in Taiwan requested investigation of an outbreak of hand ulcers among workers. Ten enamel department workers (13.5%) who developed such 'chromium ulcers' were identified between 1 January and 30 June 1988. Workers who handled conveyer hooks were at greatest risk (RR = 12.4; 95% CI 2.90–53.4). Workers with gloves were protected from developing ulcers (RR = 0.08; 95% CI 0.01–0.60). Analysis of hooks that had passed through the oven revealed chromium VI on their surface (Deng *et al.*, 1990).

An epidemic of paediatric traffic injuries (USA)

This study identified specific regional risk factors for the high rate of paediatric pedestrian trauma in Florida. Of the 29 cases studied, 3 (10%) occurred near ice-cream trucks and 13 (45%) involved 'dart-outs'. Recommendations included an engineering change for a dangerous intersection, and a recommendation to equip ice-cream trucks with extending stop signs (Hameed *et al.*, 2004).

An outbreak of piranha attacks on humans (Brazil)

There are many tales describing ferocious schools of piranha attacking humans, but few scientific data supporting such behaviour. These predacious fish do occasionally injure bathers and swimmers in lakes and rivers and an outbreak of piranha bites was reported in a dammed river in southeast Brazil. The report focused on epidemiological and clinical aspects as well as piranha biology to gain a better understanding of the natural history of such outbreaks (Haddad and Sazima, 2003).

(continued)

Box 12.2 (*continued*)

An outbreak of influenza aboard a commercial airliner
A jet liner with 54 persons aboard was delayed on the ground in Anchorage,
Alaska, for three hours because of engine failure during a takeoff attempt.
Most passengers stayed on the aeroplane during the delay. Within 72 hours,
almost three quarters of the passengers became ill with symptoms of cough,
fever, fatigue, headache, sore throat and myalgia. One passenger, the
apparent index case, was ill on the aeroplane, and the clinical attack rate
among the others varied with the amount of time spent aboard. Virus
antigenically similar to A/Texas/1/77 (H3N2) was isolated from 8 of 31
passengers cultured and 20 of 22 ill persons tested had serologic evidence of
infection with this virus. The aeroplane ventilation system was inoperative
during the delay and this may account for the high attack rate (Moser *et al.*,
1979).

A cluster of Creutzfeldt–Jakob disease (CJD) (Australia)
Six confirmed sporadic cases of CJD were recognized in 13 years in persons
who had been long-term residents of a moderate-sized rural city; the
expected number was less than one. An extensive investigation could not
find any point-source or case-to-case transmission links. This occurrence
was highly statistically significant ($p = 0.003$) and remained significant
($p < 0.02$) when only the cases that arose after the cluster had been
recognized were taken into account. However, a more conservative analysis
suggested that, when the whole country is taken into consideration, such a
grouping could have arisen by chance (Collins *et al.*, 2002).

and this causes great difficulty for health officials who are asked to respond to
the problem. Interpreting the data is not straightforward and pitfalls include the
fact that cluster analyses are usually done *post hoc*, without prior hypotheses.
Rare diseases will inevitably be distributed in small numbers, thus in small areas
their frequency will fluctuate widely due to chance. In a country like the USA
with a large population and a large area it is inevitable that numerous small-
area clusters will arise for rare diseases and it is difficult to determine whether
this is due to chance. This is particularly true for investigations prompted by
reported clusters of disease because the cases may represent a much larger population than that in the immediate vicinity of the cluster. For example, several
of the cases that occur in a large state may just happen to occur in one corner
of that state by chance. Community members are likely first to note the cluster,
then to look for possible causes, including any nearby environmental contamination, and then they may well attribute the cluster to the potential source. They

will draw boundaries around the cluster after noting it, not before, and there is a danger of overestimating the disease rate through 'boundary shrinkage' of the population from which the cases are assumed to have arisen (Olsen *et al.*, 1996).

Investigating such clusters has rarely led to conclusive evidence as to the cause and usually reveals that the cluster is most probably a chance effect due to variation of small expected numbers. This might not be considered a satisfactory answer, especially if people have formed their own hypotheses as to the cause.

Some public health authorities have developed education tools to help them address the problem of rare disease clusters. For example the US Centers for Disease Control (CDC) have issued their own guidelines for investigating clusters (http://www.cdc.gov/nceh/clusters). They note that, in many cases, what appears to be a cluster of cancer cases does not represent any more disease than might be expected by chance, but that it is more likely to indicate a genuine local risk if the cancers are of a single rare type or have occurred in an unusual age group. In 1990 a conference on the topic noted the large volume of work these clusters impose on regional health departments (AJE, 1990). More recently the Royal Statistical Society in the UK revisited the topic (Editorial, 2001). Statisticians are developing new methods for analysing space–time clusters and the field continues to evolve. In 2006 the journal *Statistics in Medicine* devoted a special issue to disease cluster investigation (Volume 25, Issue 5), with emphasis on statistical modelling and the detection of clusters within surveillance systems. However, many epidemiologists remain concerned that the resources consumed by investigation of rare disease clusters, especially if political pressure is applied, may far exceed the benefits gained. Such expenditure may deprive the community of public funds needed for other activities, including environmental clean-ups that should be done anyway. Ultimately, the final public health decisions are often based on expert opinion and prudent judgements and do not depend on *p*-values and associated mathematical models (Coory, 2008).

Epidemiology of infectious diseases

When would we describe a disease as infectious or communicable? In the *Dictionary of Epidemiology*, it is defined as follows:

Communicable disease (synonym: infectious disease) An illness due to a specific infectious agent or its toxic products that arises through transmission of that agent or its products from an infected person, animal or reservoir to a susceptible host, either directly or indirectly through an intermediate plant or animal host, vector, or the inanimate environment. (Porta, 2008, p. 46)

During the last four to five decades, infectious diseases have not generally been considered a major cause of mortality in developed countries. The production of powerful antibiotics (1950s), polio vaccine (1950s) and measles vaccine (late 1960s) were major milestones along the road to this stage of human history. However, it is worth noting that, in the West, most of the fall in death rates from infections such as TB, pneumonia and diphtheria occurred long before specific clinical treatments or vaccinations were available. Nonetheless, there is no doubt these medical interventions helped speed a further decline in mortality, lowered morbidity, and have since helped maintain this situation (see also Figures 14.1, 14.2). In some countries, notably in South East Asia and South America, a fall in infection mortality (which is still under way) came later and was greatly accelerated by medical and public health interventions. The development and deployment of good vaccines or other effective interventions for diseases that still account for much of the infectious disease burden in the poorer parts of the world would make a huge difference to both morbidity and mortality rates – especially for pneumonia, diarrhoea, HIV infection, dengue, malaria and TB.

In developed countries, mortality due to acute infection is largely restricted to the very young, the elderly and the infirm, but infections remain an important cause of expensive morbidity in these richer nations. Their populations continue to experience considerable sickness and loss of productivity from common infections, notably of the respiratory tract, including influenza, and the gastro-intestinal tract, especially food poisoning. Periodically, epidemics of some vaccine-preventable diseases also recur; for example, pertussis (whooping cough), rubella and measles. In addition, there are many infections that have recently emerged or re-emerged and for some we have made little headway with prevention, or treatment, for example Hendra virus (from horses and bats) in Australia, Lyme disease in the USA (tick-borne) and varicella-zoster infection which causes shingles and is common among the elderly.

There are also new (or unsolved) problems with the old infections. Worldwide, frequent use and misuse of antibiotics produced resistant bacteria, some now unresponsive to all available drugs. Furthermore, anti-viral drugs remain very expensive, are often toxic, and are of limited utility. They are not yet helpful for transmission control or for treating many viral infections.

Infections still constitute the most important disease group in low- and middle-income countries, where they are responsible for almost one-third of the disease burden (Figure 12.1). In particular, the high incidence of pneumonia, diarrhoeal diseases (including cholera), malaria, tuberculosis and dengue in many poor countries causes much premature mortality and disability. Some populous regions in the tropics have additional problems with environments that are receptive for parasitic infections, notably schistosomiasis, trypanosomiasis, filariasis, onchocerciasis and leishmaniasis. These neglected diseases collectively cause substantial morbidity and premature mortality for a large proportion of the world population.

Figure 12.1 The contribution of infectious and chronic conditions to total DALYs in low- and middle-income versus high-income countries. (*Data source:* WHO, 2008.)

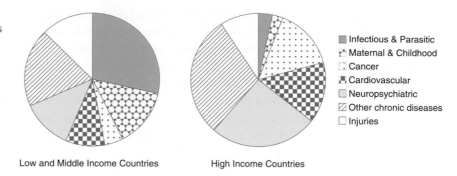

Low and Middle Income Countries   High Income Countries

Legend:
- Infectious & Parasitic
- Maternal & Childhood
- Cancer
- Cardiovascular
- Neuropsychiatric
- Other chronic diseases
- Injuries

Infections everywhere may become more important in the future as old, changed or newly encountered microbes pose threats of local or regional epidemics, or even large pandemics. Emerging and re-emerging infections have steadily become more common over the last 30 years. Many are vector-borne (usually transmitted by blood-feeding arthropods, especially mosquitoes and ticks), most are zoonotic (initially transmitted from non-human vertebrates, usually mammals or birds) and a disproportionate number are viral (especially rapidly evolving RNA viruses such as those causing HIV/AIDS, SARS and influenza). We expect this trend to continue, since it is based on many factors that are sure to persist or increase in the future including population growth, expanding trade and travel, mass-produced food, intensive livestock production, environmental change, resistance to antimicrobial drugs, human encroachment on wilderness and forest, and global warming (Sleigh *et al.*, 2006).

The SARS multi-country epidemic of 2003 was a chilling example of a global threat due to emergence of a new infectious disease. Box 12.1 at the start of this chapter describes its introduction and spread in Hong Kong and beyond. This reveals the problem posed by such lethal fast-moving epidemics of an unknown disease and in this case it involved an infection that attacked the health system itself by infecting and disabling or killing many health workers treating those who were infected. These important events, and the extraordinary global response, are described more fully in the February 2004 issue of *Emerging Infectious Diseases* (vol. 10, No. 2), which is freely available through the US CDC (www.cdc.gov/ncidod/EID/). The worldwide threat posed by new infections has continued unabated since SARS. We have confronted ongoing multi-regional ('panzootic') outbreaks of virulent avian influenza caused by a new H5N1 strain (see Box 12.2 above) and the possibility that a pandemic human variant will develop remains of great concern. And since 2009, as mentioned above, the whole world has been reached by the first wave of a new pandemic variant of human H1N1 influenza which could become more virulent in the future if it follows the pattern of previous pandemics.

Effective identification and control of outbreaks of infectious disease remains an important and complex component of public health. Epidemics are bad news and bad news is always a valuable commodity for the media, so their investigation and control is often conducted as a health emergency under the public eye. Sometimes epidemic alerts trigger worldwide alarm and politically complex national and international responses, as has been noted over the last decade for cholera in South America, plague in India, avian influenza in Asia, SARS in Asia and Canada and pandemic H1N1 influenza worldwide. Increasingly, small or large outbreaks threaten economically important industries, as seen with Hendra virus in Australia (1994, horse racing), Nipah virus in Malaysia (1998–9, pig farming), SARS in Hong Kong (2003, services and tourism) and avian influenza in Asia (1997 and 2003–4, poultry). All of the diseases on this short list of economically devastating epidemics involve zoonotic infections from livestock or wildlife and it is increasingly recognised that human and animal health epidemiologists need to work together. Each new event moves this integration further along under the banner of 'One Health' (http://www.onehealthinitiative.com/) and the responsible national agencies are already sharing expertise and approaches. This integration is also occurring at the international level involving WHO, the OIE (Organization for Animal Health) and FAO (Food and Agriculture Organization).

Infection *eradication* (removal from all human populations), *elimination* (removal from defined areas) and *control* (reduction below the threshold of public health significance) have made substantial progress over the last 50 years but there is a long way to go. The declaration of smallpox eradication by the WHO in 1980 was probably the most important achievement in terms of global health last century. Ongoing programmes to eradicate polio and leprosy and, in some West African countries, to eliminate onchocerciasis are now being attempted. The global Guinea worm eradication programme is close to final success in East and West Africa but is being impeded by civil wars. There has been moderate success in controlling HIV/AIDS among special risk groups in Australia, New Zealand, North America and Europe over the last decade, and more recently in some other countries (notably Thailand), but elsewhere the global AIDS pandemic, the most lethal in human history, continues to spread at an alarming rate, especially among the general populations of many parts of Asia and sub-Saharan Africa.

A causal model

Simple ecological models of the 'agent–host–environment' interplay have served infectious disease epidemiology well, providing a neat structure for linking the variety of factors that determine whether disease occurs. Figure 12.2 is a straightforward version that shows the interaction between an infectious agent and its potential host, the transmission process (how the disease is spread) and

Figure 12.2 The relationships among agent, host, transmission and environment.

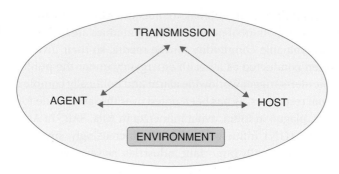

how all of these may be influenced by the environment. We will use its axes to organise our more detailed examination of the links between exposures to infectious agents and disease occurrence.

Although we did not invoke such a model when dealing with causality in Chapter 10, its relevance to most causal circumstances is readily apparent. The *host* mobilises a variety of genetically directed and other adaptive responses against a particular agent; the *agent* can be any infectious or non-infectious risk factor, some of which have a variety of modes of *transmission*; and the *environment* includes the background social, economic and ecological circumstances that surround the host and determine the community risk level.

What influences the spread of infectious diseases?

Before moving to deal with epidemics and their management, it is helpful to consider briefly the biology of infectious agents. Infectious diseases have one distinguishing attribute. They involve one living organism preying on another. Some parasite life cycles even involve two or more hosts and such intersection of biological lifelines is intrinsically complex. Furthermore, within environmental constraints, interacting organisms must evolve elaborate defence or attack mechanisms to maintain their life cycles. Consequently, although infectious diseases may be relatively easy to define (on the basis of presence of the organism and the typical host response), infections are often difficult to understand biologically or epidemiologically. Like many harmful exposures, they have a wide range of host effects, varying from inapparent infection (acute or chronic) to severe disease and death. Also, as environments change, both agents and hosts may be affected, impeding or promoting transmission.

The aims of infectious disease epidemiology reflect those of epidemiology in general: to describe and explain the occurrence and distribution of infections and the relationship of infection to disease. To do this it is necessary to understand the *properties of the agent*, to know (or discover) the *sources of infection* and the existence of any *biological reservoirs* of infection, to clarify the *pathway* or process whereby the agent is transmitted, via the environment, and to know how the *host reacts* to an infectious challenge. Our knowledge of infections has become far more detailed since the development of bacteriology and the germ theory of disease at the end of the nineteenth century, but the agent–host–environment circumstances frequently change and new organisms continually emerge. The relationships are always dynamic and usually extremely complex; it is rarely possible to understand every step of the process, often difficult to assess the probability that infection will occur, and always a battle to keep pace with changes and stay half a step ahead, or even just one step behind.

Exposure variation will often influence the risk of infection. For example, tuberculosis (TB) infection is usually contracted by breathing air contaminated with the organism *Mycobacterium tuberculosis*, but crowded, poorly ventilated environments are not always risky for TB. While there would be a high risk of exposure in a crowded, poorly ventilated area such as a prison in a highly endemic country, the risk in comparable circumstances in a developed country would be much lower. This is one aspect of the crucial role played by the background environment, the population-level influences on individual risk.

Environments also change and this in turn alters infection risks in numerous ways: directly, via effects on humans or agents, or indirectly, via effects on intermediate hosts or infection vectors. This is the basis for recent interest in the effects of global warming on the distribution and incidence of infections. The most obvious effect of warming is the potential increase in the geographical range of vectors or intermediate hosts associated with transmission and a possible shortening of the phase of the life cycle associated with the invertebrate host. Dengue fever is one example of an infection that could be greatly influenced by climate change if the range of the mosquito vector increases (Hales *et al.*, 2002). Another example is schistosomiasis in China and Figure 12.3 shows how its potential range could increase if intermediate host snails could thrive in areas that are currently unaffected (Zhou *et al.*, 2008). However, it should be noted that environmental effects are exerted through multiple drivers and a focus on temperature will show changes in the potential range but cannot predict actual outcomes. For example, the distribution of the snail hosts in China depends on many factors besides temperature including suitable soil chemistry, the presence of other vegetation and appropriate moisture, with needs varying across the life cycle (Seto *et al.*, 2002).

Host factors also come into play. If a person is infected with TB, various personal attributes (such as malnutrition, HIV infection and diabetes) then modulate their risk of developing subsequent *disease*. Such agent–host interactions vary enormously, altering risks of many infectious diseases. In an area highly endemic for malaria, partially immune adults often have detectable blood parasites without becoming ill; but in a less endemic area, or in young children with little or no immunity, detectable parasites in the blood stream would almost

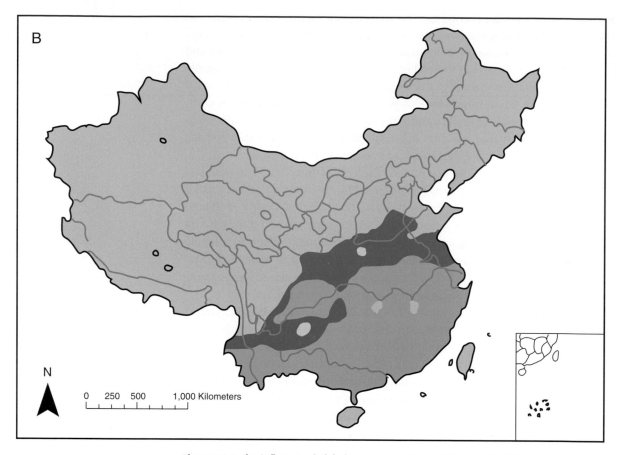

Figure 12.3 The influence of global warming on the predicted distribution of schistosomiasis risk in China in 2050 (mid-blue denotes the risk area in 2000, dark blue denotes predicted additional risk areas in 2050). (*Source*: Figure 3B from Zhou *et al.*, 2008, reproduced with permission.)

always cause symptoms, including fever. This shows how acquired host defences can alter clinical manifestations of infection, often affecting the ability of epidemiologists to detect cases accurately.

Finally, the *agent* also varies frequently. As they evolve, microbial agents that appear to be similar may vary considerably over time or place, with powerful or subtle effects on transmission, host responses, treatment and control. Some, such as influenza virus, are constantly changing their structure as part of the quest for survival; TB, and many other bacteria, have evolved to resist antibiotics. Sometimes agent effects and disease manifestations are simply a reflection of the intensity of the infection, particularly with multicellular parasites such as hookworms, schistosomes and filaria. Morbidity due to these parasites relates directly to the worm burden – more worms for more time produces more disease.

Overall, whether infection occurs depends on factors influencing the probability and result of contact between an infectious agent and a susceptible host. Some of these factors are described below.

The infectious agent

There are many different types of infectious agent: bacteria, viruses, fungi, protozoa, helminths (parasitic worms), etc. In almost every natural habitat there will be agents potentially infectious to humans. Animal contact is particularly important in the genesis of human infections and many (perhaps most) infections afflicting us have been traced back to the beginnings of agriculture and animal farming.

What then is **infection**? It is the entry of a microbial agent into a higher-order host and its multiplication within the host. When a lower organism lives on an external surface of another (usually higher) organism it is called an **infestation** rather than an infection; examples of infestations include lice and scabies. Infections do not necessarily lead to overt disease and the principal characteristics of microbial agents that influence their ability to cause disease are defined below.

Infectivity is the ability of an organism to invade and multiply in a host. It is the proportion of exposures that result in infection. One measure of infectivity is the **secondary attack rate**, which measures the number of cases of infection that develop among the susceptible contacts of an infected case. **Pathogenicity** is the power of an organism to produce overt illness among those infected. It is measured as the proportion of those exposed to infection who develop clinical or overt illness. **Virulence** is the ability of an organism to produce serious disease and is measured by the proportion of those who are infected (determined by immunoassay) who develop severe disease. If death is a criterion of severity, this can be measured by the **case–fatality ratio** (CFR, see Chapter 2).

One highly *infectious* agent is the polio virus. If a source of polio infection enters a community of susceptible people, it is likely that the majority will eventually become infected. However, only a small proportion will develop even mild disease; i.e. the polio virus has low *pathogenicity*. An even smaller proportion will develop symptoms of paralysis and only a small percentage of these will have permanent sequelae; i.e. the virus is of relatively low *virulence*. Like polio, measles also has a very high infectivity; secondary attack rates for measles approach 100%, but, unlike polio, the measles virus demonstrates a high degree of *pathogenicity* because most of those infected will develop symptoms. In the very young, or in malnourished children, measles causes serious disease and is thus also highly *virulent*. Typhoid is a disease with variable virulence. Under the best circumstances of early diagnosis and rapid treatment the CFR may be less than 1%, but late presentation, in the absence of high-quality treatment, often results in CFRs of 10%–15%.

Intensity of infection is especially important for helminth infections. Generally a few parasitic worms (such as hookworms or schistosomes) will not cause detectable disease, but when individual worm burdens reach the hundreds (or thousands), the outcome is often serious debility and premature death.

The natural habitat of the agent is known as its **reservoir** and this may be human, animal or environmental. Agents with human reservoirs include the pertussis bacterium, the malarial parasite and the roundworm. With some agents it is not clear where their reservoir is. There is still debate, for instance, about the environmental reservoir of the cholera bacterium – where does it hide between annual epidemics in the Indo-Gangetic delta? We have also searched for the reservoir of the SARS virus, since we did not know whether certain animals found to be infected (such as civet cats) actually acquired it from another source; it now appears they may have acquired the infection from bats (Lau *et al.*, 2005).

The **source** of an infectious agent is the person, animal or object from which the host acquires the infection. The source may be another human who is sick or convalescent. Infected persons may become long-term carriers of infection without being clinically sick themselves, as with hepatitis B, typhoid and HIV. One of the best-known examples of a long-term carrier is 'Typhoid Mary', who worked as a cook in New York, USA. She is thought to have caused 10 outbreaks of typhoid fever with a total of 51 cases and 3 deaths before her own death in 1938. She was a poor woman and moved from household to household aware that the infection seemed to follow her around but unaware, at least initially, of her own role, and also unaware of the preventive measures needed (scrupulous hygiene).

The host

The host is the human or animal to which an agent acquires entry and in which it multiplies. A host's reaction to infection can be extremely variable, depending on the interplay between the characteristics of the agent, including the dose received, and the specific and non-specific immune status of the host.

The immune response of the very young (especially pre-vaccination) and the old is not as protective as that of a young healthy adult. Most influenza mortality, for example, occurs in the elderly; but this is not always the case and the lethal pandemic of influenza in 1918–19 killed millions of young adults. If the host has been exposed to the agent before, there may be residual natural immunity, or immunity may be induced artificially by vaccination. A person who is susceptible to a particular agent is often referred to simply as a 'susceptible'.

These factors, and others to do with the biology, maturation and replication of the agent, influence the **incubation period**. This is the time between initial infection (entry into host) and the onset of clinical disease (symptoms). For control of infectious diseases it is also important to know the **latent period**; this is defined as the time from entry into the host until the onset of infectiousness and it may be longer or shorter than the incubation period. If it is shorter then infected persons may pass on the infection before they become ill (as with influenza) and if it is longer they will be ill before they are very infectious (as with SARS). This timing is an important determinant of infection dynamics. Infections transmitted before becoming ill (or without becoming ill) are the most difficult to control and the most likely to cause explosive epidemics in susceptible populations. These features are known for the majority of infectious diseases. They are useful tools in the investigation and control of epidemics and are always the focus of attention for new infections such as SARS.

Transmission

Transmission of an agent is its spread from a reservoir or source to a new host by one or more of three possible routes – *direct*, *indirect* or *airborne*.

Direct transmission

This arises from 'close personal contact' by touching infectious secretions or excreta. This includes touching or inhaling the large (10–100 micrometres) respiratory droplets produced by sneezing, coughing or talking by a person suffering from a patent respiratory infection. These heavy droplets contain mostly water and pass through the air to fall on surrounding objects within 1–2 metres of the source. Examples of direct transmission include sexual, skin, eye, congenital and most respiratory infections, including measles and influenza. Sometimes *vertical transmission* (direct from mother to unborn child) is distinguished from *horizontal transmission* (direct or indirect) among persons already born.

Indirect transmission

This always involves a **vehicle**. It may be inanimate, such as bedding, clothes or utensils (collectively called 'fomites'), food or water (many intestinal infections), or the soil (a reservoir for many infectious fungi, Legionella and diphtheria bacteria, and required to complete the life cycle of protozoan Toxoplasma parasites shed by cats and for common human helminths such as ascaris and hookworm). Or the vehicle may be alive and considered a **vector** (e.g. mosquitoes that transmit malaria and dengue, ticks that transmit Lyme disease and lice that transmit typhus) or an obligatory intermediate host (such as snails for schistosomiasis). Most faecal–oral infections, such as polio, typhoid, cholera and many forms of gastroenteritis, are transmitted indirectly (via food or water), but some, such as bacillary dysentery, can also be transmitted via direct contamination of hands and mouth.

Airborne transmission

This became an outmoded concept in the nineteenth century after Snow had shown that London cholera was water-borne, disproving the prevailing theory of an infectious airborne 'miasma' rising from the river. Later, Pasteur and others demonstrated the existence of germs and showed that they could be transmitted directly. The laboratory production in the 1930s of 'bioaerosols' of tiny infectious droplet nuclei that could be inhaled as well as careful epidemiological studies on TB and Q fever in the 1940s and 1950s eventually resurrected the concept of airborne infection as an important mode of transmission (Langmuir, 1961). Bioaerosols may also be produced in abattoirs when cutting open body cavities of infected animals, in air-conditioning cooling towers, or by germ warfare. Droplet nuclei are particles less than 5 micrometers in diameter that are dried-out residuals of large droplets and which remain infectious in air over a long distance and time. The WHO now classifies airborne transmission as *obligate* (pathogens only transmitted by droplet nuclei under normal circumstances, for example TB) and *preferential* (pathogens that can infect by multiple routes but are mostly transmitted by droplet nuclei, for example measles and chickenpox) (Atkinson *et al.*, 2009).

It is important to remember that the type and mode of transmission of an agent are key factors for designing control strategies and that some agents may have several modes of transmission. For example, SARS is usually transmitted by (large) respiratory droplets reaching close contacts, but a few cases spread infection to scores of persons, some of whom had only fleeting contact with cases or no direct contact at all (Li *et al.*, 2004); this raised questions about airborne infection in certain circumstances, such as after intubation and in very confined spaces. The presumed mode of transmission profoundly affects the management of infections, since in hospitals precautions against (heavy) respiratory droplets (ordinary masks and gloves, clean nearby surfaces) are much less exacting than precautions against airborne infection (special masks or respirators, eye shields, negative-pressure ventilation).

The environment

The environment has a strong influence on the transmission of infectious diseases. The physical environment or climate has obvious influences, sometimes for reasons we do not understand well. In temperate zones, influenza and rotavirus appear in the colder winter months, times of close human contact. On the other hand, Ross River fever usually occurs in hot humid months, reflecting the importance of an abundance of mosquitoes for transmission of that disease. Other environmental influences include levels of sanitation, air pollution, water quality, population density, overcrowding, poverty, housing conditions and food availability, to name but a few. The environment affects survival both of arthropod vectors (such as mosquitoes) and of the vertebrate hosts of disease. The environment is, in turn, affected by the agents and, of course, the host. Human behaviour often creates environments suitable for infections. Frequently this is due to imposed ecological circumstances, such as unsanitary households due to lack of clean water and poverty; sometimes it is due to human folly or ignorance, such as creation of mosquito breeding sites in domestic environments in tropical areas and lack of preventive measures to defend against infections such as Q fever in abattoirs. It can also be due to necessity, such as wet-rice farming to produce a crucial food staple that also creates breeding sites for the intermediate host snails of schistosome infections.

Epidemics or outbreaks

There are two principal types of epidemic. Distinguishing between these can help to narrow an epidemic investigation, leading quickly to the cause of the outbreak and to its control.

Point-source epidemics

This type is sometimes called a common-source (or common-vehicle) or extended-source epidemic, the latter implying that the exposure may be spread over a period. This type of epidemic occurs when many people are suddenly exposed to the same source of infection, leading to a clear increase in incidence of disease. We can study the progress of an epidemic by plotting the distribution of cases in relation to the date of onset, producing what is known as an epidemic curve. Figure 12.4 shows the typical shape of the epidemic curve for a point-source outbreak. The number of cases of disease (defined by the onset of symptoms) is plotted against the time since exposure. In this way we

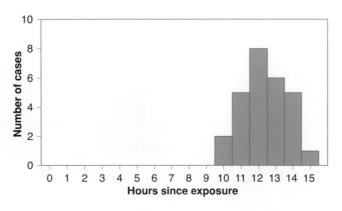

Figure 12.4 The epidemic curve for a point-source epidemic.

can assess the average incubation period, which in this case will be between 12 and 13 hours. This is the typical pattern of an outbreak of food poisoning and shows the distribution of incubation periods in differently susceptible people. Figure 1.3 showed an actual point-source epidemic that you met in Chapter 1.

In practice, the epidemic curve for a common-source outbreak might not be as clear as these examples. A common source like the polluted River Thames in nineteenth-century London could lead to an outbreak of cholera that started at different times in different places, giving a much more complex and drawn-out curve.

Propagative (contagious) epidemics

This type arises from the introduction of an infection into a susceptible population with subsequent transmission from person to person and a progressive increase in incidence. The pattern in Figure 12.5 is typical of a propagative epidemic. On 12 May there was a single case, referred to as the *index* or primary case (there may be more than one). Eight to eleven days later we see another cluster of cases, sometimes referred to as *secondary* cases, which have arisen from the index case by person-to-person transmission. A further eight to thirteen days later there is a third generation of cases, serially infected by the secondary cases. If the spread of incubation periods is wide, the gaps between the peaks progressively close as long-incubation cases for one generation merge with short-incubation cases for the next generation, producing a fluctuating pattern of continuous cases.

Figure 12.5 The epidemic curve for a propagative epidemic.

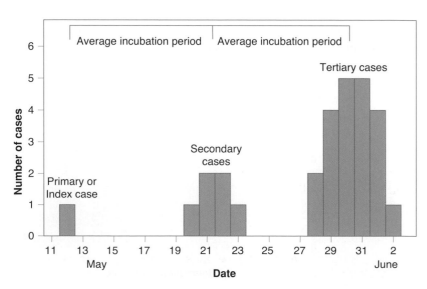

Common conditions for the occurrence (and cessation) of an outbreak

There are numerous agent–host–environment states that might change and precipitate an outbreak. Some of the more common circumstances are

- the *new appearance or sudden increase of an infectious agent*, which may arrive in a human or animal host, a plant, or in an inanimate environment such as soil, and can come from any part of the world by trade, travel or natural spread;
- an *increase in susceptibles* in an environment that has an endemic pathogen; this could be by immigration or birth, or by a drop in immunisation rates in a community; and
- the *introduction of an effective route of transmission* from source to susceptible, e.g. climatic change bringing a new species of mosquito, or a new process of food preparation or storage.

An epidemic will end or diminish when contrary conditions hold, i.e. anything that leads to a large drop in the number of susceptibles and when each case reproduces on average less than once. This may occur through immunisation (including 'natural' immunisation whereby people actually catch the disease and then become immune) or prophylaxis, by removing the source of infection, or by breaking the transmission cycle (e.g. by spraying mosquito breeding sites to lower vector density, by isolating people while they are infectious, by adopting personal protection measures such as gloves and masks in hospitals, or by treating infectious persons early). We see here another complex causal web with the same demands as for any other disease: the need to identify the most cost-efficient response to the short-term threat together with longer-term planning to lower risk overall.

Investigating outbreaks

As with any epidemiological study, the investigation of an outbreak must be systematic. Going back to first principles, we need to look at the distribution of disease by person, place and time in the early stages of the outbreak, and use those observations together with knowledge of relevant preliminary disease characteristics to formulate rapidly initial hypotheses on which early action can be based.

The 2003 SARS epidemic was a perfect example of the urgent interplay of investigations across many disciplines. The studies were conducted successfully during an epidemic that was killing frontline health-system staff and spreading rapidly in many countries. Laboratory scientists quickly defined the organism, its survival in the environment and its susceptibility to antiseptics. Hospital doctors and nurses tested various treatments and instituted exceptional measures to protect hospital staff. Epidemiologists determined the incubation period, the usual mode of transmission, the variable (and usual) infectiousness and the effective control achieved by personal protective measures in hospitals, early isolation of cases and quarantine of contacts. Information managers, computer experts and statistical modellers helped to track the epidemic and analyse control effects. In Hong Kong even the police service played a vital role, collaborating with the Department of Health for contact tracing and identification of high-rise buildings with multiple cases for disinfection teams. This first 'Internet-assisted' global effort for epidemic control led to rapid and complete control of the disease. The overall SARS experience suggests that tools available to combat epidemics are, at least so far, evolving just fast enough to match the increasing demands. Many of those tools have been deployed again, along with considerable input from the Organization for Animal Health and the Food and Agriculture Organization, in the response to H5N1 influenza (2003–). The response to H1N1 pandemic influenza began in 2009 and continues, with emphasis on worldwide monitoring of human susceptibility, disease virulence, drug sensitivity and molecular evolution as well as rapid development of a safe and effective vaccine.

The following series of steps is essential in any outbreak investigation but, with the possible exception of the first three, it is rare to follow them in a neat order as listed below; usually several steps proceed at once.

Provisional case definition. A clear 'working' or 'provisional' case definition is an essential first step. This may be changed or refined – ideally to an aetiological diagnosis – at a later stage in the investigation. For a new or as yet undiagnosed infection a syndromic definition based on some combination of epidemiology (potential exposure), symptoms and signs, and key laboratory information (e.g. elevated white-cell count or radiological evidence of pneumonia) must be developed.

Confirm that the epidemic exists. This will be obvious if there is an abnormally high number of cases of a particular disease, concentrated in time or space or with unique clinical features. With common diseases like influenza or measles you would compare current incidence with background rates in the time before the outbreak, or during the same period or season in previous years. Remember the definition: ' . . . clearly in excess of that expected'.

Assess the extent of the outbreak and its essential epidemiological features. Serious cases might not be a problem to identify since they are likely to present to hospital, but the mildly or moderately ill may be hard to find. Inapparent infections can be discovered only afterwards, usually by serology. A rapid initial survey (by phone and/or record searching) of local hospitals, clinics and doctors will give a preliminary estimate of the size. If the outbreak seems to be widespread, a random household telephone survey might be considered. In addition to clinical and sociodemographic data, the person–place–time approach must be tailored to the situation at hand. Depending on the working hypotheses, it may be necessary to collect details from the patients' workplaces or to obtain evidence of current

Table 12.1 An example of a line list used for recording data in an epidemic following a lunch on December 21 2003.

ID	Age	Sex	Time of lunch	Onset of symptoms (date – time)	Sea-food salad	Oysters	Cured ham	Pizza bread	Pavlova	Coffee with milk
01	34	M	1.15	21/12 – 20.30	Y	N	Y	N	Y	Y
02	23	F	1.10	21/12 – 21.15	Y	N	Y	Y	Y	N
03	65	M	1.20	21/12 – 19.30	Y	Y	Y	N	N	Y
04	47	M	1.40	21/12 – 22.00	N	N	Y	N	Y	N
05	61	F	2.10	None	Y	Y	Y	Y	N	Y
06	58	M	1.15	21/12 – 20.10	Y	N	Y	Y	Y	Y
07	39	F	1.00	21/12 – 19.00	Y	N	Y	Y	Y	N
08	43	F	1.30	21/12 – 21.40	Y	Y	Y	Y	Y	Y
09	47	M	1.25	21/12 – 21.15	Y	N	Y	Y	Y	N
10	51	F	2.15	None	Y	Y	Y	Y	N	Y
etc.										

immunisation status, for example, as well as gathering appropriate biological samples for laboratory testing.

Define the population 'at risk' (the denominator). One task is to define those who have been, may have been and have not been exposed to the agent of the particular outbreak. It is sometimes an impossible task, but for other situations it is more straightforward. These data provide us with denominators for calculating *attack rates.*

Formulate working hypotheses. A number of tools can help with the formulation of some initial hypotheses.

- Draw up a list of all potential cases early on, and for each list crucial data, along the lines of Table 12.1. Refine this to include only definite cases as the investigation proceeds.
- Does the case definition need modification? Is there a definitive diagnosis?
- Draw a spot map, looking for clustering of cases or a link to some point source. Maps by site of residence, occupation or education may be informative.
- Draw the epidemic curve, because its shape will reflect both the time distribution of exposure and the distribution of incubation periods and this can lead to hypotheses on the aetiology.
- Note any interesting anomalies. They sometimes hold the key and are worth investigating in detail. (Remember Snow (1855) at the Broad Street pump.)

Test hypotheses. Additional data may be required to test the hypotheses as outlined below. For example, if a meal is suspected to be a common source, it is essential to try to identify which foods are implicated, as in the example in Chapter 1. If one or two specific foods are linked to high attack rates then it is important to attempt to obtain samples of them in order to try to isolate the agent.

Study design and analysis

Most outbreak investigations are carried out retrospectively, although some may be partly prospective. If the source is known or strongly suspected, a retrospective cohort of all people thought to have been exposed, and at least a sample of those not exposed, can be assembled. From the data we can calculate the **attack rate** in those exposed to the source and compare it with the attack rate in those not exposed. Recall that the attack rate is a specific measure of cumulative incidence that is often used for particular groups being observed for a limited period of time and under special circumstances (such as an epidemic). In propagative epidemics it may also be of interest to calculate the **secondary attack rate**. This is the number of cases among the contacts of a primary case that occurred within the likely incubation period following exposure, as a proportion of the total number of exposed contacts. The attack rates in the exposed and the unexposed can then be compared to give the **relative risk** (risk ratio) of catching the disease if exposed.

If the source of infection is not known, a case–control study can be used to investigate exposure to a variety of possible events and sources of infection. This allows calculation of an **odds ratio** to estimate the association between the source and disease in the usual way (see Chapter 5).

Epidemic management

Dealing sensibly with the media is always an important element in controlling the wider social effects of a real or perceived outbreak. For alarming and lethal outbreaks, such as SARS in Hong Kong in 2003, the skills required in dealing with the media are very particular: panic can be induced, or prevented; scapegoating is easily aroused and tensions can rise rapidly. In such situations media briefings are best left to senior staff, or those specially trained in media skills. The contrast between media management for SARS in China (initial denial) and Hong Kong (candid accounts) was striking; management within China itself changed enormously towards the end of the emergency when all officials were instructed to disclose the situation. Media problems also arose in other affected areas, not just Asia. Large, lethal and mysterious epidemics are always going to make dealing with the media an unavoidable and vital management issue.

There are several other managerial tasks for public health workers responding to an epidemic. Treatment of cases may need to be organised. This will depend on the type of illness, its severity and the number of cases involved. Can local health facilities cope with additional patient loads or will outside help be required? Are there severe cases who may need to be transferred to a tertiary referral centre? Will cases need to be isolated or staff (including any investigating epidemiologists) protected? It may also be necessary to organise collection, transport and reception of specimens for laboratory investigation. These must be handled carefully and others must not be exposed to any risks. For example, collection of throat specimens from potential SARS cases is a risky procedure unless a protective mask, gown, goggles and gloves are used.

In parallel, control measures, both short- and long-term, need to be initiated, particularly if there are signs of a continuing epidemic. These can be aimed at eliminating or controlling the source of the agent, such as contaminated foods. Alternatively, it may be more efficient to reduce transmission of infection, especially if there is a known vector. It may also be necessary to set up a local surveillance system to monitor further cases of the disease, which may facilitate early prevention measures and avoid a further outbreak. The full investigation of an epidemic may be a protracted affair. Confirmation of diagnoses often depends on serology; vectors may need to be collected and identified and there may be need for further, more formal epidemiological studies.

Finally, it is important to ensure that all aspects of an outbreak are reported accurately. The primary reporting responsibility of an epidemiologist investigating an outbreak is to the health authorities but, as the examples above show, the media and public are also vitally interested in such occurrences and need to be kept informed of the situation as clearly and simply as possible.

Epidemic prevention

In an ideal world we could both anticipate and prevent epidemics and that remains the public health goal for all serious infection threats. Even novel infections can be partly anticipated and we can be ready to rapidly detect and investigate them when they appear. To be 'ready' we need to develop and maintain substantial human and laboratory resources, have a suitable system of surveillance, be able to manage the media effectively, and have a clear institutional framework within which surveillance, interdiction and response can operate. (We will discuss surveillance in more detail in the next chapter.) The increasing frequency of emerging and re-emerging infections is ensuring that in many countries the systems are developing to respond more effectively, with less emphasis on politically attractive 'border control' and more emphasis on 'early detection' and 'rapid response'. Improved building, water, food and hygiene standards, and the production and use of vaccines, along with health education, have already lowered the risks for many of the old infections like pertussis, diphtheria, typhoid and plague. But we cannot escape the need to invest in preparation so we can be ready for the new challenges that will certainly emerge. The signs over the last 30 years have been very clear. We must expect the unexpected and be ready for it.

Tuberculosis: a case study

The following case study was adapted and condensed with permission from a teaching exercise devised by Dr Donald Hopkins (The Carter Center, USA). It is based on a pioneering report on the transmission and natural history of an outbreak of tuberculosis (TB) at a Danish school in 1942–3. The approach to the study and the information that emerged remain valid today. The investigation was completed before the availability of anti-TB drugs such as streptomycin (1949) and isoniazid (1952) that would have altered the natural history observed. Few epidemiological studies have had a greater influence on concepts and action for an important infection. The natural histories of primary and post-primary TB were documented, the risks were quantified, and the mode of transmission clarified – all essential information for improving control of the infection.

Background

In the 1940s, the pathogenesis and epidemiology of pulmonary TB was controversial. The mode of spreading was assumed to be prolonged intimate contact but it was not known whether this involved contamination of the environment (e.g. cups or surfaces), direct contact with infectious secretions, or contact via air. Emphasis for control was on contact examination and follow-up, isolation of those with active pulmonary TB and improving home and public hygiene, especially the control of spitting. Use of BCG vaccination was (and remains) of uncertain utility.

The epidemic of tuberculosis in a Danish girls' school, 1942–3

Between December 1942 and March 1943 an epidemic of an acute febrile disease, first thought to be influenza, occurred in a community public school for girls in Denmark. Over a period of 11 weeks 53 cases occurred among the 368 pupils (Figure 12.6).

During the middle of the epidemic, eight cases of erythema nodosum (small, painful skin nodules) were noted and this suggested a diagnosis of primary pulmonary TB. Investigations included tuberculin skin testing of all apparent

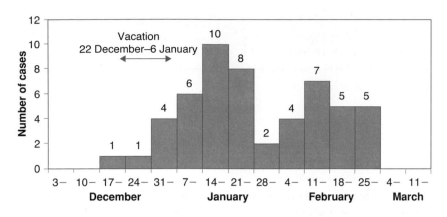

Figure 12.6 The epidemic curve for the Danish tuberculosis outbreak 1942–1944. (*Data source:* Hyge, 1947.)

non-cases, gastric lavage and culturing of skin-test converters, and the taking of chest X-rays of all the students.

The school was already under observation because one year earlier (October 1941) there had been three cases of pulmonary TB with no further spread. Vaccination (BCG) was offered at the time to those who were skin-test negative. On 7 December 1942 a regular follow-up had revealed that 130 pupils were naturally tuberculin positive, 133 had converted after the BCG and 105 were negative (i.e. overall 71.5% were positive). The negatives included those who had refused BCG and new girls who had entered the school in autumn 1942. Thus, coincidentally, the tuberculin status of the school was surveyed just before the 1942–3 outbreak.

The source of infection and mode of transmission

Tuberculin tests performed again in March 1943 revealed that 70 (66.7%) of the 105 previously tuberculin-negative pupils had converted to positive. Of these 53 had suffered from a flu-like illness (with or without erythema nodosum) and 17 were apparently asymptomatic.

School classes moved from room to room on a regular schedule throughout the day. The school building was at ground level except for several rooms 'in the basement which were small and dark . . . in particular the physics room of the middle school which also served as the air-raid shelter. This was a permanently blacked out cellar . . . Any ventilation was practically out of the question because of sand bags piled up in front of windows . . .' (Hyge, 1947).

A search for the source of infection begun in March 1943 included X-ray examination of all teachers and employees. Only one teacher showed distinct changes, but the findings were the same as on preceding examinations. She nevertheless became a suspect source of infection.

This female teacher taught a total of nine separate classes in the physics room spending 'all of her hours at the school in these basement rooms'. Four other classes with different teachers were also held in the basement early in the

Table 12.2 Tuberculin conversion rates between December 1942 and March 1943 among known tuberculin-negative pupils by degree of exposure to suspect teacher.

| | | Tuberculin status | | |
| | | Negative | Positive | % |
Group	Degree of exposure	Dec 1942	Mar 1943	Converted
A	Taught by suspect teacher	53	46	86.6
B	In basement classrooms with other teacher	41	24	58.5
C	In basement classroom prior to arrival of suspect teacher	6	0	0
D	Not in basement	5	0	0
Total		105	70	66.7

(*Data source:* Hyge, 1947.)

morning before the suspect teacher arrived at the school. Three classes did not normally enter the basement rooms.

The tuberculin conversion rates among the pupils who were negative in December 1942 are shown in Table 12.2, according to their exposure to the suspect teacher.

The suspect teacher was placed on leave on 5 March and 'after some objection she was persuaded to submit to gastric lavage on April 6'. (Persons with post-primary infectious pulmonary TB often swallow their sputum and TB organisms may be found in the stomach contents.) The culture revealed four colonies of tubercle bacillus, human type. On careful inquiry 'this teacher stated, as was also confirmed by others, that she had a cold from about the middle of December 1942, when the infection became more aggressive'.

'Very frequent tuberculin tests on the remaining 35 tuberculin-negative pupils who kept attending school' were performed. No new infections appeared after the tuberculin survey in March.

Short-term infection outcomes

All of the 70 converters were repeatedly examined by X-ray and by culturing of gastric lavage specimens. More than half (41) were shown to have a positive culture (5), a positive X-ray (4), or both (32), as evidence of primary pulmonary tuberculosis. The 263 pupils who were found to be tuberculin positive in December 1942 (130 naturally positive and 133 BCG-induced) were also given X-ray examinations in March 1943. 'None was found to show any evidence of active pulmonary tuberculosis.'

Table 12.3 The occurrence of progressive pulmonary tuberculosis in a Danish school for girls, 1943–55.

Tuberculin status	Number of pupils	Total cases of progressive tuberculosis	
		3-year follow-up	12-year follow-up
Naturally positive in December 1942	130	4	9
BCG-induced positive in February 1942	133	3[a]	3[a]
Converters between December 1942 – March 1943	70	6	14
Negative[b]	35	0	0
Total	368	13[a]	26[a]

(*Data source:* Hyge, 1957.)

[a] One mild case of tuberculosis developed in a BCG vaccinee whose tuberculin test had reverted to negative in December 1942

[b] Those who escaped infection during the epidemic.

Follow-up studies and natural history of TB infection

All 368 pupils in the school were followed at regular intervals over the course of the next 12 years for the development of progressive pulmonary TB. The findings are summarized in Table 12.3. Among the 130 pupils who were naturally positive before the outbreak a total of 9 cases of progressive TB developed. Among the 133 who received BCG, 3 cases developed within the first year and none subsequently. Among the 70 who became infected during the epidemic, 6 cases developed within 1 year with a total of 14 cases over the 12-year period (20%).

Implications of the study

Because this study had a defined population and a clear exposure event, we can infer the mode of transmission. In addition, the long follow-up before the advent of specific therapy reveals the natural history of the infection, which is an always important but often elusive component of infectious disease epidemiology. We also note the effectiveness of BCG in that setting, and the 12-year cumulative incidence of progressive (post-primary) TB among four important host categories: recent tuberculin converters, persons naturally infected at an earlier date, BCG vaccinees and tuberculin negatives. The information has implications for post-exposure surveillance of TB and for its prevention and control.

The incubation period for primary pulmonary TB had not been defined accurately because point-source outbreaks with single exposures were rare and the dates of onset of first symptoms were often vague because the symptoms are relatively mild (flu-like). This epidemic is one of the few with onsets specified to weeks. Experimental animals take 1–3 months for tuberculin conversion after inoculation. These girls developed acute primary TB after inhaling TB organisms that lodged in their lungs. Primary TB is usually self-healing and the organisms become dormant in the lungs. The usual situation is that, months to years later, post-primary pulmonary TB may develop with chronic coughing and, in some cases, production of infectious aerosols, usually related to the development of lung cavities connecting to the airway. This is the debilitating and frequently fatal condition generally called 'tuberculosis'.

Conclusion

To conclude this chapter we reiterate that while we have focused on infectious diseases to introduce their special features which had not been covered by the predominantly chronic disease examples used in other sections of this book, the principles used apply to all disease outbreaks, communicable or otherwise. In the next chapter, we will go on to consider another practical public health application of epidemiology that has largely developed from systems originally established to monitor endemic and epidemic infectious diseases, namely the process of **surveillance**. This process provides us with much of our information regarding changes in morbidity and mortality that might signify the emergence of a new health problem (or the resolution of an old one).

Questions

The Public Health Training Network of the US Centers for Disease Control and Prevention has developed some excellent computer-based exercises in outbreak investigation. These are freely available from http://www.cdc.gov/eis/casestudies/casestudy-list.htm.

The following questions relate to the TB case study described at the end of the chapter.

1. Use the epidemic curve in Figure 12.6 to help estimate the probable time of exposure and the incubation period.
2. Were the initial investigations in March 1943 (Table 12.2) based on a case–control or cohort approach to investigating an epidemic? What sort of study was the subsequent 12-year follow-up (Table 12.3)? What biases or confounders could have arisen?
3. What types of measure (cumulative incidence, prevalence, attack rates or other estimates) are shown in the last column of Table 12.2?
4. Comment on the absence of tuberculin in groups C and D of Table 12.2. Do you think these groups are really different from groups A and B (i.e. is the difference likely to be statistically significant), or are the numbers of students in these two groups too small to warrant confident conclusions?
5. From the information yielded by this outbreak, would you prefer your tuberculin status to be:

- naturally positive, i.e. infected at some unidentified time in the past;
- BCG-induced, i.e. converted by receiving BCG after a negative test result;
- recently converted; or
- tuberculin negative?

6. What has this report shown about the mode of transmission of TB?

REFERENCES

AJE (*American Journal of Epidemiology*). (1990). Volume **132**, supplement.

Atkinson, J., Chartier, Y., Pessoa-Silva, C. L., Jensen, P., Li, Y., and Seto, W. H. (Eds). (2009). *Natural ventilation for infection control in health-care settings*. Geneva: WHO

Benenson, A. S. (Ed.) (1990). *Control of Communicable Diseases in Man*, 15th edn. Washington DC: American Public Health Association.

Chan-Yeung, M. and Yu, W. C. (2003). Outbreak of severe acute respiratory syndrome in Hong Kong Special Administrative Region: case report. *British Medical Journal*, **326**: 850–852.

Collins, S., Boyd, A., Fletcher, A. *et al.* (2002). Creutzfeldt–Jakob disease cluster in an Australian rural city. *Annals of Neurology*, **52**: 115–118.

Coory, M. (2008). Statistical inference is overemphasised in cluster investigations: the case of the cluster of breast cancers at the Australian Broadcasting Corporation studios in Brisbane, Australia. *Internal Medicine Journal*, **38**: 288–291.

Deng, J. F., Fleeger, A. K. and Sinks, T. (1990). An outbreak of chromium ulcer in a manufacturing plant. *Veterinary and Human Toxicology*, **32**: 142–146.

Editorial. (2001). Disease clusters and ecological studies. *Journal of the Royal Statistical Society*, **164**: 1–2.

Haddad, V. and Sazima, I. (2003). Piranha attacks on humans, in southeast Brazil: epidemiology, natural history, and clinical treatment, with description of a bite outbreak. *Wilderness and Environmental Medicine*, **14**: 249–254.

Hales, S., de Wet, N., Maindonald, J. and Woodward, A. (2002). Potential effect of population and climate changes on global distribution of dengue fever: an empirical model. *Lancet*, **360**: 830–834.

Hameed, S. M., Popkin, C. A., Cohn, S. M. and Johnson, E. W. (2004). The epidemic of pediatric traffic injuries in South Florida: a review of the problem and initial results of a prospective surveillance strategy. *American Journal of Public Health*, **94**: 554–556.

Hyge, T. V. (1947). Epidemic of tuberculosis in a state school. *Acta Tuberculosea Scandinavica*, **XXI**: 1–57.

Hyge, T. V. (1957). The efficacy of BCG vaccination. Tuberculosis epidemic in a state school with an observation period of 12 years. *Danish Medical Bulletin*, **4**: 13–15.

Langmuir, A. D. (1961). Keynote address. Epidemiology of airborne infections. *Bacteriological Reviews*, **25**: 173–181.

Lau, S. K. P., Woo, P. C. Y., Li, K. S. M. *et al.* (2005). Severe acute respiratory syndrome coronavirus-like virus in Chinese horseshoe bats. *Proceedings of the National Academy of Sciences*, **102**: 14040–14045.

Li, Y., Yu, I. T. S., Xu, P. *et al.* (2004). Predicting super spreading events during the 2003 severe acute respiratory syndrome epidemics in Hong Kong and Singapore. *American Journal of Epidemiology*, **160**: 719–728.

Moser, M. R., Bender, T. R., Margolis, H. S., Noble, G. R., Kendal, A. P. and Ritter, D. G. (1979). An outbreak of Influenza aboard a commercial airliner. *American Journal of Epidemiology*, **110**: 1–6.

Olsen, S. F., Martuzzi, M. and Elliott, P. (1996). Cluster analysis and disease mapping – why, when, and how? A step by step guide. *British Medical Journal*, **313**: 863–866.

Peiris, J. S., Yu, W. C., Leung, C. W. *et al.* (2004). Re-emergence of fatal human influenza A subtype H5N1 disease. *Lancet*, **363**: 617–619.

Porta, M. (Ed.) (2008). *A Dictionary of Epidemiology*, 5th edn. New York: Oxford University Press.

Seto, E., Xu, B., Liang, S. *et al.* (2002). The use of remote sensing for predictive modeling of schistosomiasis in China. *Photogrammetric Engineering and Remote Sensing*, **68**: 167–174.

Sleigh, A. C., Chee, H. L., Yeoh, B. S. A., Phua, K. H. and Safman, R. (2006). *Population Dynamics and Infectious Diseases in Asia*. London: World Scientific.

Snow, J. (1855). *On the Mode of Communication of Cholera*, 2nd edn. London: Churchill. (Source: http://www.ph.ucla.edu/epi/snow/snowbook.html.)

WHO (World Health Organization). (2008). *The Global Burden of Disease: 2003 Update*. Geneva: WHO.

Zhou, X. N., Yang, G. J., Yang, K. *et al.* (2008). Potential impact of climate change on schistosomiasis transmission in China. *American Journal of Tropical Medicine and Hygiene*, **78**: 188–194.

Watching not waiting: surveillance and epidemiological intelligence

Description Chapters 2–3	**Association** Chapters 4–5	**Alternative explanations** Chapters 6–8	**Integration & interpretation** Chapters 9–11	**Practical applications** Chapter 13: Surveillance

Box 13.1 A timeline of events during the identification of the 2002–3 SARS epidemic

November 2002: two GOARN (Global Alert and Response Network) partners, the WHO Global Influenza Surveillance Network and the US Global Emerging Infections Surveillance and Response System, noted media reports of influenza in China.

December 2002: an influenza B epidemic was virologically confirmed by Chinese authorities. In retrospect those early media reports were probably also the first indication of SARS, which also erupted at that time as seemingly unrelated clusters of atypical pneumonia in the south of China (atypical pneumonia is common in that region each winter).

20 February, 2003: Hong Kong confirmed two human cases of much-feared avian influenza (H5N1). This was soon after the Chinese government had

(continued)

Box 13.1 (*continued*)

reported that the atypical pneumonia had been unusually lethal in many cases.

21 February, 2003: just as the WHO prepared for an influenza pandemic, a Chinese doctor was admitted to a local Hong Kong hospital; staff adopted strict precautions against bird influenza but he had already infected several people at the hotel he occupied the night before. They spread the virus to other hospitals, the Hong Kong community, Canada, Vietnam and Singapore.

12 March, 2003: GOARN had gathered enough data from those countries and Hong Kong for the WHO to issue its first global alert.

15 March, 2003: the disease was given the name severe acute respiratory syndrome (SARS). GOARN then linked laboratory scientists, clinicians and epidemiologists all over the world.

July 2003: the causative agent, incubation period, infectious period and usual modes of transmission had been determined, good diagnostic tests and surveillance and control programmes had been devised and implemented, and human transmission ceased.

(From Heyman and Rodier, 2003.)

Box 13.1 summarises the timeline of a critical global health incident – the SARS (sudden acute respiratory syndrome) epidemic – which prompted an unprecedented rapid and collective global response, leading to early effective surveillance and control. Without the ability to gather timely information on such emerging and changing health problems, public health can be paralysed or at best inefficient. In this chapter we will discuss the design and use of the special information systems that allow health officials to detect new risks and diseases such as SARS promptly, track known problems, and generate data needed for effective health planning and resource allocation. This is the population health surveillance system. It is complex in practice but simple in its aims – to generate timely and useful information on the occurrence of health events. It covers infections, chronic diseases and injuries, as well as many of the exposures known to cause ill-health. It is inter-connected within and among regions and has grown much more accessible since the advent of the Internet. Surveillance is the eyes (and ears) of public health.

The word surveillance, meaning 'the constant watching of subversives', came into use during the time of the Napoleonic wars. The modern epidemiological meaning is consistent with the idea of constant watching, but usually of diseases rather than suspects:

Public health surveillance is the ongoing, systematic collection, analysis, interpretation, and dissemination of data regarding a health-related event for use in public health action to reduce morbidity and mortality and to improve health. (CDC, 2001)

However, surveillance of people does still occur for public health purposes; for example, close contacts of infectious persons who have been isolated (or quarantined) to interrupt community transmission are observed until the end of the incubation period for that infection. Similarly, those emerging from a zone with an ongoing epidemic may be monitored; for example, the temperature (thermal screening) and respiratory symptom checks (by questionnaire) of travellers arriving at airports during the 2003 SARS and 2009 H1N1 influenza (often inappropriately described as 'swine flu') epidemics. During the SARS epidemic even high-rise apartment buildings were placed under watch in Hong Kong if two or more cases of SARS occurred there.

Dynamic surveillance data on population risks, morbidity and mortality are the key indicators for epidemiological intelligence on community health. When surveillance data vary from the expected they may provide a justification for investing in basic or strategic research to respond to the anomalies. Surveillance is used to detect outbreaks of new or old diseases and, over recent years, has increasingly been recognised as a crucial component of national and global defences against catastrophic epidemics. Globally, regionally and locally, it also provides evidence and data for health planning and evaluation. Surveillance detects and quantifies the occurrence of important or potentially important health risks or outcomes, revealing their distribution, incidence and prevalence. For many infections (such as HIV/AIDS, TB, malaria, meningitis and dengue) local and regional transmission rates are of central interest in deciding whether to activate and justify control programmes or to monitor their effects. For other infections (such as new strains of influenza) the surveillance data lead to rapid global responses.

The essential features of a surveillance system are:
- practical, clear case definitions for each disease;
- workable, uniform and continuous data collection methods; and
- rapidity of collection, analysis, interpretation and dissemination of data.

Ultimately, the purpose of surveillance is disease control and prevention. Practical intermediate goals include identifying and monitoring outbreaks, limiting transmission of infectious agents, prompt treatment of illness, evaluation of disease control programmes and planning health services.

The scope of surveillance

Traditionally the term surveillance has been applied to monitoring acute infectious diseases and although this remains a major focus, its scope has widened substantially. Today, surveillance also covers morbidity and mortality for many non-infectious diseases (e.g. congenital malformations, injuries and cancer); hospital discharges; use of vaccines and prescription drugs and their adverse reactions; and even environmental hazards in the workplace and the general environment (air, water, soil). Although not demanding such an immediate response, the principles underlying these newer extensions of the concept to chronic disease are the same: unless we monitor trends we cannot identify emerging problems. In addition, health information systems are beginning to extend surveillance to risk factors themselves, an interest reinforced by *The World Health Report* in 2002 which highlighted the need to reduce risks in order to lower the avoidable burden of disease. The WHO identified the ten leading risk factors accounting for over one-third of all deaths worldwide: being underweight; unsafe sex; high blood pressure; tobacco consumption; alcohol consumption; unsafe water, sanitation and hygiene; iron deficiency; indoor smoke from solid fuels; high cholesterol level and obesity (WHO, 2002). It is not possible to tackle these risks without good surveillance to monitor their trends and distributions. Some of these are monitored by specialised units while others are rolled into general health service information collections.

At the same time as a risk-oriented re-focusing has occurred in public health, there has been growing awareness (or rediscovery) of the role of poverty and other fundamental social determinants of health. The last decades of increasingly active research on social epidemiology have brought the concern with health inequities into the consideration of many health ministries. Surveillance and geo-social mapping of these socioeconomic trends is in its infancy but is growing quickly. This development involves partnerships between the health and social service sectors, as well as with national statistics offices and treasuries, information technologists and statisticians.

Finally, useful contributions to health surveillance activities can also come from many other types of information. This could include, for example, reports on climatic conditions, which could be of interest with respect to patterns of respiratory disease, mosquito-borne infections or even heat- or cold-induced thermal stress. Information on animal health is also an important component of public health surveillance. Contemporary examples include avian influenza, Q fever and leptospirosis – all subject to surveillance in animal populations. Historical examples in developed countries since World War II include surveillance for brucellosis, tuberculosis in dairy herds (to control human TB in the 1950s) and then tuberculosis in beef cattle (to protect abattoir workers). Today, meat inspection remains a very important component of all infectious-disease surveillance systems intended to protect human populations from zoonoses – infections that cross from animals to humans.

Notifiable diseases

What issues do you think should be considered before a disease is included on a notifiable list as a disease to be watched?

In the first instance, this is a matter of assigning a level of public health importance to a disease. When doing this, the first issue to be considered is the incidence of the disease (if it is of long duration, its prevalence might be more appropriate). How many people are affected and how many more are likely to be? How severe is the illness? What is its expected mortality? Infectivity? Other pertinent factors include the degree of preventability of the disease, the potential effects on productivity and medical costs, media exposure and political and economic costs. The recent global focus on the explosive SARS epidemic of 2003 was driven by a powerful combination of its high case–fatality ratio (10% overall), mysterious origins and cause, apparent rapidity of long-distance spread and the severe consequences for the travel industry. Furthermore, although there were eventually only 8,422 cases worldwide, 1,706 (21%) of those affected were healthcare workers and in some areas (such as Hong Kong and Canada) the case–fatality ratio was as high as 17%. Once the outbreak was recognised, global surveillance was adopted and SARS was made a notifiable disease. The experience with SARS helped improve the global surveillance and notification system and in 2007 WHO member states adopted new International Health Regulations (WHO, 2008). These include an expanded list of diseases that must be notified to WHO and the requirement to report any event that could become a public health emergency of international concern, including events that do not involve infections. The appearance of a new low-virulence variant of pandemic influenza (H1N1) in 2009 tested the new regulations in ways that had not been anticipated, as WHO had to balance well-prepared responses against a public heath impact that was less severe than expected.

Clearly, any schedule of notifiable diseases should be reviewed regularly. Are there new problems we need a handle on? Have laboratory advances meant that we need to review the case definitions? Also, in a system that relies heavily on the co-operation of busy clinicians, is everything being done to maximise co-operation? This includes keeping the list of notifiable diseases as short as possible (in practice it seems to be a lot harder for a disease to 'leave' a list than to join it!); using simple reporting forms or procedures (electronic forms are increasingly common); and giving timely feedback to show how the data collected are used to enhance healthcare.

Sometimes surveillance information is available within the health system but there is a slow response (or no response) or further dissemination is actually suppressed; combinations of system failures and/or misguided political judgement can compromise the utility of the best data collection protocols. Response fail-ures have been shown to lead to much avoidable national morbidity and mor-tality for infections such as plague, cholera, Ebola haemorrhagic fever, West Nile virus and SARS. It is even worse when the infection spreads to multiple coun-tries, or around the world. Early responses to outbreaks of lethal transmissible infections, or to diseases caused by new exposures to environmental toxins, may save many lives. However, over-response is also an issue and public health offi-cials need good judgement to balance the response against the risk. Once an emergency is declared trade, travel, schools and many facets of normal life and the economy are quickly disrupted. The situation that unfolded with pandemic H1N1 influenza in 2009–10 has tested the ability of public health leaders to get it right and it will take several years before judgements can be made about the appropriateness of the global response.

Types of surveillance

Surveillance systems fall into three broad types, all of which may co-exist in a single geographical area or health system: passive, active and sentinel systems.

Passive surveillance

As the name implies, a passive surveillance system depends on the discretion or whim of the healthcare provider, even where notification is required by law. Although a passive system is likely to be inexpensive, it may not be complete because not all events will be reported. An exception to this might be the report-ing of a condition with a high level of media coverage at a particular time (e.g. SARS, dengue haemorrhagic fever, Ebola, haemolytic–uraemic syndrome and anthrax).

Media-driven alerts can also assist passive surveillance of non-infectious dis-eases. An example is the spectacular epidemic of eosinophilia–myalgia syn-drome (a rare autoimmune disease) in the USA. Over 1,500 cases and more than 25 deaths were detected in 1989 and 1990. This painful and mysterious non-infectious condition was investigated epidemiologically by contacting many cases detected by the passive surveillance system. The cause was found to be the chemical composition of a single source of L-tryptophan, a common over-the-counter dietary supplement for which the method of manufacture had been altered just before the epidemic began (Jimenez and Varga, 1991).

Surveillance of the majority of notifiable diseases in many countries relies heavily on a passive system, whereby the diagnosing doctor initiates a report to the monitoring authority (although often only a minority of cases is actually reported). In addition, laboratories notify the authority when they come across an individual with any one of a specific set of diseases for which notification is required by law (including cancer as well as infectious diseases). These laboratory reports are likely to be much more complete than the primary care-initiated reports.

Absolute figures from passive surveillance frequently underestimate the true illness burden. It is likely, however, that patterns and changes over time, across regions and among differing groups of people (age, sex, ethnicity) will still be informative. It is also possible to perform 'active' surveillance (see below) in representative sub-sets of a passive-surveillance population and thus derive multipliers to convert the passive rates into more accurate estimates. Of course this is cheaper than a population-wide active surveillance system but it will miss small outbreaks and other sub-regional variation if those areas were not included in the active-surveillance samples.

Active surveillance

Active surveillance is based on specific collection of data from healthcare providers or institutions, both as a need arises and in the longer term. Unlike passive surveillance which relies on healthcare providers remembering to report events, in active surveillance the organisation conducting the surveillance actively seeks the relevant information. It is used, for example, during outbreaks of food-borne pathogens or measles when healthcare providers are contacted and asked to provide details of any cases they have seen. Laboratory data defining strains of prevalent organisms are used for forward planning (e.g. choosing the right influenza vaccine for the next winter epidemic); and knowledge of patterns of resistance to antibiotics can influence local choices of treatment for bacterial diseases. A further example is the requirement that hospitals provide data on all discharges. Expansion to non-infectious diseases has come with legal requirements to report incidence of cancers in many countries, establishing high-quality networks that permit research as well as monitoring (see Chapter 3).

Active surveillance may also include household surveys to detect ongoing transmission of infections. For example, this can be done serologically for malaria in at-risk areas if incidence rates are low and reports by health workers are unreliable. It may also be done for TB or schistosomiasis, by using skin tests to detect past infection, or for polio, by searching for floppy paralysis. Active surveillance may extend to environmental assessment for ongoing, reappearing or even new disease risks, including the presence or abundance of relevant vectors of infection such as specific species of mosquitoes or snails.

Active surveillance can produce more complete data of better quality than that provided by other systems. However, it is resource-intensive to maintain, especially to produce timely output of information. In those jurisdictions that permit it, and when the technology makes it feasible, active surveillance can be done

Box 13.2 Post-marketing surveillance of the safety of the drug cimetidine

Almost 10,000 patients who took cimetidine (mostly for peptic ulcer) between 1977 and 1980 were followed for 15 years to observe their long-term health outcomes. The findings were reassuring, providing no evidence of any long-term adverse effects of cimetidine (at least not ones that could be detected by monitoring mortality rates). The data arising from this surveillance have also been used to examine the possible positive relationships between ingestion of aluminium and Alzheimer's disease, and *H. pylori* infection and ischaemic heart disease, but no significant relationships were found (Beresford *et al.*, 1998).

using *record linkage* to link records from different sources to extract information that would otherwise be sought by passive surveillance systems. Examples include the use of clinical and treatment records to detect iatrogenesis (illness as a result of treatment by a physician), especially adverse reactions to drugs as shown in Box 13.2. This can be taken further by establishing systems to anticipate such events even before they occur (e.g. when potentially adversely interacting drugs are prescribed but before they are dispensed), so linking surveillance with prevention in a most direct manner.

Sentinel surveillance

Sentinel surveillance relies on the reporting of cases of specific diseases or risk factors that may indicate that a particular preventive or therapeutic activity is not working as planned. Examples of sentinel health events would include a case of poliomyelitis, which might indicate that there has been a breakdown in the vaccine cold chain (such that a batch of vaccine has not been stored correctly) or that vaccination coverage has fallen to a low level (see Box 13.3); or a case of mesothelioma linked to a past history of exposure to asbestos. In some countries (Australia and the UK to name two), there is also a network of sentinel primary care practices that report a number of diseases on a regular basis. Their list of diseases reported varies from year to year but typically includes things such as influenza-like illnesses, culture-confirmed influenza, chickenpox and shingles. Sentinel surveillance of the staff in large hospitals that treat cases arising from an epidemic in the community can also be useful. For example, annual influenza trends among staff in large Hong Kong hospitals amplify early trends in the community and could be used as an early warning system, provided that staff members are not vaccinated against influenza (and many are not). Similarly, presentations of community-acquired pneumonia to such hospitals can be monitored to discern trends of respiratory illness in the community, detect unusual pathogens

Box 13.3 Polio eradication – surveillance and progress in India

By 2001, polio had largely been limited to two states in India, with only 268 new cases that year, but in 2002 there was a major resurgence with 1,600 new cases. In 2003, a network of 248 medical officers trained in surveillance assisted Indian health authorities with surveillance for acute flaccid paralysis (AFP), the critical clinical marker of polio. The WHO criteria for assessing the quality of polio surveillance require that

- *non-polio* AFP should be detected at a rate of ≥ 1 per 100,000 in the population aged <15 years (to ensure that 'background' AFP cases are being detected at a level showing good coverage) and
- adequate stool specimens should be collected from $\geq 80\%$ of people with AFP for polio diagnosis.

India had been meeting these criteria since 2000, but in 2003 the non-polio AFP rate was <1/100,000 in seven small states and stool specimens were inadequate in 11 states (covering 35% of India's population). During 2002, the proportion of infants aged less than 1 year who received three or more routine doses of oral poliovirus vaccine was only 21% in some states. Following this effort, vaccination increased again in 2003 and only 225 wild poliovirus cases were reported that year, the lowest level yet (Anonymous, 2004).

and track incidence rates for year-to-year comparisons and early detection of epidemics. At the most active end of the scale internationally, the CDC Division of Emerging Infections and Surveillance Services website reports a complex array of current US sentinel and active surveillance programmes (http://www.cdc.gov/ncpdcid/deiss/index.html).

Surveillance in practice

The most developed surveillance systems can be found in the USA. There the Centers for Disease Control and Prevention (CDC) provide an excellent example of integrated disease surveillance and Table 13.1 gives a brief history of the development of the current system. The CDC website (http://www.cdc.gov/DataStatistics/) also lists many surveillance activities, related scientific data (e.g. injury maps and information on hazardous materials), health statistics (including the National Center for Health Statistics database) and up-to-date laboratory information on disease organisms. Sixteen surveillance programme categories were listed in March 2004; this list has expanded to over 50 in 2010, with just over 20 specifically for infectious diseases, and new elements including an Enhanced Terrorism Surveillance Network – the '8 Cities Project'. Box 13.4

Table 13.1 A brief history of the US National Notifiable Diseases Surveillance System.

Year	Events
1878	Congress authorised the US Marine Hospital Service, the forerunner of the Public Health Service (PHS), to collect morbidity reports regarding cholera, smallpox, plague and yellow fever from US consuls overseas. This information was to be used for instituting quarantine measures to prevent the introduction and spread of these diseases into the USA.
1879	A specific Congressional appropriation was made for the collection and publication of reports of these 'notifiable' diseases.
1893	The authority for weekly reporting and publication of these reports was expanded by Congress to include data from states and municipal authorities.
1902	To increase the uniformity of the data, Congress enacted a law directing the Surgeon General to provide forms for the collection and compilation of data and for the publication of reports at the national level.
1912	State and territorial health authorities – in conjunction with PHS – recommended immediate telegraphic reporting of five infectious diseases and the monthly reporting, by letter, of 10 additional diseases. The first annual summary of 'The Notifiable Diseases' included reports of 10 diseases from 19 states, the District of Columbia, and Hawaii.
1928	All states, the District of Columbia, Hawaii, and Puerto Rico were now participating in national reporting of 29 specified diseases.
1950	State and Territorial Health Officers authorised a conference of state and territorial epidemiologists whose purpose was to determine which diseases should be reported to PHS.
1961	The Centers for Disease Control (CDC) assumed responsibility for the collection and publication of data concerning nationally notifiable diseases.
2010	More than 50 infectious diseases are listed as notifiable.

(From http://www.cdc.gov/ncphi/disss/nndss/nndsshis.htm, accessed 23 January 2010.)

gives some examples of the many programmes running as at January 2010 – you have already met one of these, the Behavioral Risk Factor Surveillance System (BRFSS), as this was the source of the obesity data shown in Figure 3.4.

The CDC integrates surveillance with its Public Health Information Network (PHIN) and uses on-line and other methods to enhance the system. A current initiative is the National Electronic Telephonic Surveillance System (NETSS) (http://www.cdc.gov/ncphi/disss/nndss/netss.htm) which promotes integrated systems of reporting at federal, state and local levels.

The WHO is the leading international agency for disease surveillance. It compiles global data and is the central resource for monitoring infectious diseases and detecting and reporting outbreaks. The WHO is especially important for helping resource-poor areas respond to epidemics. Since 1997 it has operated the Global Alert and Response Network (GOARN). This network includes 120 partners throughout the world and identifies and responds to over 50 national outbreaks per year in developing countries. It includes tracking of media reports in its surveillance strategies and has found that it is helpful to monitor and plot rumours of outbreaks as well as respond to reports from member

Box 13.4 Examples of surveillance programmes in the USA (2010)

8 City Enhanced Terrorism Surveillance Project
Assisted Reproductive Technology (ART) Success Rates
Behavioral Risk Factor Surveillance System (BRFSS)
Birth Defects Surveillance
Early Warning Infectious Disease Surveillance (EWIDS)
HIV/AIDS Statistics and Surveillance
National Diabetes Surveillance System
National Notifiable Diseases Surveillance System (NNDSS)
National Oral Health Surveillance System (NOHSS)
Pediatric Nutrition Surveillance System (PedNSS)
Pregnancy Nutrition Surveillance System (PNSS)
Pregnancy Risk Assessment Monitoring System (PRAMS)
Registry of Toxic Effects of Chemical Substances (RTECS®)
Sexually Transmitted Diseases
Traumatic Injury Surveillance
Tuberculosis Surveillance Reports
United States Cancer Statistics
Vaccine Adverse Event Reporting System (VAERS)
Workplace Safety and Health Surveillance
                    (From http://www.cdc.gov/DataStatistics, accessed 17 January 2010.)

countries or its network. The utility of GOARN for multi-country epidemics was revealed by the SARS emergency in 2003 (see Box 13.1 at the start of the chapter).

Like the CDC, the WHO also conducts surveillance for risk factors. In 2003 the Non-Communicable Diseases and Mental Health team at the WHO launched the first 'SuRF' report on Surveillance of Risk Factors related to non-communicable disease, with a second more comprehensive report in 2005 (https://apps.who.int/infobase/surf2/start.html). These reports assembled existing data on the prevalence of major risk factors related to non-communicable diseases for WHO member states for the first time, using information from the WHO Global NCD (non-communicable disease) Infobase. The WHO has since introduced a stepwise system for surveillance (STEPS) to help member countries collect comparable information using the same standardised questions and protocols (http://www.who.int/chp/steps/en/). The risk factors reported are tobacco and alcohol use, patterns of physical inactivity, low fruit/vegetable intake, obesity, raised blood pressure, and raised blood cholesterol levels, as these make the major contribution to mortality and morbidity from chronic diseases, can be changed by primary interventions, and can be easily measured in populations.

Figure 13.1 Evolution of
surveillance for measles, mumps
and rubella in England and
Wales: providing the platform
for evidence-based vaccination
policy. (From Vyse *et al.*,
Evolution of surveillance of
measles, mumps and rubella in
England and Wales,
Epidemiologic Reviews, 2002;
24: 125–136, by permission of
Oxford University Press.)

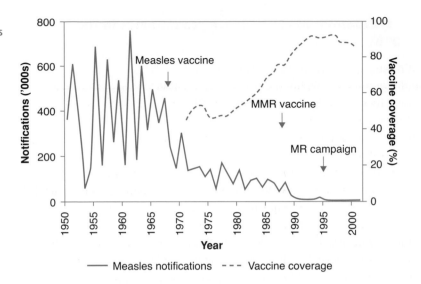

A national example – surveillance for MMR (measles–mumps–rubella) in England and Wales

Box 13.5 shows the historical development of measles, mumps and rubella (MMR) surveillance in the UK. It is a good example of the extension of a basic passive surveillance system with sophisticated use of several complementary data sources in order to plan, evaluate and update the evolving vaccination strategy. The original article (Vyse *et al.*, 2002) shows elegantly how each element contributed to the increasingly subtle analyses required as vaccine coverage has improved, local disease rates have declined (causing more misdiagnosis), imported disease has increased and vaccine resistance has emerged in some population subgroups. Figure 13.1 shows the very positive overall disease trends, but the continuing challenge is to maintain and extend control of these diseases. The WHO is committed to eliminating measles as a global problem, but, as demonstrated by this example, this will not be easy.

Describe the overall pattern of measles occurrence. Comment on the likely role played by vaccination in its control.

The graph shows a regular see-saw of epidemic peaks (with hundreds of thousands of extra cases) and troughs from 1950 through to the commencement of measles vaccination in 1968, although their amplitude was already lessening somewhat. Thereafter there is an initial sharp drop in the number of notified cases (even though vaccine coverage expanded slowly at first), followed by a general pattern of steady decline interrupted by occasional peaks. The switch to MMR vaccination and extra coverage pushed notifications down

Box 13.5 Surveillance of MMR (measles–mumps–rubella) in England and Wales

Methods of monitoring vaccine coverage

(i) Estimate *vaccine coverage* in 2- and 5-year olds (since 1960s for 2-year olds); done quarterly, using sentinel antigens with rapid feedback to immunisation services.

(ii) Introduce *statutory notification* of clinical measles (1940), mumps (1988) and rubella (1988).

(iii) Widespread *laboratory confirmation* of clinical reports (since 1994) – a critical addition because with the falling prevalence, only 20% of clinical diagnoses were actually confirmed as cases (also genotyping for diagnosis and outbreak tracing).

(iv) *Antibody prevalence monitoring* of MMR (1986) in residues of general specimens submitted to public health laboratories; plus *sentinel laboratory monitoring* of rubella susceptibility in antenatal women (1984).

(v) Supplementation by other data sources: death certificates, hospital admissions, primary care surveillance of mumps (sentinel practices), and congenital abnormality surveillance for rubella.

Vaccine policy

Guided by modelling based on the above data and vaccine availability, delivery strategies moved through a number of stages:

1968: measles vaccine introduced (80% coverage by 1988);

1970: rubella vaccine introduced for schoolgirls and susceptible women (>95% protection of young adult women by 1988);

1988: combined MMR vaccination of infants commenced (plus initial catch-up for 2–4-year-olds and selective vaccination of older females susceptible to rubella);

1994: one-off measles–rubella campaign in 5–16-year-olds to head off possible measles epidemic and 'top up' rubella coverage;

1996: two-dose MMR strategy implemented (second dose before school entry).

(Vyse *et al.*, 2002.)

sharply again towards zero (this would show better on a logarithmic scale); and the 1994 campaign does look as if it might have killed off a possible small epidemic. This is a very successful public health intervention that has required a lot of thought and hard work, in particular very active surveillance via a variety of data sources as outlined in Box 13.5, to implement.

A regional example – disease surveillance in Queensland, Australia

As a fairly standard example of a practical overall surveillance scheme at a regional level, we describe below the Queensland (Australia) notifiable-diseases system. Queensland is a geographically large state (seven times the area of the UK) but has a population of only about 4.5 million. Queensland Health conducts surveillance for approximately 80 conditions, primarily using passive surveillance based on combinations of clinical and laboratory notifications. Data are collated centrally and then disseminated to the local Public Health Units for action. Regular improvements to the underlying information technology aim to enhance the system's sensitivity, timeliness, uniformity and acceptability. Giving good feedback to clinicians and increasing their involvement in the process are also expected to add substantially to the system's quality. Some case studies give examples of the varied ways in which surveillance data are used, which are often a function of the nature, severity and frequency of the disease concerned.

> *Hepatitis C.* Most notifications are of chronic (i.e. prevalent) infections (acute clinical presentations are rare), so reported numbers give no idea of incidence. There is no active public health response to a notification, and the data are used for health planning only.
>
> *Poliomyelitis.* This is now a very rare disease (as in most developed countries). Apart from local needs, this viral illness is monitored as an element of the WHO programme to eradicate polio. There is enhanced surveillance seeking all cases of acute flaccid paralysis (clinical diagnosis) with very strict guidelines on laboratory samples and testing. There is a direct public health response to every case notified.
>
> *Ross River virus.* Queensland has large annual outbreaks of this often debilitating mosquito-spread viral illness. Actual notifications received are only a small proportion of cases, and there is a lag time in notification reflecting both the long incubation period of the disease and the time needed for confirmatory laboratory testing. The data are used for health planning, including responses at the local government level (mosquito control), and in public awareness campaigns.

Rumour surveillance

An important practical aspect of surveillance is the surveillance of rumours. In 2004, news of a possible outbreak of avian influenza or 'bird flu' (H5N1) in Vietnam led to an 'epidemic' of reports of avian influenza from around the world. Rumours of outbreaks of disease cause anxiety, especially when the disease is poorly understood, and can lead countries to impose travel and trade restrictions with inevitable social and economic consequences. An important component of the H5N1 surveillance program was thus the identification and investigation of such rumours so that false rumours could be countered as quickly as possible. Media reports and web/email-based public health discussion groups were accessed on a regular basis to identify rumours of cases and these rumours were then followed up by the local WHO country office. Of a total of 40 rumours identified from 12 different countries only nine were found to be correct (Samaan *et al.*, 2005). The importance of this aspect of disease surveillance – the verification of reports of disease from unofficial sources – is now recognised in the latest edition of the International Health Regulations (WHO, 2008) which states:

Article 10 Verification

WHO shall request, in accordance with Article 9, verification from a State Party of reports from sources other than notifications or consultations of events which may constitute a public health emergency of international concern allegedly occurring in the State's territory. In such cases, WHO shall inform the State Party concerned regarding the reports it is seeking to verify.

Evaluation of surveillance

Surveillance systems have (or should have) stated goals and objectives. These are the logical starting points for evaluations and the following attributes should be the focus.

1. Is the system detecting what it is supposed to detect?
   The surveillance system data need to be compared with data produced by another detection mechanism set up especially for evaluation.
2. Is the system producing data in time for appropriate responses?
3. Can the system cope with anomalies and changes?
   The disease, or our knowledge of it (or both), may be changing quickly. A surveillance system should be able to adapt to such changes and should not rigidly adhere to outdated definitions or criteria. A good system needs to have a mechanism to enable such flexibility.
4. Is the system as simple and cheap as possible?
5. Are the public health responses timely and appropriate?
   Any system that does not lead to appropriate responses is flawed. Evidence that the responses are appropriate should be sought.

Summary

Surveillance is an important tool for public health, and routine surveillance data are available in regular reports produced by national and international sources all over the world (we discussed some of these in Chapter 3). Any system that provides for the rapid collection, analysis and interpretation of data in order to prevent disease is highly valuable, but here is a word of caution from one of the world's pre-eminent epidemiologists, the late Sir Richard Doll. In an article on 'Surveillance and monitoring' (1974), he warned that 'It is almost as easy to be drowned in useless information as it is to be starved of essential elements'. The growing lists of surveillance targets noted above show that this caution is more relevant today than ever.

This and the previous chapter have largely focused on the control of infectious diseases, through prevention and other strategies, and the monitoring and evaluation thereof. In the next chapter we will move on to a broader consideration of disease prevention in general.

REFERENCES

Anonymous. (2004). Progress toward poliomyelitis eradication – India, 2003. *Morbidity Mortality Weekly Report*, **53**: 238–241.

Beresford, J., Colin-Jones, D. G., Flind, A. C. *et al.* (1998). Postmarketing surveillance of the safety of cimetidine: 15-year mortality report. *Pharmacoepidemiology and Drug Safety*, **7**: 319–322.

CDC (Centers for Disease Control and Prevention). (2001). Updated guidelines for evaluating public health surveillance systems: recommendations from the guidelines working group. *Morbidity and Mortality Weekly Report*, **50** (No. RR-13): page 2.

Doll, R. (1974). Surveillance and monitoring. *International Journal of Epidemiology*, **3**: 305–313.

Heyman, D. L. and Rodier, G. (2003). Global surveillance, national surveillance, and SARS. *Emerging Infectious Diseases*, **10**: 173–175. Available from www.cdc.gov/ncidod/EID/vol10no2/03–1038.htm.

Jimenez, S. A. and Varga, J. (1991). The eosinophilia–myalgia syndrome and eosinophilic fasciitis. *Current Opinion in Rheumatology*, **3**: 986–994.

Samaan, G., Patel, M., Lolwokure, B., Roces, M. C., Oshitani, H. and the World Health Organization Outbreak Response Team. (2005). Rumor surveillance and avian influenza H5N1. *Emerging Infectious Diseases*, **11**: 463–466.

Vyse, A. J., Gay, N. J., White, M. E. *et al.* (2002). Evolution of surveillance of measles, mumps and rubella in England and Wales: providing the platform for evidence-based vaccination policy. *Epidemiologic Reviews*, **24**: 125–136.

WHO (World Health Organization). (2002). *The World Health Report 2002. Reducing Risks, Promoting Healthy Life*. Geneva: World Health Organization.

WHO (World Health Organization). (2008). *International Health Regulations (2005). Second Edition*. Geneva: World Health Organization.

Prevention: better than cure?

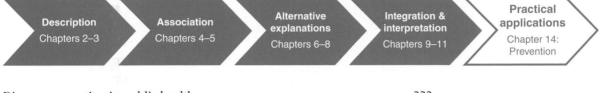

'Prevention is so much better than healing, because it saves the labour of being sick.' (Adams 1618)

While in population health we would prefer that people did not become ill in the first place, this largely remains a remote goal, so achieving disease control through more effective treatments remains a core public health strategy. But prevention is still our ideal, and epidemiology underpins much of our work in this area. In particular, it is central to identifying causes of disease that we can change; it provides quantitative measures of relative and absolute risk that help direct preventive action; and it plays a major role in evaluating whether preventive programmes might actually work in practice. Additionally, what we might term the 'epidemiological perspective' is helpful in conceptualising both the practical and the ethical elements of prevention.

Disease prevention in public health

When we speak of prevention, we usually mean **primary prevention**, which aims to prevent disease from occurring in the first place, i.e. to reduce the incidence of disease. Vaccination against childhood infectious diseases is a good example

Figure 14.1 Age-standardised death rates from tuberculosis in England and Wales, 1840–1968. (From McKeown, *The Role of Medicine. Dream, Mirage or Nemesis?* (1979), with permission from Blackwell Publishing.)

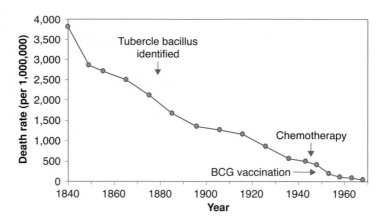

Figure 14.1 Age-standardised death rates from tuberculosis in England and Wales, 1840–1968. (From McKeown, *The Role of Medicine. Dream, Mirage or Nemesis?* (1979), with permission from Blackwell Publishing.)

of primary prevention, as is the use of sunscreen to prevent the development of skin cancer.

Figure 14.1 shows tuberculosis (TB) mortality over time in England and Wales. This is a disease that had all but disappeared from developed countries but is now re-emerging elsewhere as a worldwide scourge.

Considering the figure, how important do you think the BCG vaccine and new therapy were in promoting the decline in TB mortality?

Figure 14.1 and other historical trends make it clear that major health gains were made before the advent of any sophisticated medical therapies and preventive measures. Social and cultural changes such as improved housing, sanitation, general hygiene and nutrition have had a major influence on TB mortality, presumably both by reducing incidence and by increasing survival. The effects of such 'upstream' effects on disease incidence are sometimes termed *primordial prevention*, because they are remote from the more proximal causes that medicine and (conventionally) public health usually deal with. Our view is that the upstream and proximal causes are inter-related and in practice it can be difficult to distinguish the two; any intervention that lowers incidence is thus sensibly termed primary prevention.

So, should we dismiss the value of the proximal strategies for TB control? (Note that BCG vaccination was introduced later in the UK than in Denmark, as shown in the example at the end of Chapter 12.) On the absolute scale of Figure 14.1 their contribution does seem marginal. But would mortality have declined less quickly if there had been no BCG vaccine and no chemotherapy? Consider Figure 14.2, which shows the same information plotted on a log scale so that a 50% reduction in mortality looks the same regardless of whether the drop is from a death rate of 4,000 to 2,000 per million or from 40 to 20 per million, i.e. Figure 14.2 depicts the *rate of change*. We now see a slow and steady fall in mortality across

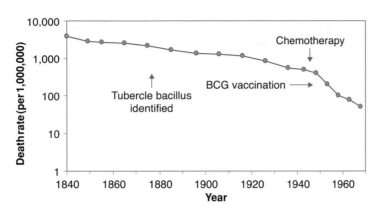

Figure 14.2 Age-standardised death rates from tuberculosis in England and Wales, 1840–1968, plotted on a logarithmic scale.

the first 80 years that quickens slightly around 1920. The slope steepens just after the introduction of chemotherapy and continues to fall following the introduction of BCG vaccination. These are hardly definitive evaluations of the benefits of these advances, but the acceleration of the fall in mortality around 1950 implies that something has changed, and the introductions of vaccination and treatment are the best candidates. And here, as elsewhere, when evaluating the 'big-picture' population effects of interventions we have to realise that such apparently simple descriptive data are often going to be the main basis on which our judgements rest.

While the principal goal of public health should first and foremost be primary prevention, as suggested above, for many diseases we do not have enough information (biological and/or epidemiological) to mount such a programme effectively (or cost-effectively). Even when we do have the knowledge, the barriers to implementation may be substantial (e.g. financial, cultural, social, ethical). For example, we know already that ensuring everyone has access to clean water would prevent a large proportion of infectious disease, but for many countries the practical and financial implications are enormous. Similarly, by persuading more people to stop smoking, stay out of the sun, lose weight, exercise more and eat better we could prevent much of our present burden of chronic disease, but changing behaviour remains a major challenge.

Additional strategies are therefore required in order to enhance disease control and, rather confusingly, some of these have also been labelled as prevention. So-called *secondary prevention* is directed towards reducing morbidity and mortality by improving the outcomes of disease that has already developed. Generally this means early diagnosis by **screening**, allowing earlier (and hopefully more effective) intervention; we will take this up in more detail in the next chapter. What is sometimes called *tertiary prevention* is even more remote from the everyday concept of disease avoidance, usually implying limiting disease progression or providing better rehabilitation to enhance quality of life in the longer term.

Table 14.1 The role of epidemiological knowledge in disease control: a case of two cancers.

Intervention	Accepted utility for widescale use	
	Lung cancer	Breast cancer
Prevention	YES. Smoking cigarettes is *the* strong risk factor; and exposure is modifiable by actions at personal and community levels.	NO. Many weak risk factors, most not readily modifiable (although limiting alcohol intake and, post-menopause, weight control and limiting use of hormone therapy are possibilities).
Screening	NO. Even the newest tests (computed-tomography lung scans) yield very limited survival benefits.	YES. Substantial good evidence (from RCTs) of lower mortality due to population screening programmes for over 50s.
Improved treatment	NO. Minor survival improvements only with newer treatments.	YES. Results from RCTs show that a survival advantage can be achieved with appropriate chemotherapy/radiotherapy.

In terms of *disease control* then it seems more useful to emphasise the fundamental distinction between preventive interventions (primary prevention) and all other actions that lead to improved clinical outcomes once disease occurs. The former lower disease incidence and hence limit the clinical burden from a disease, while the latter (e.g. screening) can actually lead to large increases in clinical activity to bring about additional reductions in morbidity and mortality.

Decisions as to the most appropriate approach for disease control need to be disease-specific: less disease is most desirable, but might not be attainable if causal knowledge is limited. Screening may be a good second choice in some circumstances if advancing diagnosis really does produce better outcomes (not as straightforward as it might seem, as you will see in the next chapter). Finally, improvements in treatment remain an important avenue for enhancing survival and quality of life for affected individuals. Table 14.1 contrasts two cancers with markedly different control profiles, showing epidemiological and other research findings.

The solution to the lung cancer epidemic is obvious, and concerted multi-level efforts to reduce smoking rates (ranging from targeting individual behaviours to banning advertising and legislating for smoke-free public space) have made big inroads on lung cancer rates in many countries (see Figures 3.5 and 3.6). Nonetheless, it remains a common disease, so efforts to improve clinical outcomes through early detection and better treatments are also important, although their yield to date has been slight. Valuable extra benefits have come from smoking control programmes as noted in Box 14.1, but the other examples point to the need to consider the balance of *all* effects – positive and negative – of any intervention before deciding if it should be introduced widely.

Box 14.1 Choosing a preventive strategy: the whole story

An important aside to the lung cancer story is that anti-smoking campaigns have also greatly reduced the incidence of other respiratory disease and heart disease. While causal research is primarily disease-specific, preventive interventions manipulate exposures that may have many consequences. Thus we need good information on the full array of effects of any exposure we plan on modifying: a strong association with one disease is generally insufficient in itself. Immunisation campaigns against infectious diseases would seem an obvious exception to this, but they have lowered incidence so dramatically that fewer lives are now saved and the occasional severe side-effects of immunisation start to take a more prominent place on the balance sheet. Although virtually every consequence of decreased exposure to cigarettes is positive and thus the total benefit-to-cost ratio is huge, counter-examples abound where complexity is the rule. For example, moderate alcohol consumption is linked to *lower* heart disease but *higher* breast cancer rates and, at high intakes, it is associated with an array of other health and social problems.

How do we combine the different effects on morbidity and mortality for various diseases? Does the benefit of avoiding one non-fatal stroke obtained by long-term aspirin use outweigh the risk of three new life-threatening gastric bleeds? Measures such as DALYs and QALYs provide a more quantitative method of doing this and, although they are still rarely used in primary research publications, they are increasingly reported by health agencies as you saw in Chapter 2. (Note: there are many guides available to aid decision-making in the clinical setting; see, e.g., Steyerberg, 2009.)

With breast cancer we see the reverse situation. Quite a lot is known about its aetiology, but there is no strong established causal factor, as we have with cigarettes and lung cancer, that offers a basis for widespread intervention. However, recent sharp drops in use of postmenopausal hormones have probably lowered incidence in a number of countries (Parkin, 2009), and reducing alcohol intake and, in postmenopausal women, weight could also yield some preventive benefits. Fortunately, dual approaches to decreasing morbidity and mortality, namely population screening by mammography to detect early lesions and more effective non-surgical treatments, have paid off. Despite incidence rates that have, until recently, been constant or even increasing, there have been downturns in mortality from breast cancer in a number of countries from the early 1990s, with an example from the USA shown in Figure 14.3. This suggests that the improved outcomes predicted by tightly controlled clinical trials have transferred reasonably effectively to the community setting. Note again the use

Figure 14.3 Breast cancer mortality rates per 100,000/ year age-standardised to the 2000 USA population, for women in the USA, 1979–2006. (*Data source:* CDC Wonder (US DHHS), accessed 9 January 2010.)

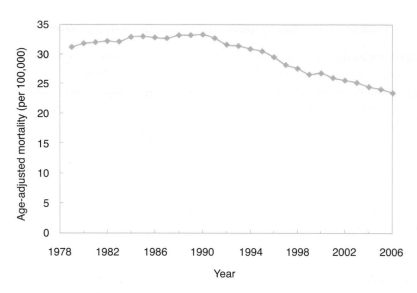

of routine descriptive data to evaluate the effects of interventions in the community; but also that this alone cannot separate out the relative contributions of early diagnosis and improved treatment. However, as this is important knowledge for setting the cancer control agenda, there have been a number of attempts to address the question by comparing disease characteristics and survival in eras with different screening and treatment interventions (Webb *et al.*, 2004) and by statistical modelling (Berry *et al.*, 2005).

We will not consider clinical contributions to disease control any further here – instead our discussion will focus largely on the applications of both epidemiological data and epidemiological thinking to disease prevention and screening. In relation to disease prevention, we will concentrate on the conceptual underpinnings of the preventive approach and some current practical concerns and challenges, as well as looking at the utility of using population attributable fractions (PAFs) to target potential 'high-yield' interventions. In Chapter 15 we will go on to consider screening in terms of its underlying logic, and the major challenges to evaluating its contributions to the control of any given disease.

The scope for preventive medicine

Our earlier examples of disease variation by person, place and time have shown that there are large differences between groups, suggesting that much disease should be preventable if only we could lower everyone's risk to that of the lower-risk populations. Another striking example comes from an investigation seeking an explanation for the three-fold excess of cardiovascular disease (CVD)

Table 14.2 A comparison of prevalence of CVD risk factors between Finnish and Chinese village populations aged 20–64 years.[a]

Risk factor	Men		Women	
	Finns (%)	Chinese (%)	Finns (%)	Chinese (%)
Being overweight	63	21	61	24
Obesity	19	2	24	5
Hypercholesterolaemia	34	3	28	6
Hypertension	49	32	35	28
Smoking	26	73	7	37

[a] All differences were statistically significant ($p < 0.001$, except $p < 0.05$ for hypertension among women) (Hu *et al.*, 2001).

mortality in Finland compared with China. Surveys carried out in rural villages in the two countries over the same time period revealed quite different profiles of CVD risk factors (Table 14.2). The first three factors, all more prevalent in Finland, could be taken as related to over-nutrition, and possibly to the fat content of the diet. Given China's history of major famines in the mid twentieth century it is not surprising that differences remain so profound, at least in rural populations. Countries undergoing the *health transition* away from a predominance of infectious diseases and problems of marginal nutrition are, in principle, well placed for intervention to prevent the emergence of Western lifestyle diseases, many of which are related to over-consumption and inactivity. However, social engineering is challenging, and the pace of development and industrialisation in Chinese cities suggests that the risk-factor profiles of the urban populations there are already less favourable than those in rural China. This is also true for other countries in transition, as can be seen in Thailand, where obesity was 50% more common among younger Thai adults who were life-long urban dwellers compared to those who maintained rural residence (Banwell *et al.*, 2009). Table 14.2 also reflects the different attitudes to control of smoking, with predictable negative consequences for China that are already emerging in the rising lung cancer and CVD rates there.

Population versus individual risk

There is a tendency in medicine and epidemiology to try to divide people into two groups – those who have a high risk of developing a particular disease and those at low risk. For instance, a woman of child-bearing age with high blood pressure, who smokes and has a family history of blood clotting would be considered at high risk of complications if she took the oral contraceptive pill and

Figure 14.4 Distribution of systolic blood pressure in a population of middle-aged men. (Adapted from Figure 2.1, *The Strategy of Preventive Medicine*, G. Rose (1992), by permission of Oxford University Press.)

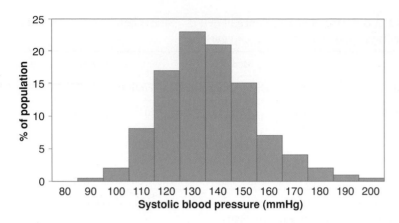

this would not be prescribed. In population terms, however, the benefits of the pill are well recognised to outweigh harms, and it is widely prescribed – although not primarily for the prevention of disease (it does, however, prevent ovarian and endometrial cancers).

So, how should we think about our approaches to preventing ill-health? Should we devote most of our attention to the high-risk groups? This has been the basis of the vast improvements in occupational health and safety since the industrial revolution, and remains an appropriate approach for other specifically disadvantaged or exposed groups, including many indigenous peoples. However, risk of disease is not a simple high–low phenomenon and there are few well-defined natural borders between clearly different levels of risk. As an example, consider the relationship between blood pressure and risk of fatal cardiovascular disease (CVD). Figure 14.4 shows the wide range of 'usual' blood pressure levels in a population. Individuals do not fall sharply into two separate groups with low and high blood pressure and do not, therefore, have a clear-cut 'low' or 'high' risk of heart disease.

As discussed by Rose (1992), the Whitehall cohort study of British public servants showed that the age-adjusted risk of dying from CVD over the 18-year follow-up period increased with increasing blood pressure. The results are shown in Figure 14.5.

In Figure 14.5, is there any level of systolic blood pressure that is not 'riskier' than the one below it?

Looking at Figure 14.4 and 14.5, how many men in a population of 10,000 would have a systolic blood pressure of 150 mmHg? What is the risk (cumulative incidence) of dying from CVD in this group?

So how many men with a blood pressure of 150 mmHg will die from CVD? What about those with a blood pressure of 170 mmHg?

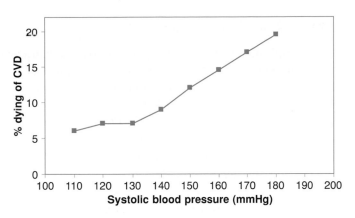

Figure 14.5 The relationship between systolic blood pressure and risk of fatal coronary heart disease or stroke over 18 years of follow-up. (From Figure 2.2, *The Strategy of Preventive Medicine*, G. Rose (1992), by permission of Oxford University Press.)

From Figure 14.5 we can infer that the risk of dying from CVD at any level of blood pressure is greater than that at the level below. The risk increases slowly up to 130 mmHg and then increases more sharply and linearly from there. From Figure 14.4 we can estimate that 15% or 1,500 of a population of 10,000 men would have a blood pressure around 150 mmHg, and from Figure 14.5 the risk of dying of CVD in this group is 12% over the 18 years of follow-up. We would, therefore, expect about 12% × 1,500 = 180 CVD deaths in this group. Similarly, 4% or 400 of the population would have a blood pressure of 170 mmHg and they have a 17% risk of dying of CVD. We would therefore expect about 17% × 400 = 68 CVD deaths in this group. Thus, although the risk of dying of CVD is greater for those with higher blood pressure, over twice as many actual CVD deaths will occur among the much larger number of people with intermediate blood pressure. Targeting prevention at only those with very high blood pressure will not, therefore, address the majority of deaths (but see Box 14.2 on the next page for a clinical perspective).

Figure 14.6 shows a concrete example of the close overlap in risk-factor distributions (in this case serum cholesterol level) between those who did and did not subsequently die from ischaemic heart disease (IHD; if the disease terminology here is becoming confusing, check back to Box 2.6). The whole curve for those who died from IHD is clearly shifted to the right compared with those who did not die, but the two overlap considerably and the cut-off point identifying the extreme upper 5% of the 'healthy' cohort identifies only 15% of those who will develop IHD. So again, screening for high-risk individuals according to their cholesterol level is not a good preventive strategy for the whole population.

Strategies for prevention

Choosing the best way to intervene in order to lower disease risk in a specific population will often be a challenge. We present below some brief comments

Box 14.2 A clinical perspective

The example in the text shows the population perspective on prevention: at the community level more CVD deaths would be prevented by focusing on the larger numbers of people at intermediate risk than on the few at high risk. But let us focus on the individual for a moment. Lowering an individual's blood pressure from 150 to 120 mmHg would reduce their risk of CVD from 12% to about 7%, an absolute risk reduction of 5%. This then translates to a 'number needed to treat' (NNT) of 20 (1 ÷ 0.05) in order to prevent one CVD death. Similarly, lowering an individual's blood pressure from 170 to 120 mmHg would reduce their risk of CVD from 17% to about 7%, an absolute risk reduction of 10%, which gives an NNT of 10. At the individual level, therefore, the benefits are greatest for those at highest risk. This highlights that what is best for the individual is not necessarily best for the population and vice versa.

Figure 14.6 Relative distributions of serum cholesterol levels in men who subsequently died of ischaemic heart disease and men who did not. The shaded areas indicate the proportions of the population above a cut-point that identifies the top 5% of the healthy cohort. (Reproduced from Wald and Law, *BMJ*, 2003; 326: 1419–1425, with permission from BMJ Publishing Group Ltd.)

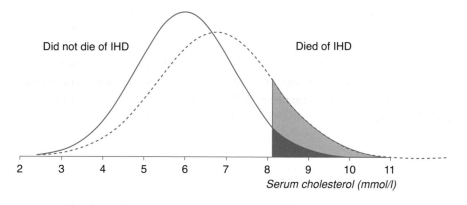

on the theoretical extremes of practice, the *high-risk* and the *mass* or population strategies. Although we have seen why the mass strategy is widely considered to be preferable, it might not always be practical. To borrow from an old definition of politics, skill in the art of identifying the possible is needed. To reinforce this point, we also show a 'middle path' showing the value of considering detailed patterns of risk factor–disease associations to guide intervention targets and strategies.

The high-risk strategy

Classically, preventive medicine takes a high-risk approach; that is, a targeted rescue operation for vulnerable individuals. First, those individuals in special need are identified (e.g. intravenous drug users). The preventive process then

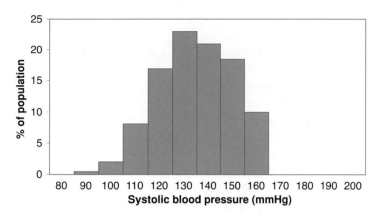

Figure 14.7 The hypothetical distribution of systolic blood pressure in middle-aged men after applying a 'high-risk' screening strategy. (Adapted from Figure 4.1, *The Strategy of Preventive Medicine*, G. Rose (1992), by permission of Oxford University Press.)

takes the form of controlling the level of exposure to a cause (e.g. introduction of a needle-exchange programme) or providing protection against the consequences of the exposure (e.g. vaccination against hepatitis B) in this high-risk group.

Another example can be found in the blood pressure problem we discussed earlier. We might decide that the high-risk patients are those with a systolic blood pressure over 160 mmHg. The high-risk strategy would then involve screening out those individuals with high blood pressure, followed by intervention to ensure that their blood pressure is brought below this level. This remains a common approach in clinical practice and, if fully applied, might lead to a population blood pressure distribution like that in Figure 14.7. If we compare this graph with Figure 14.4, we can see that those who were in the upper tail have lowered their blood pressure, and thus presumably their CVD risk, but the main group (among whom most cases will occur) is unaffected.

High-risk strategies appeal for a number of reasons. The intervention is well matched to individuals and their concerns (e.g. a needle-exchange programme is a specific and tailored response to a tightly defined group), and thus should also improve the benefit-to-risk and benefit-to-cost ratios. Furthermore, avoiding interference with the non-needy group and adopting a 'magic bullet' approach to the target group are readily accommodated within the ethos of the medical care system.

So, can the high-risk strategy play a useful preventive role? Of course it remains highly appropriate and desirable in clinical practice. If, at the community level, a problem is confined to an identifiable minority and can be successfully controlled in isolation, then the high-risk approach can also be appropriate. Apart from the well-documented benefits that can come from targeting various occupational groups, for example hepatitis vaccination for those who work with blood products, others where this approach has current relevance include refugees, other migrants and many indigenous peoples. However, on its

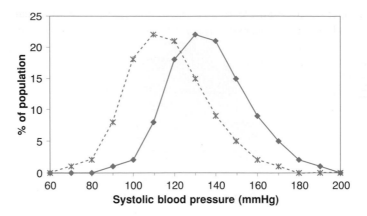

own it is an inadequate response to a common disease or a widespread cause and we need to be very cautious in claiming that a risk really is sufficiently limited to the so-called high-risk group. For example, screening only older pregnant women, who are known to be at highest risk of conceiving a child with Down's syndrome, will miss the majority of afflicted fetuses, which are conceived by younger women in whom most pregnancies occur.

The mass strategy

In the case of a common disease or widespread cause, the extreme alternative approach is the mass or population strategy advocated by Geoffrey Rose (1992). This starts with the recognition that the occurrence of common diseases and exposures reflects the behaviour and circumstances of society as a whole. The mass strategy thus aims to reduce the health risks of the entire population.

Using the blood pressure data again we can illustrate a mass-strategy approach to this problem. Instead of targeting only those people with the highest blood pressure, we would aim to reduce everybody's blood pressure by a smaller amount. This would shift both the blood pressure and the CVD risk of the population to a lower level (Figure 14.8). This is a much healthier situation for the whole group (although perhaps not for some highest-risk individuals) than the truncated distribution we saw in Figure 14.7.

Other examples of the mass strategy are immunisation programmes, water fluoridation and the legislated use of seat belts (together with effective enforcement, as without this a number of countries have failed to realise the true benefits from introducing seat belt laws). Imagine the problems of implementing a 'high-risk' approach to seat-belt use by targeting only male drivers under the age of 25 years who are at the greatest risk of dying in a motor-vehicle accident... In many countries, other background and personal aspects of the 'causal web' for motor-vehicle-related deaths and injuries have also been effectively targeted at the population level with, for example, better road and barrier engineering, car structural safety and legislation backed by enforcement to curb speeding and drink-driving.

 In Box 14.3 we show an example of a 'middle-road' approach that sits somewhere between the mass and high-risk approaches, reminding us of the need to

Box 14.3 Weight and diabetes: a 'middle-road' strategy

Brown and colleagues (2007) used data from the Australian Longitudinal Study on Women's Health to model the effects of different patterns of weight reduction on risk of hypertension and diabetes. As predicted, for hypertension they found a larger benefit for a mass approach than for a targeted high-risk approach (Table 14.3). However, the pattern was somewhat different for diabetes, where the high-risk approach was more effective, largely because unlike risks of hypertension, which increase linearly with increasing BMI, the risks of diabetes are more concentrated at the higher end of the distribution. But for both outcomes, a 'middle-road' approach aiming for a moderate reduction in weight in the top half of the population gave the greatest reductions in risk. Ultimately though, the predicted benefits have to be balanced against the costs and acceptability of each approach. For example, while targeting only a fifth of the population via a high-risk strategy may save money initially, achieving and maintaining the greater weight loss required to deliver the full benefit may prove impractical in the longer term and aiming for a more modest weight loss in a greater proportion of the population may be more cost-effective.

Table 14.3 Effects of different intervention approaches on risk of hypertension and diabetes in an Australian population.

		Risk reduction	
Approach	Intervention	Hypertension	Diabetes
Mass	Modest reduction in weight (1 BMI unit) across whole population	10%	13%
High-risk	Larger reduction in weight (3 BMI units) in heaviest 20% of the population	7%	17%
Middle-road	Moderate reduction in weight (2 BMI units) in heaviest 50% of the population	12%	23%

(*Data source:* Brown *et al.*, 2007.)

test our presumptions and prejudices against the known data before proceeding with a particular approach to implementing a prevention programme. Indeed Rose made it clear that careful attention must be paid to the patterns of association between risk factor and disease (e.g. a linear increase in risk versus an exponential one – see Box 14.3 for example). The prevalence of the high-risk exposures is also important, as seen for blood pressure and CVD above, and it is for this reason that the population attributable fraction (PAF) that you met in Chapter 5 can be useful in identifying optimal preventive interventions. We will look at this further in the next section.

The population attributable fraction as a guide to prevention

As you saw in Chapter 5, one useful way to estimate the burden of disease in a population that can be attributed to a particular risk factor is to calculate the **population attributable fraction** (PAF):[1]

$$\text{PAF} = P_{e(\text{cases})}\frac{(\text{RR} - 1)}{\text{RR}}$$

where P_e is the prevalence of exposure to the risk factor of interest *in those with disease* and RR is the relative risk of disease for the exposure of interest. The PAF also represents the maximum percentage reduction in the burden of disease (or death) that might be expected if we could remove the exposure completely.

However, this formula assumes that exposure is dichotomous: people are either exposed to a risk factor or they are not. For instance, if we are interested in the PAF of CHD or stroke due to high blood pressure we could set a cut-off point at 140 mmHg to define 'high blood pressure'. But we know that while the highest risks of CHD and stroke are seen at blood pressures above 140 mmHg, there is also some increase in risk between 110 and 140 mmHg (Figure 14.5). We also know that most of the population have values below 140 mmHg (Figure 14.4), so using that simple cutpoint would underestimate the total amount of disease due to elevated blood pressure. Moreover, if we uniformly apply one average value of RR for the effects of having any systolic blood pressure over 140 mmHg, we ignore the dramatic increases in risk above that level. This is a major issue if we want to make comparisons between populations because their prevalences of high and very high blood pressures are likely to differ.

This was a particular problem for the World Health Organization when it set out to estimate cross-national burdens of disease due to a range of risk factors

---

[1] Note: as you saw in Chapter 5, there are several different formulae for calculating the PAF. This version is the most flexible as it is still valid when we need to use adjusted relative risks to allow for confounding.

as a basis for identifying preventive strategies (the *Comparative Risk Assessment* study; Murray *et al.*, 2003). Their practical solution was to develop an approach which could account for several different levels of a risk factor by summing the effects across these levels to produce an overall PAF for the risk factor.

A second challenge for the WHO was to determine what the unexposed or *reference* level should be for a particular risk factor to allow sensible comparisons to be made between risk factors and preventive strategies to be chosen accordingly. For risk factors with an obvious zero exposure level (e.g. smoking, air pollution) it makes intuitive sense to use that level as the reference. However for risk factors such as blood pressure, body mass and serum cholesterol there is no zero exposure so, for these factors, the reference value was taken to be that level of exposure which would give the minimum disease/injury burden (Murray and Lopez 1999). The **attributable burden** of disease due to a risk factor is thus *the amount of disease due to levels of exposure above the defined reference level* and the **attributable fraction** is the *proportion of that disease which can be attributed to the risk factor.*

To gain the maximum future benefit from a preventive intervention we would have to reduce exposures to their reference level, e.g. by eliminating smoking or air pollution completely. This of course is infeasible, particularly for an exposure like smoking because once someone has smoked they can never return to being a never smoker, so more realistic estimates are needed. A *plausible minimum* for tobacco exposure might be the low smoking prevalence in Sweden (16%); however, even this might not be realistic for the near future and a more *feasible* target might be to reduce smoking prevalence by 5%, say from 25% to 20%.

Figure 14.9 on the next page shows the hypothetical effects of reducing levels of current exposure (time T_0) on the future burden of disease (time T_x). The dark blue area represents the burden of disease *attributable* to prior exposure; at time T_0 this is equal to 'a' and the attributable fraction is therefore $a \div (a + b)$. The dashed arrows represent the effects on the burden of disease of different reductions in exposure at T_0: 0% (no change), 25%, 50%, 75% or 100% (complete elimination). Thus if we were to reduce the prevalence of exposure by 50% at time T_0 the amount of disease *avoided* at time T_x would be that indicated 'c' and the avoidable fraction is $c \div (c + d)$. Note that the burden of disease *not* attributable to the risk factor of interest (the spotted area) may be decreasing, constant or increasing over time (as shown in the figure).

Attributable and avoidable disease

Figure 14.9 also shows the difference between the *current burden* of premature death and disability due to past or current exposure (dark blue) and the *future*

Figure 14.9 Attributable and avoidable burden. (Adapted from Murray *et al.*, 2003.)

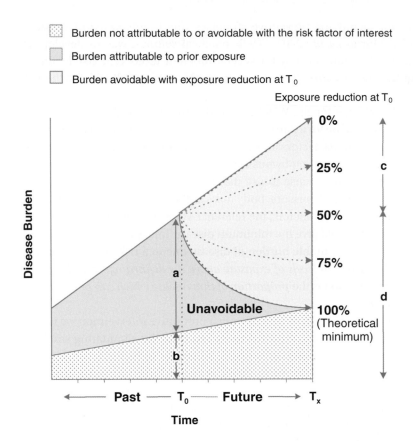

burden due to current and future exposure (light blue). The **attributable burden** is the amount of the current burden that can be attributed to past exposure, and thus would not have been observed if past levels of exposure had been zero (the amount of disease *a* in Figure 14.9 at time T_0). The **avoidable burden** is the amount of *future* disease that could be avoided if current and/or future levels of exposure are reduced to a specified level. The figure shows the predicted effects of reducing exposure by 25, 50, 75 and 100%.

For a real-life example see Figure 14.10. This shows standardised lung cancer mortality rates in Australia from 1979 to 2001, with projections to 2021. The dark blue area shows the unavoidable burden of lung cancer attributable to past smoking, the light blue area predicts the amount of future disease that would potentially be prevented if smoking levels had dropped to zero in 2001, and the dashed line shows the effects of a 50% reduction in smoking in 2001. Of course we must always keep in mind the uncertainty of all such forward projections as they are highly dependent on all of the other factors that affect population behaviours.

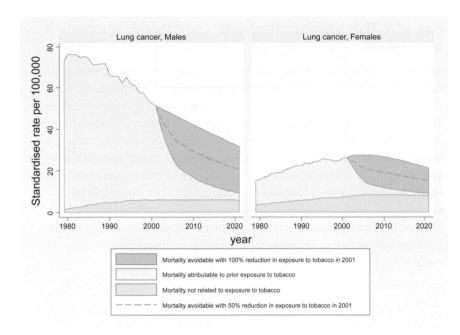

Figure 14.10 Attributable and avoidable lung cancer mortality due to tobacco (standardised rates), Australia 1979 to 2021. (*Source:* Stephen Begg, Queensland Health, reproduced with permission.)

Prevention in practice

Box 14.4 on the next page describes an innovative population-wide suicide-prevention programme that was developed explicitly from Rose's ideal model of population change.

How highly would you rate this study design for evaluating such a programme?

How easily can we generalise from these findings to, say, the US population as a whole?

The actual study design used is a simple pre–post-intervention comparison of suicide rates (i.e. very straightforward descriptive data). It would be nice to have RCT data on this issue but, for pretty obvious reasons, it is very difficult to conduct such a trial on this scale. Furthermore, since the interventions have to be applied to an entire community, not just to individuals, it would have to be a cluster randomised trial with only a few large groups and so would miss out on the core benefits of individual randomisation. A trial would, however, avoid the possible confounding of pre–post studies when there are underlying time trends in suicide rates that are independent of any intervention. (In this particular situation the unexposed and exposed cohorts, pre- and post-intervention, are likely to have been quite similar with regard to potential confounders.) While the summary figures indicate the programme's likely benefit, we can see from

Box 14.4 Flying higher: the US Air Force suicide prevention programme

Suicide rates in the US Air Force increased notably in the early 1990s, leading to a concerted effort by senior staff to halt and reverse this trend. A multilayered population-based prevention programme was introduced in 1996 to reduce risk factors and enhance protective factors among the more than 5 million personnel. The intervention focused on removing the stigma from mental health problems, enhancing understanding of mental health, and changing policies and social norms. Strong and continuing endorsement of the initiative by senior leaders was a critical element. The approach adopted was explicitly a population-oriented risk-reduction approach. Its effectiveness was measured by comparison of suicide rates among US Air Force personnel before and after the intervention: overall suicide was reduced by 33% (Figure 14.11) (Knox *et al.*, 2003).

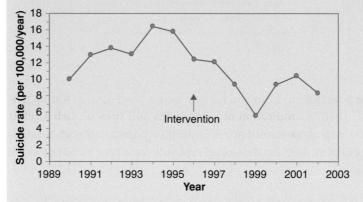

Figure 14.11 Suicide rates in the US Air Force before and after the population-based intervention in 1996–1997. (*Data source:* Knox *et al.*, 2003.)

Figure 14.11 that the pattern of change for suicide is not simple to interpret. It would be helpful to see the longer-term pattern before 1990, and future rates will also be telling.

Generalising the specific findings to the whole population is more problematic, not the least because air force personnel and the air force environment are likely to be very different from the general US population; however, the underlying theories may well be quite generally applicable. Taken at face value, these results suggest that the mass strategy is capable of addressing the underlying social, economic and political determinants of ill-health in a population, and need not be restricted to immediate causes. It is also a desirable approach to intervention because it aims to change not only the risk factors, but also the

Reprinted with permission.

Frank and Ernest

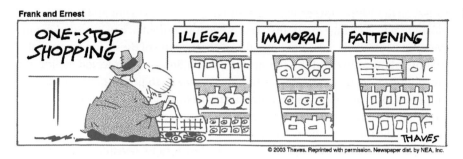

© 2003 Thaves. Reprinted with permission. Newspaper dist. by NEA, Inc.

context in which they are embedded: it is easier to seek help for a problem, or give up smoking, for example, if the rest of the population is supportive.

Naturally, simpler solutions to preventive interventions are appealing – immunisations for infectious diseases and some cancers (cervix, liver) are notable and valuable examples. But the search for other 'magic bullets' continues; the editor of the *British Medical Journal* speculated that the 28 June 2003 edition might be 'The most important *BMJ* for 50 years' (Smith, 2003). He referred to an article by Wald and Law (2003) proposing the 'Polypill', a six-drugs-in-one cardiovascular panacea that might prevent 80% of all vascular morbidity and mortality beyond the age of 55 by reducing blood pressure (a three-drug cocktail), serum levels of LDL cholesterol (a statin) and homocysteine (folate), and clotting tendency (aspirin). Their quantification of the benefits and risks of such a pill is based on combining relevant evidence from RCTs and long-term cohort studies drawn from a series of systematic reviews and meta-analyses. They recommend implementing a population strategy aimed to shift the whole cardiovascular 'risk curve' well to the left, exactly the sort of outcome of which Rose would have approved. This achieves the same preventive end as the Air Force suicide intervention programme by moderating whole-of-population risk, but the onus on achieving the goal is shifted from society to the individual, from primary structural and behavioural change to life-long pill taking (and if compliance is not high the benefits shrink rapidly). Whether this 'medicalisation' of a society is desirable or acceptable is contentious, and the paper has engendered debate although, as of 2008, little action in the sense of formal testing of the intervention (Rogers and Patel, 2008).

Evaluation of preventive interventions in practice

The first reasonably strong evidence that intervention (adding or removing an exposure) might decrease disease incidence often comes from observational epidemiology, i.e. case–control or cohort studies. If, as this evidence accumulates, a causal relationship between exposure and disease seems likely, and if the potential for practical change exists, then this preventive potential can be tested in randomised controlled trials. You have already seen some of these, for example the trial of polio vaccine and the Physicians' Health Study which tested aspirin for preventing coronary heart disease and beta-carotene to prevent cancer (Box 4.7 on page 113). The utility (polio immunisation) or otherwise (beta-carotene) of these interventions as demonstrated by the trials will then inform the decisions regarding the implementation of a preventive programme.

However, once the programme has been shown to be feasible in a trial, and is rolled out to the wider population, it is no longer operating with the close overview that characterises most experimental research, and so it cannot automatically be assumed that it will be as effective as in the RCT setting. It now needs 'real-world' monitoring and evaluation and in the first instance this information usually comes from the 'routine' data sources that we discussed in Chapter 3, especially trends in disease-specific mortality. You have met a number of examples of this already, including figures showing mortality declines from lung cancer (Figure 1.1), heart attacks (Figure 1.7), tuberculosis (Figure 14.1) and breast cancer (Figure 14.3). Interpretation of the falling lung cancer mortality among men in the USA is fairly straightforward from consideration of Table 14.1 and Figure 3.6, and the additional knowledge that the incidence of this cancer is also falling. The multiple strategies applied to induce falling smoking rates have produced effective primary prevention of this fatal cancer, although it is hard to know exactly which elements of the anti-smoking campaigns have had most effect. We have discussed factors behind the mortality changes for TB and breast cancer above, and in the next chapter will consider the contributions of screening to controlling breast cancer in more detail.

These examples underline the critical importance of having good mortality data to monitor the effectiveness of disease control programmes whether they are attempting primary prevention or to improve treatment outcomes.

A final (cautionary) word

There are inevitably limitations to the mass strategy, especially the difficulties of effective implementation. It is quite hard to persuade the public that a health problem is a matter for concerted public action rather than simply the responsibility of the few affected individuals. If everyone wants to smoke or drive cars fast then it is not easy to stop them (the enforced changes in views on drink-driving in many societies are, however, encouraging). Population-level interventions such as water fluoridation or fortification of flour products with folate are also highly controversial as they effectively remove an individual's choice as to whether they want to receive the intervention or not. Even if we know what is desirable and the public is on side, it can still be difficult to effect a change (e.g. to reduce poverty). All change involves costs, and change on a large scale involves large-scale costs. Finally, population change is made more difficult because of what Rose dubbed the *prevention paradox*: 'a preventive measure which brings much benefit to the community offers little to each participating individual' (Rose, 1981). We all have to change our risk profile (by wearing seat belts, changing our behaviour, etc.), but the only people who really benefit are the unidentifiable minority among us whose seat belt will save them in an accident or who would have died from CVD if they had not reduced their blood pressure. In practice we often fall short of fully informing the public of the very limited individual benefits that result from mass prevention programmes (and screening programmes; see Chapter 15).

In the next chapter we will move from primary prevention to secondary prevention or screening, and will apply an epidemiological perspective to the use of population screening as a public health intervention. It often seems to be a given that early detection of disease must be a good thing but, as you will see, this is not always the case thus this assumption should never be allowed to go untested!

Question

1. Comment on the utility of relative and absolute measures of effect in assessing the benefits a community will get from a prevention program.

REFERENCES

Adams, T. (1618). *Happiness of Church*; p. 146.

Banwell, C., Lim, L., Seubsman, S.-A. *et al.* (2009). BMI and health-related behaviours in a national cohort of 87,134 Thai open university students. *Journal of Epidemiology and Community Health*, **63**: 366–372.

Berry, D. A., Cronin, K. A., Plevritis, S. K. *et al.* (2005). Effect of screening and adjuvant therapy on mortality from breast cancer. *New England Journal of Medicine*, **353**: 1784–1792.

Brown, W. J., Hockey, R. and Dobson, A. (2007). Rose revisited: a "middle road" prevention strategy to reduce noncommunicable chronic disease risk. *Bulletin of the World Health Organization*, **85**: 886–887.

Hu, G., Pekkarinen, H., Halonen, P. *et al.* (2001). Different worlds, different tasks for health promotion: comparisons of health risk profiles in Chinese and Finnish rural people. *Health Promotion International*, **16**: 315–320.

Knox, K. L., Litts, D. A., Talcott, G. W., Feig, J. C. and Caine, E. D. (2003). Risk of suicide and related adverse outcomes after exposure to a suicide prevention programme in the US Air Force: a cohort study. *British Medical Journal*, **327**: 1376–1380.

McKeown, T. (1979). *The Role of Medicine. Dream, Mirage or Nemesis?* Oxford: Blackwell Publishing.

Murray, C. J. L. and Lopez, A. D. (1999). On the quantification of health risks: lessons from the Global Burden of Disease Study. *Epidemiology*, **10**: 594–605.

Murray, C. J. L., Ezzati, M., Lopez, A. D., Rodgers, A. and Vander Hoorn S. (2003). Comparative quantification of health risks: conceptual framework and methodological issues. *Population Health Metrics*, **1**: 1. http://www.pophealthmetrics.com/content/1/1/1. Licensee BioMed Central Ltd.

Parkin, D. M. (2009). Is the recent fall in post-menopausal breast cancer in UK related to changes in use of hormone replacement therapy? *European Journal of Cancer*, **45**: 1649–1653.

Rogers, A. and Patel, A. (2008). What happened to the polypill?: why is there more heat than light concerning the polypill? *British Medical Journal*, **337**:a2162.

Rose, G. (1981). Strategy of prevention: lessons from cardiovascular disease. *British Medical Journal*, **282**: 1847–1851.

Rose, G. (1992). *The Strategy of Preventive Medicine*. London: Oxford University Press.

Smith, R. (2003). The most important BMJ for 50 years? *British Medical Journal*, **326**: un-numbered pages at the beginning of issue 7404.

Steyerberg E. W. (2009). *Clinical Prediction Models: a Practical Approach to Development, Validation, and Updating*. New York: Springer.

Wald, N. J. and Law, M. R. (2003). A strategy to reduce cardiovascular disease by more than 80%. *British Medical Journal*, **326**: 1419–1425.

Webb, P., Bain, C., Cummings, M. and Furnival, C. (2004). Changes in survival after breast cancer: improvements in diagnosis or treatment? *Breast*, **13**: 7–14.

Early detection: what benefits at what cost?

Description	Association	Alternative explanations	Integration & interpretation	Practical applications
Chapters 2–3	Chapters 4–5	Chapters 6–8	Chapters 9–11	Chapter 15: Screening

> ## Box 15.1 Just because screening should work doesn't mean it will!
>
> In the 1960s, public health practitioners were seduced by the concept of early diagnosis – give people regular health checks to identify and treat disease early. It seemed so obvious it would work that initiatives of this type started springing up in the USA and UK. The UK Ministry of Health realised that the implications were enormous, so between 1967 and 1976 a trial was conducted in London to evaluate the benefits of multiphasic screening of middle-aged adults in general practice. Approximately 7,000 participants were randomly allocated to receive two screening checks two years apart or no screening and all participants then underwent a health survey. The investigators did not find any significant differences between the two groups in terms of their morbidity, hospital admissions, absence from work for sickness or mortality. The only outcome appeared to be the increased costs of health-care – approximately £142 million to screen the entire middle-aged UK population (and that was at 1976 prices). (The South-East London Screening Study Group, 1977; reprinted in 2001 with a series of commentaries, Various, 2001.)

Up to this point we have mainly focused on the issues of how we can quantify health (or ill-health) and how to identify the factors that might be causing ill-health, with a view to preventing it in the future. In the previous chapter we alluded to what is sometimes called 'secondary prevention', where instead of trying to prevent disease from occurring, we try to detect it earlier in the hope that this will allow more effective treatment and thus improved health outcomes. This is an aspect of public health that has great intuitive appeal, especially for serious conditions such as cancer where the options for prevention are often very limited. However, as you will discover, screening programmes are usually very costly exercises and they do not always deliver the expected benefits in terms of improved health outcomes (see Box 15.1 above). In this chapter we will introduce you to the requirements for implementing a successful screening programme, and to some of the problems that we encounter when trying to determine whether such a programme is actually beneficial in practice.

Why screen?

It has been known for some time that infection with human papillomavirus (HPV) is a major, and perhaps a **necessary cause** of cervical cancer (see Chapter 10) but, until the development of HPV vaccines in recent years, we could not prevent people from becoming infected. As uptake of these vaccines becomes widespread, they may replace the current screening programmes as the preferred method for control of this disease. However, the screening programmes have shown that in the absence of primary preventives like vaccines, detecting disease before the usual time of diagnosis can provide an effective 'second level' of public health intervention.

When used as a public health measure for disease control, screening implies the widespread use of a simple test for disease in an apparently healthy (asymptomatic) population. A screening test will often not diagnose the presence of disease directly but will instead separate people who are more likely to have the disease from those who are less likely to have it. Those who may have the disease (i.e. those who screen positive) can then undergo further diagnostic tests and treatment if necessary. The improved public health outcomes we seek through screening are reduced morbidity, mortality and/or disability. The benefits of public health screening are primarily for those people who are actually screened, and generally even among this group only very few will benefit directly, but there may also be wider social benefits if overall health costs are reduced.

Screening is also used, in a slightly different fashion, to protect the general population from exposure to disease. As an example, immigrants to a number of countries are screened for HIV and hepatitis B infection; and travellers from regions with epidemic acute infectious diseases, such as SARS (severe acute respiratory syndrome) or H1N1 influenza, have been subjected to screening using health declaration cards to identify symptoms and sometimes thermal scanning to detect signs of infection at airports. The primary aim of this type of screening is not to benefit the individual who is screened, but to protect the local population from these viruses. Similarly, some occupations require regular screening; for example, airline pilots have regular medical checks in an attempt to ensure that they will not have a heart attack while flying. Insurance companies often require people to undergo health checks and screening before they offer them a life insurance policy. Here the 'screening' is done for purely financial reasons, because insurance companies charge higher premiums for people at higher risk.

The disease process

The first we know of the existence of a disease in a person is when it is diagnosed. This is usually some time after it first produces the symptoms which cause the person to seek medical care. The actual onset of disease will of course be earlier than this – how much earlier depends on the disease concerned. Figure 15.1 illustrates this point.

At some stage between the biological onset of disease and the time of usual clinical diagnosis there may come a time when early signs of disease are there, if only we could detect them. The position of this point will vary depending on the disease, perhaps occurring many years before the appearance of clinical disease

Figure 15.1 The natural history of a disease (adapted from Sackett *et al.*, 1991).

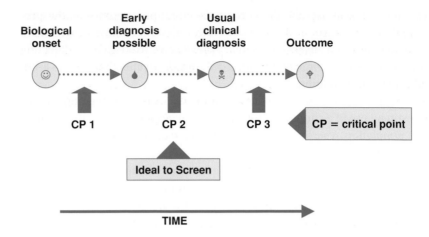

Figure 15.1 The natural history of a disease (adapted from Sackett *et al.*, 1991).

(e.g. high blood pressure, some cancers), or only shortly before symptoms appear (e.g. acute infectious diseases).

At some stage during the disease process there is also likely to be a **critical point**, after which the disease process is irreversible and treatment will confer little or no benefit. An example is the point at which a cancer starts spreading to other tissues (known as metastasis). If this 'point of no return' occurs before it is possible to detect the disease (CP1 in Figure 15.1), then advancing the time of detection will simply mean that the person knows about their disease for longer but their outcome will not be improved. Similarly, if this point occurs after the time of usual clinical diagnosis (CP3) there is no need to detect the disease any earlier, given that treatment following usual diagnosis will be effective.

Screening, then, is of greatest potential benefit when the critical point occurs at CP2 – between the time of first possible detection and the usual time of diagnosis. In this situation it may be that picking up the disease early would improve outcomes, and this is the aim of a screening programme. Unfortunately, we currently have too little knowledge of the progress of most diseases for this to have much practical value in planning screening programmes.

Screening versus case-finding

There is considerable debate about the best way to implement early detection of disease. Should the focus be on large-scale mass population screening, or are we better off pursuing opportunistic early detection or 'case-finding' when someone comes into contact with the health system for another reason? There are some parallels here with the mass versus high-risk approach to primary prevention that we discussed in the previous chapter, but they are not exact. The terms 'screening' and 'case-finding' can also have quite different meanings to different practitioners. We think it is most useful, and best accepted, to use the term 'screening' for organised population-wide approaches and 'case-finding' for more opportunistic attempts at early detection. If systematically applied, case-finding can nonetheless form the basis for quite good population coverage. If a large proportion of the people visit a primary care physician every year or two, this contact could permit early detection of risks (e.g. from cigarette smoking, high blood pressure) in a setting that allows good follow-up.

The requirements of a screening programme

Screening differs from diagnostic testing in that it is performed *before* the development of clinical disease. Thus, those who undergo screening are free, or appear to be free, of the disease of interest. They are not seeking care because they are sick, but are instead persuaded to be screened by the health service. The requirements of a screening test are, therefore, quite distinct from those of a diagnostic test, which is performed only when someone is suspected to have a disease. The suitability of a *disease* for screening has to be considered explicitly; the quality and acceptability of the *screening test* must be demonstrated; and the whole *programme* must be shown to confer a net benefit to the community. We will explore these issues further below.

The disease

We need to consider the following characteristics of a disease before deciding whether screening for it is desirable.
- The disease should be severe, relatively common and perceived as a public health problem by the community.
- We must understand the natural history of the disease sufficiently well that we can be reasonably sure that earlier detection will give a better outcome.

Prostate cancer shows us the importance of this. It appears to occur in a number of biological forms that we cannot tell apart, and it is probable that many men in whom a cancer could be detected by screening (e.g. with a prostate specific antigen (PSA) test) would never develop symptoms or suffer from the disease (and therefore would not otherwise be diagnosed). To detect and treat these men would be wholly harmful and, largely for this reason, screening for prostate cancer is generally not recommended, even though there are tests that could be used (and which are used quite widely in some countries, e.g. the USA, on an *ad hoc* case-finding basis). Research is under way in a number of countries in an attempt to shed light on this dilemma to allow a more informed judgement to be made.

- In general, there should be a high prevalence of pre-clinical (early-stage) disease.

This criterion becomes less important as the severity of the disease increases. For example, it may be of benefit to screen for a fairly uncommon disease if not treating it has severe consequences – an example is the use of screening for phenylketonuria (PKU) in newborns. Babies born with this condition lack an enzyme that metabolises the amino acid phenylalanine. When they eat proteins containing this amino acid, the end-products accumulate in the brain, leading to severe mental retardation. By simply restricting the phenylalanine in their diet this can be prevented. Although only about one in 15,000 babies is born with this condition, the availability of a simple, accurate and inexpensive test makes it worthwhile to screen all newborn babies (Wilcken *et al.*, 2003).

- Screening is likely to be more effective if there is a long period between the first detectable signs of disease and the overt symptoms that normally lead to diagnosis (the **lead time**).

If a disease progresses rapidly from the pre-clinical to clinical stages then it is much harder to detect the disease while it is still at an early stage and, consequently, early intervention is less likely to be of benefit. (Clearly, metabolic conditions of early life, such as PKU, are exceptions to this).

The screening test

The next requirement for a worthwhile screening programme is that we have a test that will enable us to detect the disease before the usual time of diagnosis. Any such test must meet the following criteria.

- Firstly it should be **accurate**.

As discussed in Chapter 7, accuracy reflects the degree to which the results of the test correspond to the true state of the phenomenon being measured. In practice, accuracy can be influenced by the standardisation or calibration of the testing apparatus and by the skill of the persons conducting or interpreting the test. Maintaining high standards of testing in a service setting is thus crucial for a screening programme to reach its full potential.

So what should we expect of a screening test in relation to its accuracy? We would expect it to be:

sensitive – ideally it would identify *all* people with the disease; in practice, it should identify *most* of these people.

specific – ideally it would identify *only* those with that particular disease and those without the disease should test negative; in practice, *most* of those without the disease should test negative.

- It must be safe and acceptable to the population being screened.

Since we are advising apparently well people to undergo screening, we should not offer them a test that might adversely affect their health. The only exception might be for those at very high risk of developing a serious disease, when a slight risk from screening might be outweighed by a large benefit of early diagnosis (e.g. regular colonoscopy for people with ulcerative colitis, who develop large bowel cancer at a high rate). Social and cultural acceptability are separate issues and are seldom related to the safety of the screening test. For example, persuading people to take a sample of their faeces to test for blood as an early indicator of colon cancer is unpalatable to many. Likewise, cervical cancer screening is not immediately appealing in many societies and in some it may be prohibited, particularly if the health professional is male.

- It should be simple and cheap.

If we wish to screen a large proportion of the population any test used should be relatively cheap to administer and simple to perform or it would be too costly to perform large-scale screening.

Mammography is neither simple nor cheap. Why then do you think that mammographic screening to detect early breast cancer is recommended?

Although mammography is neither simple nor cheap, breast cancer is a severe disease of substantial concern to many communities. It occurs relatively commonly and, if detected early, is usually highly treatable.

Test quality: sensitivity and specificity

We can evaluate the performance of a test by comparing the results with a 'gold standard' method that ideally would give 100% correct results (but more commonly is just the best test available). This standard might be a more costly or time-consuming test, or perhaps a combination of investigations performed in hospital that is reliable for diagnosis but unsuitable for routine use in screening.

For example, children in many countries undergo a simple hearing test in their first year at school. Any who fail this screening test are retested at a later date and/or referred to a hearing clinic for further, more extensive tests to identify whether they have a real hearing problem. Imagine that in a group of 500 children, 50 have a genuine hearing problem. Of these, 45 fail the school hearing test, as do 30 of the children with normal hearing (perhaps they had a cold on the day of the test). We could summarise the results of the test as in Table 15.1.

There are four possible outcomes for a child, as shown in Figure 15.2. A child with a real hearing problem may either fail the screening test (**true positive**; group 'a' in Figure 15.2) or pass the test, suggesting falsely that they do not have a problem (**false negative**; group 'c'). Similarly, a child without a problem may

Table 15.1 Hypothetical results from a school hearing test programme.

School hearing test	True hearing status		
	Hearing problem	Normal	Total
Fail (positive test result)	45	30	75
Pass (negative test result)	5	420	425
Total	50	450	500

Figure 15.2 Possible outcomes from a screening test.

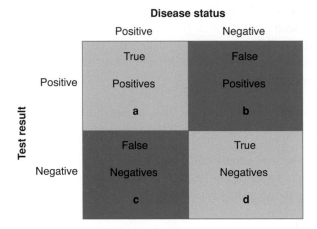

pass the test (**true negative**; group 'd') or fail, falsely implying that they do have a problem (**false positive**; group 'b').

For a test to be accurate it should produce few false-positive and false-negative results. So how good is the school hearing test? There are two issues to consider: how well has the test identified the children who do have a problem; and how well has it classified the normal children as normal?

What percentage of children with a real hearing problem failed the school test?

What percentage of children with normal hearing passed the school test?

Looking at Table 15.1, we see that 90% (45 ÷ 50) of children with a hearing problem failed the school test and 93% (420 ÷ 450) of children with normal hearing passed the test. These measures of a test are known respectively as its **sensitivity** and **specificity**.

The **sensitivity** of a test measures how well it classifies people with the disease as sick. It is the *percentage of people with the disease who test positive* (90% in the example above). It is calculated by dividing the number of true-positive results

(a) by the total number of people with disease $(a + c)$ from Figure 15.2:

$$\text{Sensitivity (\%)} = \frac{\text{True positives}}{\text{All with disease}} \times 100$$

$$= \frac{a}{a + c} \times 100 \qquad (15.1)$$

The **specificity** of a test measures how well it classifies people without the disease as healthy. It is the *percentage of people without disease who test negative* (93% in the above example). To calculate it, we divide the number of true negative results (d) by the total number of people without disease $(b + d)$:

$$\text{Specificity (\%)} = \frac{\text{True negatives}}{\text{All without disease}} \times 100$$

$$= \frac{d}{b + d} \times 100 \qquad (15.2)$$

A combination of high sensitivity and high specificity is essential for a good screening test – in this regard the school hearing test works quite well.

Note that it is necessary to do a special study, as discussed in 'Diagnostic studies' in Chapter 4 (Box 4.2), to assess the sensitivity and specificity of a test. In the usual service setting only those who test positive (groups 'a' and 'b' from Figure 15.2) will be followed up with formal diagnostic testing to determine the true positives. Unless there is a specific plan to do so (which usually is possible only in a research setting), those who test negative are commonly not followed up, so the proportion of false negatives is not known and we cannot measure either the sensitivity or the specificity of the test.

Test performance in practice: positive and negative predictive values

Two other measures, the **positive** and **negative predictive values**, are sometimes given as test criteria, but they really measure how well a test performs in a given population. In practice we would not know whether a child did have a real hearing problem – we have to predict this from the screening test result. We need, therefore, to know how well a positive test result (i.e. failing the hearing test) predicts that a child does have a hearing problem and, conversely, how well a negative test result (i.e. passing the hearing test) predicts that their hearing is normal.

What percentage of children who failed the school hearing test had a real hearing problem?

What percentage of children who passed the school hearing test really did have normal hearing?

Out of 75 children who failed the school hearing test, 45 (60%) had a real hearing problem. Out of 425 children who passed the school test, 420 (99%) really did have normal hearing.

These measures are known respectively as the **positive** and **negative predictive values** (**PPV** and **NPV**) of the test *in that situation*. Unlike the sensitivity and specificity, they are not fixed properties of the test because, as you will see below, they also depend on the prevalence of disease in the population being tested. However, the PPV and NPV give us crucial information as to how well the test is performing in that population.

The **positive predictive value** (**PPV**) tells us how likely it is that a positive test result indicates the presence of disease. It is the *percentage of all people who test positive who really have the disease* (60% in the example). It is calculated by dividing the number of true-positive results (a) by the total number of positive results $(a + b)$:

$$\text{Positive Predictive Value (\%)} = \frac{\text{True positives}}{\text{All positives}} \times 100$$

$$= \frac{a}{a + b} \times 100 \qquad (15.3)$$

The **negative predictive value** (**NPV**) is the *percentage of all people who test negative who really do not have the disease* (99% in the example). To calculate it, simply divide the number of true-negative results (d) by the total number of negative results $(c + d)$:

$$\text{Negative Predictive Value (\%)} = \frac{\text{True negatives}}{\text{All negatives}} \times 100$$

$$= \frac{d}{c + d} \times 100 \qquad (15.4)$$

These measures of test performance are best thought of as operational measures of the overall programme. They reflect both the *accuracy of the test* (sensitivity and specificity) and the *disease prevalence* in the population tested. Even a superb test (very high sensitivity and specificity) will yield a low positive predictive value if the disease is rare.

An example – testing blood donors for HIV infection

It is routine practice in most countries to screen all blood donors for HIV, but what is the probability that someone who tests positive really does have HIV?

To answer this we must calculate the positive predictive value of the test. Assume that we are using the test to screen a high-risk population of intravenous drug users in New York City who have an HIV prevalence of 5,500 per 10,000.

How many in a group of 10,000 intravenous drug users would you expect to have HIV infection?

Of these, how many would test positive if the test had a sensitivity of 99.5%, and how many would falsely test negative?

How many of the drug users will not be HIV-positive and, of them, how many would test negative if the test had a specificity of 99.5%? How many would falsely test positive?

What proportion of the people who test HIV-positive would truly have HIV infection?

Given the known prevalence of HIV infection in this group, we would expect 5,500 of the 10,000 intravenous drug users to be HIV-positive and the remaining 4,500 would be HIV-negative. Of the HIV-positive group, 99.5% or 5,473 would correctly test positive and the remaining 27 would falsely test negative. Among the HIV-negative group 99.5% or 4,478 would correctly test negative and the remaining 22 would falsely test positive. From Table 15.2, we can see that this means that we would expect a total of 5,495 positive test results and that, of these, 5,473 or 99.6% would be true positives. Similarly, of the 4,505 negative test results, 4,478 or 99.4% would be true negatives. The test therefore performs very well in this high-risk population.

Now repeat the calculations for a low-risk population of new blood donors where the prevalence of HIV is only 4 per 10,000.

Table 15.2 Positive and negative predictive values of an HIV test in high- and low-risk populations.

Test	True HIV status		
	Positive	Negative	Total
Intravenous drug users			
Positive	5,473	22	5,495
Negative	27	4,478	4,505
Total	5,500	4,500	10,000
New blood donors			
Positive	4	50	54
Negative	0	9,946	9,946
Total	4	9,996	10,000

$PPV = 5{,}473 \div 5{,}495 = 99.6\%$
$NPV = 4{,}478 \div 4{,}505 = 99.4\%$

$PPV = 4 \div 54 = 7.4\%$
$NPV = 9{,}946 \div 9{,}946 = 100\%$

Table 15.3 Variation in the positive predictive value of a test with prevalence of disease and accuracy of test.

Prevalence (%)	Sensitivity and specificity[a]			
	99%	95%	90%	80%
20	96.1%	82.1%	69.2%	50.0%
10	91.7%	67.9%	50.0%	30.8%
5	83.9%	50.0%	32.1%	17.4%
1	50.0%	16.1%	8.3%	3.9%
0.1	9.0%	1.9%	0.9%	0.4%

[a] Assuming that sensitivity and specificity have the same value.

Among the blood donors we would expect only about 4 out of 10,000 people to be truly HIV-positive and the remaining 9,996 would be HIV-negative. All four of the HIV-positive people should correctly test positive (Table 15.2). Among the HIV-negative group 99.5% or 9,946 would correctly test negative and the remaining 50 would falsely test positive. This means that we now have a total of 54 positive test results but, of these, only 4 or 7.4% are true positives. This means that 93% or more than 9 of every 10 positive test results would be false positives! Thus, even with a very high sensitivity and specificity, the same test performs badly in this low-risk population. The profound influence of changes in disease prevalence and test accuracy on the positive predictive value of a test is shown in Table 15.3. In practice, the lower values for sensitivity and specificity included in the table are often encountered, and for most diseases of consequence the prevalence in the general population is also quite low; for example, recent Australian data suggest the prevalence of breast cancer among women aged 50–69 who attend for mammographic screening (the target age group) is around 0.3% (AIHW and NBOCC, 2009).

The prevalence of prostate cancer in 60-year-old men is approximately 1%. Using Table 15.3, how accurate would you want a screening test to be before you would consider starting a screening programme to detect early prostate cancer?

With such a low prevalence, even a test with 99% sensitivity and specificity would give a positive predictive value of only 50%; i.e. half of all positive test results would be false positives. While this is less than ideal, in practice this is not necessarily the sole consideration in initiating a screening programme. For example, most studies of screening mammography have demonstrated that it achieves a positive predictive value in the range of only 10%–20% for women aged between 50 and 69 years. However, the reduction in breast cancer mortality

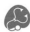

Box 15.2 Accuracy and predictive values of diagnostic tests

A red tympanic membrane is generally considered a good predictor of acute otitis media (AOM) or middle-ear infection in children. However, in a study conducted to determine the accuracy of this sign compared with the results of the 'gold standard' test, myringotomy (incising the tympanic membrane), the sensitivity and specificity were found to be only 18% and 84%, respectively (Karma *et al.*, 1989). If we assume a **pre-test probability*** or prevalence of AOM of 50%, this means that only 53% of children with a red tympanic membrane will actually have AOM (the PPV or **post-test probability**); the other positive test results will be false positives. Similarly, 49% of those who do not have a red tympanic membrane will have AOM (false negatives). On its own, then, this is not a very accurate marker of AOM, but if seen together with other signs such as bulging and reduced mobility of the tympanic membrane the accuracy of diagnosis improves. Clinical decision rules based on the presence or absence of several known clinical features of a condition are useful tools to enhance diagnostic accuracy.

* Note that this is another situation in which clinical epidemiologists tend to use different terms to describe the same things. In clinical epidemiology the term '*pre-test probability*' is often used synonymously with *prevalence*. It represents the probability that the patient had the condition on the basis of information available before the test was undertaken, i.e. the prevalence of the condition and the patient's clinical picture. Similarly, the predictive values, which represent the probability that the patient has (or does not have) disease on the basis of test results, are often called '*post-test probabilities*'.

associated with screening women over the age of 50 is deemed to outweigh the consequences of the large number of false positives that inevitably result.

Before we move on, it is also important to note that the aspects of accuracy and predictive values that we have just discussed in relation to screening also apply to all **diagnostic tests** as shown in Box 15.2.

The trade-off between sensitivity and specificity

Let us assume that we have developed a new blood test that will screen people for a debilitating but treatable disease. The test involves measuring blood levels of a marker M and is far less invasive than the 'gold standard' test. To evaluate the new test, levels of M were measured in 225 people believed to be at moderately high risk for the disease and the results were compared with the 'gold standard' test, which each person underwent independently of the blood test. For the blood test, the 'criterion of positivity' was set at an M level of 20 mg/l or more; i.e. those with M levels at or above this were said to have the disease. Figure 15.3 shows the distribution of M levels in people with and without the disease as diagnosed

Figure 15.3 Distribution of M levels by disease status according to the 'gold standard' test.

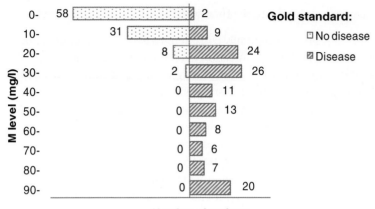

by the 'gold standard' test. The light bars on the left represent the 99 people who truly do not have the disease and the dark bars on the right represent the 126 people who truly do. When compared with the 'gold standard' results, 115 of 126 with disease tested positive (M levels ≥20 mg/l) as did 10 of 99 without disease; the remaining 11 with disease and 89 without had negative test results. We can summarise the data as shown in Table 15.4.

How accurate is the M test? *(i.e. what are the sensitivity and specificity?)*

How well has the test performed in this population? *(Here we can extract some useful information from the predictive values of the test.)*

Using a cut-off of ≥20 mg/l to classify people as positive or negative we can calculate the following:

$$\text{Sensitivity} = \frac{115}{126} \times 100 = 91.3\%$$

$$\text{Specificity} = \frac{89}{99} \times 100 = 89.9\%$$

Table 15.4 A summary 2 × 2 table for M test with a cut-off point of 20 mg/l.

M test	True disease status		
	Positive	Negative	Total
≥20 mg/l (positive)	115	10	125
<20 mg/l (negative)	11	89	100
Total	126	99	225

$$\text{PPV} = \frac{115}{125} \times 100 = 92.0\%$$

$$\text{NPV} = \frac{89}{100} \times 100 = 89.0\%$$

These look pretty good, but ideally we would like to have all of these values as close to 100% as possible. The M test has, for instance, incorrectly diagnosed 11 people who truly had the disease as not having it because their M values were less than 20 mg/l. So what if we were to lower the cut-off point to 10 mg/l? Looking again at Figure 15.3, this would mean that 9 of the 11 false-negative people would now be correctly diagnosed as having the disease, but it would also mean that an extra 31 people without the disease would be included in the diseased group.

Calculate the sensitivity, specificity and PPV for this new cut-off point. (Hint: first use Table 15.4 as a guide to how to lay out a 2 × 2 table for the new cut-off point)

How do the values compare with those obtained using the higher cut-off point (20 mg/l)?

If we change the cut-off point to 10 mg/l the results are now as shown in Table 15.5. We can calculate the new sensitivity, specificity and PPV as we did above:

$$\text{Sensitivity} = \frac{124}{126} \times 100 = 99.4\%$$

$$\text{Specificity} = \frac{58}{99} \times 100 = 58.6\%$$

$$\text{PPV} = \frac{124}{165} \times 100 = 75.2\%$$

$$\text{NPV} = \frac{58}{60} \times 100 = 96.7\%$$

Table 15.5 Results of the M test using a cut-off point of 10 mg/l.

M test	True disease status		
	+	−	Total
≥10 mg/l (positive)	124	41	165
<10 mg/l (negative)	2	58	60
Total	126	99	225

By changing the criterion for positivity to ≥ 10 mg/l the sensitivity is now excellent and there are very few false negatives, but the specificity has markedly decreased. With the drop in specificity, the PPV of the test has fallen from 92% to 75% because there are now far more false positives (41 instead of 10).

Looking at the distribution of M levels in the two groups of people (Figure 15.3), we find that, although they are clearly different, there is some overlap between the two. Where we decide to make the cut-off to try to differentiate between 'disease' and 'no disease' determines how many false-positive and false-negative test results we find. *There is, therefore, a trade-off to be made between sensitivity and specificity.* For any disease, the optimum point has to be selected depending on the consequences of missing a few positives if the cut-off point is set higher, or falsely classifying more negatives as positive if the cut-off point is set lower. If early detection greatly reduced mortality from the disease and if false positives could be identified fairly quickly and cheaply, then clearly we would set the criterion for positivity lower than if the reverse were the case.

The screening programme

Although a disease appears suitable for screening and there is a valid and acceptable test, there is still no guarantee that the public will benefit from a screening programme. Some major concerns beyond predictive values should be that

- the programme is demonstrably effective in practice, i.e. all its elements work near enough to plan that lives are saved and/or morbidity is reduced, and the cost is acceptable;
- the healthcare system can cope with the flood of extra diagnostic testing and treatment due to finding prevalent disease as well as false positives.

We thus have to measure the outcomes of a screening programme in practice, and also consider some of the logistics of maintaining quality as outlined below.

Facilities required

Before embarking on a screening programme it is important to assess the infrastructure that will be required to support it. Facilities are obviously required for the screening process but, equally importantly, they are also needed for the subsequent confirmatory testing and diagnosis, treatment and follow-up of those who test positive. Estimates are needed as to the likely uptake of screening, the total number of positive test results (including false positives) expected (on the basis of the prevalence of the disease and the sensitivity and specificity of the test) and the likely effect that this will have on the demand for medical services. *It is of no use, and is indeed unethical, to initiate a screening programme if the resources required in order to act upon the results are not available.*

Treatment

The proposed treatment must be effective and early initiation of treatment must improve the disease outcome. If it does not, then by diagnosing the disease earlier we will simply lengthen the time a person is aware of, and worrying about, the disease.

Cost

When a screening programme is introduced we must consider not only the financial cost, but also the emotional cost of both the screening and subsequent treatment for those who test positive and then weigh this against the costs of treating those who develop disease later. A positive balance is required between the costs of screening and the consequences of not screening.

Evaluation of a screening programme

The fact that a screening programme ought to work does not mean that it will in practice (see Box 15.1 at the start of the chapter). No mass screening should be introduced without convincing evidence of its likely effectiveness, and it is imperative that the programme be evaluated as a whole. We will now look at the initial research that should precede the introduction of any full-scale population screening, and provide some subsequent comment on the necessary practical in-service monitoring that should follow its introduction.

It can be difficult to assess whether a programme will work. There are some relatively simple early *process measures* that can give an idea of how things are going, but ultimately we also have to show that the programme delivers improved *outcomes*.

To see whether we have succeeded in detecting disease earlier than usual, we can compare the *stage of disease* in patients whose disease was detected at screening with the stage of disease in those in whom it was detected in the normal way. If cases identified at screening are less advanced, then at least the potential for benefit has been demonstrated. If this is not so, then the programme can be abandoned without any need for outcome evaluation.

Another simple check on the process is the positive predictive value of the screening test being used. A high PPV reflects a good combination of an accurate test and an appropriate population (reasonably high prevalence); a low PPV implies that the programme may be in trouble. Why is this so? As you saw above, a low PPV indicates that, of all the positive test results, only a few reflect true instances of disease, and the large number of false positives will lead to unnecessary concern and expense for those individuals. Since virtually all diseases considered serious enough for screening in the general population will have a fairly low prevalence, the PPV of any test will be less than optimal however high its sensitivity and specificity (refer back to Table 15.3). Health authorities and the general public need to agree explicitly on what level of false positives is acceptable, in the light of what these people will suffer. The community should also be given the chance to declare that they believe that a large benefit for a minority (some of the 'true positives') outweighs the smaller losses (and the costs) suffered by a much larger group (the 'false positives').

Turning to *outcome evaluation*, the ultimate judge of the potential value of a screening programme, there are four areas we need to address:

- the target outcomes to be considered
- potential sources of bias in the evaluation of a screening programme
- the design of an evaluation study, and
- the negative consequences of screening.

Target outcomes to be considered

For fatal conditions such as cancer, a reduction in mortality is the most important outcome to be gained from a screening programme. However, mere prolongation of life might not adequately justify screening if the quality of the additional life is poor. Thus we should also consider absence or reduction of serious morbidity and improvement in quality of life as essential target outcomes for a screening programme. The quality-adjusted life years or QALYs that you met in Chapter 2 can help with this. Other sensible endpoints need to be set for other non-fatal conditions: for example, we would want to know that detecting impaired hearing in school children led to some measurable benefits of consequence – perhaps improved performance at school. Attention also needs to be given to assessing the harms that inevitably ensue from a screening intervention and we will consider this aspect in some detail below.

Potential sources of bias in the evaluation of a screening programme

At first glance, it would seem that all we need to do is follow up people who have and have not been screened to see what effects the screening has on their morbidity and mortality. However, such simple cohort comparisons are unreliable as bias is a major problem and, as you will see, what we really need is evidence from randomised trials. There are three major sources of bias to be dealt with in any evaluation of the effects of screening: *volunteer bias, lead-time bias* and *length bias*.

Volunteer bias

People who attend for screening are likely to be different from those who do not. They tend to be of higher socioeconomic status, to be more health-conscious and more likely to comply with prescribed advice. Thus better results for a

Table 15.6 Volunteerism among women randomly allocated to the mammography group in the HIP study, showing that mortality was lower among women who took up the offer of mammography than among those who did not.

Women randomly allocated to mammography	Deaths per 10,000 women per year	
	All causes	Cardiovascular
Women who underwent mammography	42	17
Women who refused the offer of mammography	77	38
Total	54	24

(Shapiro *et al.*, 1985.)

screening programme of volunteers compared with disease outcomes in non-volunteers may relate to factors associated with the 'volunteerism', rather than benefits of treatment following earlier diagnosis. (This is the same volunteer bias that you saw when we discussed selection bias in Chapter 7.)

In the HIP trial of mammographic screening (described in Box 15.3 on the next page), only about two-thirds of the 31,000 women randomly allocated to the mammography group actually took up the initial offer to be screened and less than half attended all four annual examinations. After 5 years of follow-up of all women in the intervention arm, i.e. all those who were offered screening, those women who had refused breast screening had much higher mortality from all causes and from cardiovascular disease than those who were screened (Table 15.6).

Since the screening was directed only at breast cancer, why might women who came for screening have lower mortality rates for causes other than breast cancer?

The most likely reason is 'volunteer bias' – the women who took up the offer of screening were different in important ways from those who did not. (And note that Table 15.7 shows that the overall rates of total and cardiovascular mortality were essentially the same in both arms of the trial, reinforcing the fact that the mammographic screening itself did not affect these outcomes.)

The only way to avoid this type of bias is to recruit a pool of volunteers and then *assign them randomly* to receive screening or no screening, just as they did in the HIP trial (Box 15.3). It is also important to ensure that as many as possible of those assigned to screening are actually screened. The correct analysis is then by **intention to treat**, i.e. comparing the groups as they were originally randomised, regardless of whether women were actually screened. If only those who actually received the screening are compared with the rest, we lose all the benefits of the

> ## Box 15.3 Mammographic screening for breast cancer – still generating controversy
>
> Mammographic (X-ray) screening for breast cancer has been evaluated in a number of different countries. One of the first randomised trials conducted to determine its efficacy was the Health Insurance Plan (HIP) study in New York – an inspired initiative that linked the introduction of breast screening to a health insurance scheme. In this large-scale trial, 62,000 women aged 50–64 years who were members of this insurance plan were invited to participate in the early 1960s. About 31,000 women were randomly allocated to the intervention group and offered an initial mammographic (and physical) screening examination followed by three additional screening examinations at yearly intervals. Another 31,000 women were randomly allocated to the control group and were not offered the screening programme. After 18 years of follow-up, breast cancer mortality was 23% lower in the group offered screening (Shapiro *et al.*, 1985). These promising first results were the basis for many countries to consider mammography as a valuable public health tool, particularly in 50–64-year-old women.
>
> However, there are still controversial issues to be resolved.
>
> - Results of most studies have not shown a marked benefit of screening women aged under 50 years.
> - There have been criticisms of this and other core mammographic screening trials and, although these have generally been rebutted, they indicate that there are complex issues involved, both in conducting the studies and in interpreting the results.
> - The ability to implement programmes in routine public health practice which operate with the same high standards of those in the well-funded research projects is still a matter of concern for many countries. If programme standards are lowered (e.g. due to inadequate training of radiologists to read mammograms or longer screening intervals) then the balance of benefits and harms will shift unfavourably.
>
> Recent descriptive evidence shows that there has been a persistent downturn in deaths from breast cancer in a number of countries (Figure 14.3). Although the reasons for this downturn have been a subject of heated debate, as discussed in the previous chapter, it appears that both better treatment (particularly chemotherapy) and screening have played their part.

randomisation in terms of controlling for confounding and avoidance of selection bias. (As you saw in Table 15.6, those who do take up screening are likely to have inherently better health outcomes than those who do not, regardless of the screening.) This analysis is not only theoretically correct, but also reflects the

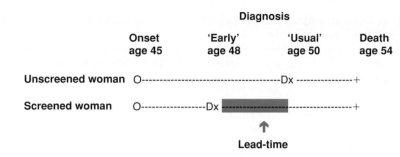

reality of public health practice, because not all of us will eagerly take up each preventive opportunity. Details of this analysis are described below, and shown in Table 15.7.

Lead-time bias

Lead-time is the period between when disease is detected by screening and when it would have become symptomatic and been diagnosed in the usual way. Consider a situation in which breast cancer starts to develop (disease onset) in two women at age 45. One attends for mammography and the tumour is detected at age 48, while the other is diagnosed at the age of 50 when she notices a lump in her breast. Both women die of their cancer at age 54 (Figure 15.4). The first woman has survived for 6 years following the discovery of the tumour while the second has lived for only 4 years following diagnosis.

Without knowledge of the time of onset of disease, the screening process appears to have increased the survival time by 2 years for the woman who was screened when in fact their disease courses were identical. Both women have lived for 9 years following the initial development of the tumour. The first woman has just known and worried about her disease, and perhaps been without one breast, for 2 years longer than the second woman. This is known as 'lead-time bias' and, if ignored, it would distort a direct comparison of survival rates in screened and unscreened groups. Conventionally, survival is calculated for a 5-year period after diagnosis of cancer: in this example the woman diagnosed clinically (unscreened) who died 4 years after diagnosis would not be in the numerator of the survival rate, i.e. she would be defined as a 'non-survivor'. However, her exact counterpart in the screened group who died 6 years after diagnosis would be included as a survivor, incorrectly suggesting a benefit from screening. If lead-time bias is ignored, the survival among women who were screened would appear to be higher than that among women diagnosed clinically, even if their disease courses were identical. A related phenomenon is the apparent transient increase in incidence seen when a screening programme is first introduced as the screening detects prevalent cases in the population earlier than they would normally have been detected.

Table 15.7 Detection of new breast cancers and mortality from breast cancer, all causes other than breast cancer and cardiovascular disease in the HIP study.

| Study group | Breast cancer cases in the first 10 years (per 1000 person-years[a]) | Deaths (per 10,000 women per year[a]) | | | | |
| | | Breast cancer | | | All other causes | Cardiovascular disease |
		Age 40–49	Age 50–59	Age 60–69		
Control	2.1	2.4	5.0	5.0	54	25
Mammography	2.1	2.5	2.3	3.4	54	24
Change	–	+4%	−54%	−32%	–	−4%

[a] Units as reported.
(Shapiro, 1989, Sackett *et al.*, 1991.)

So unless we have some idea of the actual lead-time, perhaps from previous studies, we should not use survival time after diagnosis to evaluate a screening programme. Instead, we should consider the effects on longer-term age-specific morbidity or mortality rates of the disease. These rates are less likely to be affected by early diagnosis than time-limited survival rates, and should therefore better reflect the true benefits of early treatment. Table 15.7 shows such results from the HIP study evaluating the effectiveness of mammography, based on a 10-year follow-up.

Would you implement a breast-screening programme on the basis of the data shown in Table 15.7?

Table 15.7 compares breast cancer detection rates and breast cancer mortality rates (separately for three age groups) among the group randomly allocated to mammography (regardless of whether they actually underwent the procedure) and the control group. It also shows the mortality rates for cardiovascular disease and for all causes other than breast cancer. Cardiovascular and 'all-other-cause' mortality rates were similar for the two groups (suggesting that the randomisation process had created two equivalent groups of women), but breast cancer mortality rates in women aged 50–59 and 60–69 years were lower in the group randomly allocated to screening. (Note that, over the 10 years of follow-up, the breast cancer detection rates in the two groups were identical – screening does not alter the underlying incidence of disease but simply improves the outcome after diagnosis.) On the basis of these data alone it would appear that a breast cancer screening programme for women between the ages of 50 and 64 (the maximum age of women when they entered the study) should certainly be considered. In practice, it would also be important to consider other aspects of this study, to ensure that the results were valid; and given that we are making our judgement many years after these data were published, we must also examine the results of other studies in this area, ideally through a formal meta-analysis (see Chapter 11).

Length-time bias

When we screen for disease we are also more likely to detect cases where the disease is progressing slowly. This is because rapidly developing disease will come to clinical attention sooner and so be more likely to be diagnosed outside a screening programme. These cases that are diagnosed between regular screening visits are sometimes called 'interval' cases. The 'slower' cases that are more likely to be detected by screening (remember, prevalence is a function of incidence and duration) are likely to have an inherently more favourable outcome, and the effect of this will again tend to make screening appear more favourable than it really is. **Length-time bias** refers to this over-representation of slowly progressing disease among cases detected by screening. Randomisation should give an even balance of each type of case in screened and unscreened groups, again eliminating this as a problem for comparisons of age-specific mortality.

Design of a study to evaluate a screening programme

The preceding discussion should make it clear that the initial evaluation of a novel screening programme requires a randomised trial to allay concerns about these varied threats to validity; no other design can be wholly convincing in this regard. However, it is important to note that there are situations where this is not possible, for example for ethical reasons as in the case of cervical cancer screening (see below), and in this case we will need to rely on less convincing levels of evidence. Moreover, once a screening programme has been rolled out as part of a health service's disease control activities it needs further monitoring and evaluation in that setting. As randomisation to the intervention will no longer be an option this will generally include careful assessment of the process measures we discussed above and monitoring of population-wide descriptive data including trends in incidence and mortality rates. Making sound judgements from such data is challenging, but the example of cervical cancer below gives a sense of what is achievable. However, before we look at these non-randomised designs, let us return to consider some examples of randomised studies.

Randomised studies

Secure long-term benefits of a screening programme must be documented before it can be adopted for widescale use. Ideally, this demands a number of randomised trials with persons assigned to be offered screening or not, and then followed for some time (usually many years) to assess their health. Inevitably, in the short term more disease will be found among those screened, so the real issue is whether their survival or quality of life is enhanced in the long term. The HIP study mentioned above was a landmark in this respect, with the investigators showing great foresight in realising the need for very large-scale and long-term trials to answer these questions. It included over 60,000 women and the length of follow-up was 18 years, but even so, from the point of view of obtaining reliable results, the numbers of deaths from breast cancer were not very great in the earlier years of the study. A smaller study, or one that was conducted for only a short period of time, would not have been sufficient to show with any certainty (i.e. precision) whether breast cancer screening was of benefit. Additional data from subsequent RCTs, combined in the form of a meta-analysis, have allowed even more reliable assessment of the value of mammographic screening (National Cancer Institute, 2009).

Large bowel cancer is the only other cancer for which strong evidence from randomised studies shows a consistent mortality benefit from screening using a simple test for blood in a person's stools (Ee and Olynyk, 2009). The widely accepted benefits of screening for cervical cancer by a smear test to detect abnormal cells are based on much weaker evidence (see non-randomised studies below), as it had become an accepted part of medical practice before the benefits of RCTs for assessing screening programmes were realised. And while prostate cancer screening by testing PSA (prostate specific antigen) levels in blood is widely practised in the USA, and to a lesser degree in some other countries (essentially large-scale case-finding, as there are no organised public programmes), supportive trial data are lacking – although four large RCTs are currently under way. As of 2009, two of these trials had reported interim results although these have not resolved the questions of the magnitude (if any) of any absolute benefit from screening, nor the tradeoffs (expected to be substantial, see below) in terms of extra morbidity and costs of screening (Barry, 2009).

Non-randomised studies

As you discovered in Chapter 8, non-randomised studies are much more prone to confounding than randomised trials. However, they are sometimes the only source of evidence available. Ecological studies have been used as the primary evidence to evaluate the impact of cervical screening on rates of cervix cancer and, as an example, Figure 15.5 shows changes in cervical cancer mortality rates over time in Scandinavia. Perhaps the most conspicuous feature of the graph is the fact that, until about 1975, cervical cancer mortality rates in Denmark were double those elsewhere in Scandinavia. Leaving Denmark aside for the moment, we can see that between 1965 and 1980, mortality fell more rapidly in Finland and Sweden, where nationwide screening programmes had been introduced in the early 1960s, than it did in Norway, where, at that time, only 5% of the population was covered by screening (nationwide screening was not introduced until 1995). This visual impression is reinforced by a more formal analysis that suggested

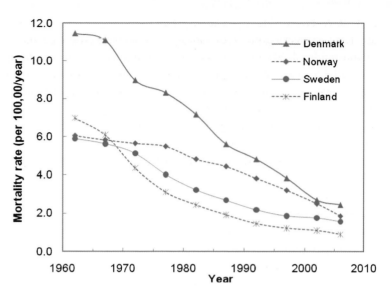

Figure 15.5 Cervical cancer mortality rates (5-year averages, standardised to the world population) from 1960–2006 in the Nordic countries. (Data source: NORDCAN, accessed via http://www-dep.iarc.fr/ NORDCAN/english/frame.asp, 3 January 2010.)

that, between 1965 and 1982, cumulative cervical cancer mortality rates fell by 50% in Finland and 34% in Sweden compared with a drop of only 10% in Norway (Laara *et al.*, 1987). Since 1980 the rates have continued to fall in all three countries.

So what about Denmark? Mortality has also fallen there, but, although the *absolute* drop is quite dramatic, the *relative* fall between 1965 and 1982 was only 25%, i.e. somewhere between that in Sweden and that in Norway, and this fits with the intermediate level of screening in Denmark – about 40% coverage of the population by 1980. Thus the data appear to support the hypothesis that screening does reduce mortality from cervical cancer, but, as you saw in Chapter 3, the results of an ecological study can be hard to interpret. For example, it has been pointed out that the fall in cervical cancer rates in some of these countries actually began before the introduction of screening, emphasising the problems of separating out other temporal effects, such as social change. It is difficult from these data to say how much of an impact the screening really had, although other evidence now supports the claim that cervical cancer screening confers a real benefit in terms of saving life.

Case–control studies have also been used to compare those with and without disease with respect to their history of screening. For example, case–control studies of bowel cancer have shown that screening sigmoidoscopy is associated with 50%–70% lower mortality from cancers in the parts of the bowel that are within reach of the sigmoidoscope, but with no difference in mortality from tumours in parts of the bowel that cannot be reached (Selby *et al.*, 1992). This design has a number of practical advantages over prospective studies, including the fact that case–control studies can often be conducted more quickly and at relatively low cost; however, considerable care must go into the design stage and interpreting the data can pose a number of additional challenges (Walter, 2003).

Non-randomised studies are also important once a screening programme has been established as a standard public health intervention, as ongoing monitoring and evaluation are required to check that the benefits shown in the research trials are actually achieved in practice. In the early stages, process measures of the sort noted above (e.g. a shift towards diagnosis of cancer at an earlier stage, high predictive values), will be prominent. In the longer term the focus needs to change to disease-specific outcomes, for example ecological-type assessments of the contributions of a screening programme to any changes in disease patterns seen, as for the cervical cancer example you saw above (see National Cancer Institute, 2009 for more examples). This need for ongoing monitoring using routine data holds for all large-scale population interventions, not just for screening programmes, and emphasises the importance of high-quality administrative data for in-service programme evaluation.

The negative consequences of a screening programme

Our prime focus in the previous discussion was how to validly assess whether screening provides a health benefit. But this is only part of the story; the potential harms that may follow screening also have to be considered and must be found to be substantially less than the benefits before screening can proceed. We therefore summarise below the sorts of problems that can follow from offering screening to healthy individuals as a counterbalance to any unbridled enthusiasm you may have developed for screening as a strategy for disease control.

The negative effects or harm that can result from screening are different for those people with positive test results and those with negative test results. Potential harm for those with a positive test result includes the possibilities of

- complications arising from investigation
- adverse effects of treatment
- unnecessary treatment of persons with true-positive test results who have inconsequential disease (this is central to doubts over prostate cancer screening, and almost certainly important for breast cancer as well (National Cancer Institute, 2009))
- adverse effects of labelling someone as having disease or early diagnosis
- anxiety generated by the investigations and treatment, and
- costs and inconvenience incurred during investigations and treatment.

For example, it has been estimated that, of 1,000 women aged less than 50 years screened by mammography, 53 women will have an abnormal mammogram (Kerlikowske *et al.*, 1993). This group will then undergo a total of 102 additional procedures, including 13 excisional biopsies, but only 2 women will finally be diagnosed as having cancer and 1 of these cancers will be ductal carcinoma *in situ*, a pre-cancerous lesion for which the benefit of surgical and medical intervention remains uncertain. This represents a positive predictive value for mammography of about 4% for all cancers and 2% for invasive cancer among women aged under 50 years. The other 51 women whose mammograms were abnormal will have undergone the stress of follow-up testing for no clear benefit. The corresponding PPVs for women over the age of 50 are 11% and 7%, i.e. approximately three times higher, thus the benefits of screening will also be higher. (Improvements in technology may improve the situation somewhat, but the fundamental problem of very low prevalence remains.) We also noted above the uncertainties that still surround screening for prostate cancer; as at 2009, the trial data show an approximate doubling of major interventions (surgery, radiotherapy, both of which have serious side effects) in the men offered screening, for at best a modest lowering of mortality (Barry, 2009).

Potential harm for those with a negative test result includes the possibilities of

- anxiety generated by the screening test and waiting for the result
- false reassurance if the result turns out to be a false negative and there is delayed presentation of symptomatic disease later, and
- costs and inconvenience incurred during the screening test.

Harm from screening programmes can therefore include the following:

(1) *Physical harm* from complications, invasive tests and/or treatments especially if falsely positive or from delayed presentation if falsely negative.

(2) *Psychological harm* from anxiety, anger or depression from waiting, distress from invasive tests or procedures, knowing a serious diagnosis earlier without improved prognosis, and from falsely negative or positive test results.

(3) *Financial harm* from the costs of tests, medical appointments, possible hospitalisation and treatments.

We detail these negatives to emphasise the need to take a balanced view of what we are really offering the public when we introduce a screening programme. If we over-emphasise the potential benefits, and neglect serious consideration of how a community might view and be impacted by the harms, we do everyone a disservice.

Summary

Screening is an inherently attractive public health strategy for controlling some diseases, particularly when no or few feasible avenues for primary prevention exist. Nonetheless, its present popularity among some segments of the public and the health professions may over-represent its capabilities. A cool-headed approach is required, and some simple questions make a good starting point when considering screening:

- Is this disease appropriate for screening?
- Do we have a truly valid test?
- How well could a screening programme work in our community?

Points to look for when evaluating the potential benefits of screening include the stage of disease in cases detected by screening, a high positive predictive value for the screening test and, most importantly, demonstrated and worthwhile improvement in outcomes in randomised trials.

These are the scientific aims. We then have to think practically and ethically. Other questions we should ask include:

- Do we have the resources to implement the programme, and to deal with the extra clinical and psychological load that will ensue?
- If we are taking resources from other public health programmes, are we sure that we are improving the overall cost–benefit ratio for the community?
- Does our community truly understand and accept the inherent trade-off – namely that there will be a large benefit for only a few and some costs (mostly smaller) for many others, and that some disease will be missed?

These are not light challenges to be faced.

Questions

1. Papanicolau (Pap) smear screening is currently the accepted method for early detection of cervical cancer and women with an abnormal Pap smear result are referred to a gynaecologist for colposcopy for definitive diagnosis. To see whether repeat Pap screening would reduce the number of unnecessary referrals, 110 women with an abnormal Pap smear were given both a second Pap smear and colposcopy. The colposcopy showed that 13 women had high-grade lesions and 97 did not. The result of the repeat Pap test was abnormal for 12 of the women with and 72 without high-grade lesions.
    (a) Construct a 2 × 2 table comparing repeat Pap test with colposcopy.
    (b) Calculate the sensitivity and specificity of the repeat Pap test.
    (c) What is the positive predictive value of the repeat Pap test?
    (d) What is the probability that a woman whose repeat Pap test gives a negative result actually has a high-grade lesion?
    (e) Could a second Pap smear be used to identify women who should be referred for colposcopy?
2. An experimental screening test for hepatitis B has a sensitivity of 82% and a specificity of 93%. The prevalence of hepatitis B in the population to be screened is estimated to be 3%.
    (a) What is the probability that an individual with a positive test result does not have hepatitis B?

(b) Using this test, what proportion of a population free of hepatitis B would falsely test positive?

3. You are considering introducing prostate cancer screening programme using the PSA (prostate specific antigen) test. You know that the test has a sensitivity of 85% and a specificity of 80% for detecting prostate cancer and that the prevalence of prostate cancer in men over 60 years of age is 4%.

(a) Among a group of 10,000 men aged over 60, how many would be expected to have prostate cancer and how many of these would be expected to have a positive PSA test?

(b) How many men would not have prostate cancer and, of these, how many would have a positive PSA test?

(c) Summarise these data in a table and calculate the positive predictive value of a positive PSA test.

(d) How useful is the PSA test in this population? Consider both the negative and positive outcomes for men who are screened.

(e) If the prevalence of prostate cancer among men older than 70 years is 15% would it be better to restrict screening to this age group?

(f) What characteristics of a disease make it one for which we would consider introducing a screening programme?

For further questions relating to screening, see an excellent case study, '*Screening for antibody to the human immunodeficiency virus*' from the Epidemic Intelligence Service of the US Centers for Disease Control and Prevention (CDC-EIS, 2003, Student Guide #871–703), which is freely available from their website: http://www.cdc.gov/eis/casestudies/casestudies.htm.

REFERENCES

AIHW (Australian Institute of Health and Welfare) and (NBOCC) National Breast and Ovarian Cancer Centre. (2009). *Breast cancer in Australia: an overview, 2009*. Cancer series no. *50. Cat.* no. CAN 46. Canberra: AIHW.

Barry, M. J. (2009). Screening for prostate cancer – the controversy that refuses to die. *New England Journal of Medicine*, **360**: 1351–1354.

Ee, H. C. and Olynyk, J. K. (2009). Making sense of differing bowel cancer screening guidelines. *Medical Journal of Australia*, **190**: 348–349.

Karma, P. H., Penttila, M. A., Sipila, M. M. and Katajs, M. J. (1989). Otoscopic diagnosis of middle ear effusion in acute and non-acute otitis media. I. The value of otoscopic findings. *International Journal of Pediatric Otorhinolaryngology*, **17**: 37–49.

Kerlikowske, K., Grady, D., Barclay, J. *et al.* (1993). Positive predictive value of screening mammography by age and family history of breast cancer. *Journal of the American Medical Association*, **270**: 2444–2450.

Laara, E., Day, N. E. and Hakama, M. (1987). Trends in mortality from cervical cancer in the Nordic countries: association with organised screening programmes. *Lancet*, **1**: 1247–1249.

National Cancer Institute. (2009). Breast cancer screening (PDQ®) Health Professionals Version. http://www.cancer.gov/cancertopics/pdq/screening/breast/healthprofessional/allpages#Section_100. Accessed 14 September 2009.

Sackett, D. L., Haynes, R. B., Guyatt, G. H. and Tugwell, P. (1991). *Clinical Epidemiology. A Basic Science for Clinical Medicine*, 2nd edn. Boston, MA: Little Brown and Co.

Selby, J. V., Friedman, G. D., Quesenberry Jr, C. P. and Weiss, N. S. (1992). A case–control study of screening sigmoidoscopy and mortality from colorectal cancer. *New England Journal of Medicine*, **326**: 653–657.

Shapiro, S. (1989). Determining the efficacy of breast cancer screening. *Cancer*, **63**: 1873–1880.

Shapiro, S., Venet, W., Strax, P., Venet, L. and Roeser, R. (1985). Selection, follow-up, and analysis in the Health Insurance Plan Study: a randomized trial with breast cancer screening. *National Cancer Institute Monograph*, **67**: 65–74.

The South-East London Screening Group. (1977). A controlled trial of multiphasic screening in middle-age: results of the South-East London Screening Study. *International Journal of Epidemiology*, **6**: 357–363; reprinted in 2001; *International Journal of Epidemiology*, **30**: 935–940.

Various. (2001). Commentaries on the South-East London Screening Study. *International Journal of Epidemiology*, **30**: 940–947.

Walter, S. D. (2003). Mammographic screening: case-control studies. *Annals of Oncology*, **14**: 1190–1192.

Wilcken, B., Wiley, V., Hammond, J. and Carpenter, K. (2003). Screening newborns for inborn errors of metabolism by tandem mass spectrometry. *New England Journal of Medicine*, **348**: 2304–2312.

A final word...

In the preceding chapters we have covered the core principles and methods of epidemiology and have shown you some of the main areas where epidemiological evidence is crucial for policy and planning. You will also have gained a sense of the breadth and depth of the subject from the examples throughout the book. To finish off we will take a step back and take a broader look at the roles epidemiological practice and logic play in improving health.

We might start by exploring the boundaries of epidemiology. The definitions given in Chapter 1 are not limiting and imply wide engagement with all influences on health – epidemiology is a 'big-picture' discipline. The proximal causes of disease (e.g. infectious agents, industrial toxins, smoking, diet) are inextricably intertwined with the social, economic and physical environments, so epidemiology must give due attention to these upstream (distal) drivers of a population's health; you have already seen examples of this in Chapter 1 and in the discussion of infectious diseases in Chapter 12 and prevention in Chapter 14.

In 1848, a year of political revolution in Germany and elsewhere in Europe, the great German medical scientist Rudolph Virchow was sent by the Prussian government to investigate an epidemic fever raging among the destitute Polish weavers of Silesia. He diagnosed it as typhus or relapsing fever, noting that such mass phenomena have mass causes (Virchow, 1985, cited by Drotman, 1998; Azar, 1997). He stunned the establishment by recommending political freedom and sweeping educational and economic reforms as the only solutions to the health problem. Although he could not then know the undiscovered proximal bacterial cause, he correctly perceived the upstream social and environmental causes: poor hygiene, malnutrition, poverty, lack of opportunity and oppression. However, without methods to establish such links, his opinion was easily dismissed as political activism rather than science, an accusation still sometimes levelled at epidemiologists who focus on sociopolitical causes of disease.

Virchow's epidemiological insight was ignored, but a few years later John Snow's epidemiological studies on water pollution and cholera (see Chapter 1) led to sanitary reforms that swept across northern Europe to combat environmental causes of infectious disease. Social causes of disease came back on to the agenda with the pioneering field studies of Goldberger and others in the first two decades of twentieth-century America (Buck *et al.*, 1988). Their work shone the epidemiological torch on pellagra, once thought to be an infectious disease but now known to be a consequence of dietary niacin (vitamin B$_3$) deficiency. They gathered meticulous data on numerous social factors, including family income, diet, food supply and food habits, and showed that there was a strong relationship between pellagra and poverty with its consequent lack of fresh meat and milk (the major dietary contributors of niacin).

The nineteenth- and early-twentieth-century health activists, like Virchow, Snow and Louis Pasteur, to name but a few, were not 'epidemiologists' but they were giants of medical science and most played a prominent role in health policy later in their lives. Much of their logic and the other tools they used are clearly recognisable as epidemiological and they broke the ground that now connects epidemiology to the allied fields of biology, natural and environmental science, economics and social and political science. Today, many of those confronting the excess burdens of disease in the developing world and Eastern Europe *are* epidemiologists, but to be effective all must operate in the wider spheres of public health and public policy. Within this partnership epidemiology provides some of the keys to causation, prevention and, particularly, health services evaluation. Specifically it emphasises *measurement* – of the size and scope of a health problem, and of the likely benefits of planned preventive or other interventions to control disease – thereby providing the quantitative basis for setting health policy.

At the other end of the causal scale, the expanding potential for genetic mapping and our growing understanding of the functional variations of particular alleles of the genes which control metabolism have opened a new avenue of 'micro-epidemiology' for studying interactions between risk factors and genes. Smoking is strongly associated with lung cancer, but nevertheless many heavy smokers do not develop lung cancer – perhaps because of a beneficial combination of genetically controlled metabolic and/or immunological responses to tobacco carcinogens. Understanding these interactions could help in predicting and modifying future disease burdens with changing patterns of smoking. It may also provide an additional tool to help current smokers to quit – the hope being that if smokers are told their genes mean that they are more likely to get lung cancer than the average smoker then this will be an added incentive to help them abandon the habit.

What does the future hold for epidemiology?

In more privileged settings such as Western Europe and North America, the explosive growth of epidemiology in recent decades has spawned negative perceptions of a developing industry in 'risk-factor epidemiology', sometimes being done more for its own sake rather than with clear and useful public health goals in mind. So is this true? Certainly the multivariable and often hard-to-measure causes of many chronic diseases, for which relevant exposures may have occurred in the distant past, do not readily yield their secrets. It may also be that the 'easier' work on chronic disease epidemiology has been done and we now confront diminishing returns – a problem that some think affects many

From www.Cartoonstock.com

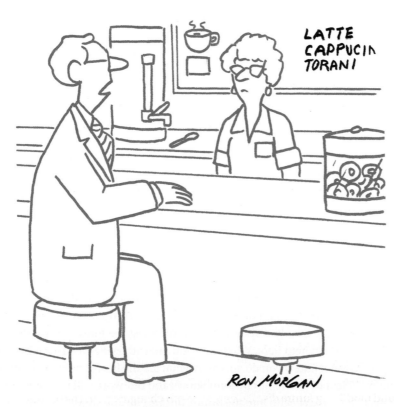

"I haven't read the health columns this morning.
Is coffee *out* or *in* today?"

areas of science (Horgan, 1996). As a result, studies are finding weak effects and different studies claim to find different effects. The end result is a flow of often contradictory newspaper headlines and journal articles depicting new panaceas or 'lifestyle' risks (although some of this information overload stems more from the economic imperatives of publicity and circulation than from flawed research). No wonder members of the public (and some epidemiologists) are becoming disillusioned. This highlights the importance of a good review to provide a balanced explanation and presentation of all relevant data as we discussed in Chapter 11. But achieving the necessary levels of restraint among editors and medical journalists so that they do not trumpet 'interesting' findings from reports of a single study, and a parallel humility among researchers who need recognition for their work to obtain ongoing funding, looks likely to be elusive in the short term.

There is also the challenge of deciding when we have enough data that we can be confident in the answer to a question or make good planning or policy decisions. There are no easy answers to this one, influenced as it must be by multiple factors, including the urgency of the issue and the quality of the data to hand – for example look back to the question of whether mobile 'phones cause brain cancer (Box 11.3). Throughout this book we have focused heavily on data quality and interpretation and we will return to these issues below. But we should also note the potential for what has been termed 'circular epidemiology' (Kuller, 1999) – excessive repetition of research into a particular question using study designs that are unlikely to truly advance knowledge. This situation can be exacerbated by policy makers who are often reluctant to act based on data from other countries, preferring to have local information despite the likely cross-border generalisability of most findings. To avoid this problem we need to ensure that new work is directed to as yet unanswered questions – ideally of practical public health relevance – as revealed by a thorough systematic review of prior work.

Thinking smarter

So what is the answer? Think smarter wherever possible. Before embarking on something new, do your homework. What has been done and where are the gaps in knowledge? Clearly a systematic review along the lines that we discussed in Chapter 11 can help here. What question are you trying to answer, how can you best answer it and, if you do answer it, what are the likely health benefits that will follow? Most of us will not be John Snows and our work will not have a dramatic effect on human health into the future, but we can and should all aim to generate new knowledge that adds to what is currently known and has the potential to move us closer to our ideal of health for all.

We have discussed the main hurdles to be overcome when conducting epidemiological research and interpreting its results – our old friends chance, bias and confounding (Chapters 6–8). We have also discussed the ways in which we can minimise these. We can never eliminate the play of *chance* from research but can ensure that studies are big enough to reduce it to acceptable levels, and should also view the results of any individual study in the context of what others have found. One result might be due to chance but similar results from different studies are unlikely to be. We also know about *confounding*, how to look for it and how to control it, always assuming that we can measure the confounders with sufficient accuracy.

Which brings us to *measurement error* – in exposure and outcome but also for confounders (we cannot control for them if they are not measured well). As you saw in Chapter 7, even a moderate amount of non-differential random misclassification can completely mask an association, so if the associations we are looking for today are better hidden than those discovered previously then we need to sharpen our tools to find them (Michels, 2001). New technologies now allow more sophisticated measurement both of exposure (e.g. serum biomarkers, DNA damage in cells) and of outcome (e.g. early cellular changes, molecular subtypes of disease based on genetic profiles). Increasing the precision and accuracy of our measurement is paramount but we also need to be more specific about what we mean by exposure and outcome. A single infectious agent may have a number of different strains, cigarettes have different levels of tar, hormone replacement therapy comes in a number of different formulations and doses and so on. Duration, intensity, pattern and timing of exposure (for example childhood versus adult) may also be important. Is someone who drinks a glass or two of wine each night getting the same 'causal dose' of alcohol as their neighbour who drinks only on Friday nights but then drinks a bottle or two? For liver cirrhosis the answer might be 'yes', but for risk of injury it would clearly be 'no', emphasising the need to be precise about the question being asked. Might diet in childhood be more important in determining risk of adult-onset disease than recent diet? This we don't know yet; but see below for attempts to address this.

Similarly, we need to be more precise about our definition of 'outcome'. Pathologists have known for years that cancers at one site can take many different forms, yet until recently epidemiologists would often treat them as a single disease. Different subtypes of cancer may have different aetiologies and, if we lump them all together in a single analysis, it is no wonder that clear patterns of risk don't fall out at our feet. This was certainly the case for uterine cancer until the mid twentieth century when cancers of the body of the uterus (or endometrium) were separated from those of the cervix (or neck of the uterus) and found to have completely different risk factors: obesity and oestrogen exposure for endometrial cancer and human papillomavirus (HPV) infection for cervical cancer. More recently, studies that have separated the different histological

Figure 16.1 Odds ratios and 95% confidence intervals (CI) for the association between human papillomavirus (HPV) infection (via HPV DNA detection) and invasive cervical cancer risk in successive molecular epidemiological studies (mostly case–control) from 1987 (top) to 2003 (bottom). Adapted from Franco and Tota, Invited commentary: Human papillomavirus infection and risk of cervical precancer – using the right methods to answer the right questions. *Am J Epidemiol.*, 2010; 171: 166, by permission of the Society for Epidemiological Research.

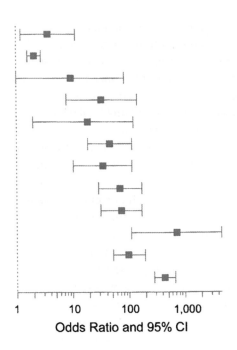

subtypes of ovarian cancer have shown that although there is little overall association with cigarette smoking, this may well be a strong risk factor for the rare subtype of mucinous ovarian cancers (Jordan *et al.*, 2006). There are almost certainly still strong associations between exposure and disease waiting to be found, but we need to be more precise about our definitions of both exposure and outcome in order to find them.

A dramatic example of the effects of clearly defining both exposure and outcome comes from studies of the relation between human papillomavirus (HPV) infection and cervical cancer. In early studies HPV was detected in 30%–60% of cases and the observed associations suggested a two- to five-fold increase in risk. Improved detection methods mean that HPV is now identified in 99% of cases and, as a result, we now see odds ratios of 100–900 for the association between the presence of specific types of HPV DNA and risk of invasive cervical cancer (Franco and Tota, 2010). The dramatic effects of this improvement in measurement on the magnitude of the observed association are shown in Figure 16.1. This precision has in turn helped identify the best targets for the recently introduced vaccines against HPV intended to prevent cancer of the cervix.

Integration

The debate over the perils of pure risk-factor epidemiology has also been valuable in forcing a re-evaluation of perspectives (Kuller, 1999; McMichael, 1999;

Rothman *et al.*, 1998; Susser, 1998). In addition to improving measurement, we believe that the key to maximising our future contributions to understanding and enhancing health lies with *integration* – from macro to micro, across lives (from birth to death) and over time. The tools and related issues that we have covered in this book are central to some of these dimensions and relevant to all of them, although other perspectives from sociology, social history, anthropology and economics may dominate on some of the larger scales.

Both macro-level ecoepidemiology (ranging from studying the health effects of climate change to the toxic sequelae of a local chemical hazard) and micro-level molecular epidemiology (perhaps to inform development of a vaccine against a parasite predicted to spread with global warming) can be relevant to the same specific goal of disease control. Whereas epidemiological analyses in the past have largely focused on a single level, individual or community, macro or micro, there is now an increasing move towards linking multiple levels of data in the one analysis. For example, one study might bring together:

- information provided by an individual that characterises their personal characteristics and exposures (e.g. smoking, diet), their social position (e.g. level of education, income) and their local environment (e.g. distance from health services);
- genetic and/or other molecular-level information from, for example, a cheek swab or blood sample provided by the individual; and
- macro-level descriptors that capture attributes of the wider community in which the individual dwells, such as indicators of disadvantage (e.g. average income, crime rate, education, accessibility of health services) and environmental challenges (e.g. air or noise pollution).

This would allow the molecular (micro) and community (macro) contexts to become part of the explanation of individual health states. Inclusion in a single analytic model allows some quantification of interactions over levels, in contrast to the more qualitative assessments that will otherwise prevail. For example a Canadian group linked *individual* data on socioeconomic status (SES) and obesity in high school children to *area-level* measures of SES including the local unemployment rate and average income derived from census data (Janssen *et al.*, 2006). They showed that childhood obesity was independently associated with both the affluence of the child's family and the unemployment rate in the local area, such that children from less affluent families who also lived in an area with high unemployment were most likely to be obese.

Another emerging and attractive, albeit challenging, approach to temporal integration is found in **lifecourse epidemiology** (Kuh and Ben-Shlomo, 2004). The aim here is explicit in the name; that is, to identify and integrate exposures and other influences across a person's life (as far back as conception) and relate them to the person's state of health. Finding out details of habits, diets and other influences in early life is mostly too much to expect from retrospective questioning in adulthood, but historical record-based data from early surveys, schools, hospitals and other institutions are opening some windows. For example, a group of Bristol epidemiologists has scoured the UK for records of past surveys that might yield early-life exposure information for people who are now adults. They identified high-quality dietary records from the 1930s for over 4,000 children, more than 85% of whom have been followed for mortality, and a proportion resurveyed six decades later (the Boyd Orr study; Frankel *et al.* (1998)). A number of pregnancy and birth cohorts have been established with collection of detailed early-life data, with the intention of life-long follow-up of the study participants (for example the ALSPAC Study; see Box 4.3). As is true for any long-term cohort study, deciding the optimal methods for analysing the mass of data generated remains daunting.

Where to now?

Which brings us back to our ultimate goal of disease control. There is no doubt that Rose's view of prevention (Chapter 14) is right, and that societies should where possible aim for changes that promote community-wide shifts in distributions of risk factors (as with the US Air Force suicide-prevention programme). However, that approach is never easy and is necessarily slow, so the potential for a 'quick fix' as an alternative or an interim measure remains appealing. We need to remove just one weak link in a causal chain for effective prevention, so seeking this at any point, proximal or upstream, makes sense. Of course trade-offs may need to be made in relation to the net balance of benefits and harms from removing a particular component cause when this affects multiple different health outcomes. As we discussed in Chapters 2 and 14, the use of PAFs and DALYs, along the lines advocated by WHO, should be increasingly helpful in this regard.

The public health argument for using vaccines against common, important infections is strongly supported by the very high population attributable fraction of these causal agents – by definition this must be 100%. However, vaccines might not be affordable for most of those who need them and many diseases that afflict the poor are neglected by research funding and still have no modern vaccine, or no effective vaccine at all – think of malaria and HIV (although both of these are actually well-funded research areas). Furthermore, when large numbers are vaccinated, the very small risks of adverse effects feature more strongly in the equation. The well-child schedule is already full of injected vaccines, to the alarm of many parents, most children and some epidemiologists concerned about risks of unsafe injections, hepatitis and HIV. Thus the 'magic-bullet' approach to prevention of infectious disease is still far away and there is much to be done now without vaccines – e.g. lessons from the West show the strong influence of an improved social environment (Figure 14.1).

For the majority of non-infectious diseases, however, we have no safe and simple solution for prevention. Here population-level change must be the key, linked to removal of harmful habits such as smoking cigarettes and inactivity via changes to the social environments that promote these habits. Such interplay between the proximal (individual) and upstream (societal) levels is well exemplified by the recent epidemic of obesity in most nations where food supply is ample. Greater relative body weight is in turn closely linked to an elevated risk of type-2 diabetes, hypertension and other conditions. While some of the causal metabolic consequences of obesity are understood, the key intervention is to reverse the pendulum swing towards increasing weight and declining physical activity – population-level phenomena. Causes operating upstream have created a so-called 'obesogenic' environment and this is where we must seek solutions – no easy task, but one being tackled by epidemiologists, nutritionists, psychologists and sociologists. We all know what a challenge this is – the parallel shifts to readily available, energy-rich refined foods and the decreased need and opportunity for physical effort both in the workplace and at home hinder attempts to redress the imbalance. Epidemiology has given us insight into the nature of the problem, but the solutions are not simple. Having said that, as a society we remain seduced by the potential of one-shot interventions such as the Polypill that you met in Chapter 14, which might allow us to improve our health forecast with minimal personal pain (although three decades of pill taking is no light task!). Other single preventive agents have been sought but, to date, most have been found wanting (see Box 16.1 on the next page).

Although we have implied that it is still uncommon to capture all desirable dimensions of health in one study, we will end with an example in which investigators are attempting to do exactly this. Many middle-income nations are currently undergoing a health transition with a shift away from a predominance of infectious diseases, high infant mortality rates and large family-size, towards the patterns of low mortality, low fertility and chronic disease seen in high-income countries. These mass population changes are driven at multiple levels by rapid political, economic, environmental and social changes. Thailand is one such country, with its own unique sociohistorical context. To capture and understand the drivers of this 'health-risk transition', a team of Thai and Australian investigators has embedded a conventional-looking cohort study of nearly 90,000 young to middle-aged Thai adults within a larger study of the social and economic history (Sleigh *et al.*, 2008). Information comes both from the participants' own experiences and perceptions across their lives (spanning two generations) and from a contemporary analysis of a number of major Thai social structures and determinants, based on documents, key informants and surveys. A further dimension is added by a historical 'look-back' survey that is charting changes in the domains of health, work, environment, diet and social structures in Thailand over the last half-century or longer. Describing and interpreting the

Box 16.1 Beta-carotene: an epidemiological tale

The history of nutritional epidemiology is based on the identification and correction of specific deficits in what came to be called vitamins, as well as the need to provide adequate energy for growth. In the second half of the twentieth century, observations from descriptive studies comparing populations with adequate energy intake led to hypotheses that much of the uneven distribution of non-infectious diseases, especially cancers and heart diseases, could be due to dietary differences between populations. This led to a flood of analytic epidemiology and parallel laboratory work as scientists tried to identify specific disease-causing agents and possible preventives.

Dietary epidemiology suggested that a number of cancers occurred less commonly among individuals and groups who ate more fruit and vegetables, and laboratory workers found (amongst many other factors) that vitamin A and related compounds (retinoids) were promising anti-carcinogens. The strands were woven together and beta-carotene, the principal dietary precursor of vitamin A, was identified as a substance that might underlie the beneficial effects of fruits and vegetables. Beta-carotene's appeal as a preventive agent was substantial: it combined a number of theoretical anti-cancer properties and appeared to be entirely safe (vitamin A itself being far more toxic at effective anti-cancer doses).

This message was captured most cogently in a paper published in *Nature* (Peto *et al.*, 1981), and several research groups were stimulated to conduct randomised trials using beta-carotene. These experiments were required to quantify precisely the 'beta-carotene effect' separately from effects of other inter-related dietary elements. But, when put to the test in this way, the hypothesis failed to stand up; and in fact beta-carotene may actually have been harmful to some smokers (ATBC, 1994).

So what has this taught us? In retrospect we know now that beta-carotene is a good marker of a beneficial diet, but insufficient on its own to provide any protection. Thus knowledge advances. We have learned that dietary epidemiology is more challenging than was initially appreciated; that we have not yet found our 'magic bullet' for cancer prevention; and that for now our public health message has to be directed towards encouraging a hearty intake of fruit and vegetables rather than supplementing our diets with specific nutrients.

interplay among these manifold influences is challenging but helped by the broad range of interdisciplinary skills contributed by the team of investigators – epidemiology, community nutrition, ecology, environmental health, anthropology, economics, demography, occupational health, psychology, sociology and

Box 16.2 The Thai Health-Risk Transition Study

In the background of this multi-level study, the researchers have noted profound social changes under way since about 1850 as peaceful, non-colonised Siam gradually abolished indentured labour, adopted wet rice agriculture, settled its frontier lands and increased its trade by steamship connection to the rest of the world (Carmichael, 2008). Since World War II the country has begun to industrialise and both rural and informal work are now rapidly decreasing, changing occupational health risks (Kelly *et al.*, 2010). Health services have expanded, birth rates fallen, and since 2001 the whole population has been insured, finally gaining universal access to modern healthcare (Yiengprugsawan *et al.*, 2009). Over the last 20–30 years, food supplies have changed and supermarkets have begun to compete with traditional fresh markets, impacting on food quality and diversity. Over the same period the attained height of young adult males has increased rapidly, biological evidence of sustained healthier childhoods (Seubsman and Sleigh, 2009).

In the foreground is the large national cohort, under observation since 2005 and with its first follow-up completed in 2009. This is revealing the major positive and negative lifestyle changes that are occurring, including increased urbanisation (Lim *et al.*, 2009), lower physical activity and an increasingly 'Western' diet (Banwell *et al.*, 2009), but also lower smoking rates as a result of improving education (Pachanee *et al.*, 2010). Early data are starting to suggest an impact of these changes on health, with increasing breast cancer rates potentially a consequence of the changes in body-size (Jordan *et al.*, 2009), and longer follow-up will show the full effects of this Thai health transition on the health of the Thai people.

statistics (See Box 16.2). This exemplifies the partnerships that epidemiology needs if it is to make a difference to understanding and influencing mass-scale health phenomena, such as the transitions currently under way in Thailand and many other countries.

A final word

We hope that by now you have a good sense of what epidemiology has offered and continues to offer the study of public health and indeed health in general. As we alluded to right at the start, perhaps epidemiology's most important role is the rigour it brings to collection, analysis and interpretation of all aspects of health data because without reliable data we cannot move forward. As you have seen, this is often not straightforward – the study of free-living people, their environment and society is necessarily highly complex. However, by applying sound epidemiological principles with a pragmatic approach that is alert to the pitfalls but also practical about assessing the likely effects of any error on the data we see, there is much we can learn and contribute to improving health.

REFERENCES

ATBC (The Alpha-Tocopheral Beta Carotene Prevention Study Group). (1994). The effect of vitamin E and beta carotene on the incidence of lung cancer and other cancers in male smokers. *New England Journal of Medicine*, **330**: 1029–1035.

Azar, H. A. (1997). Rudolf Virchow, not just a pathologist: a re-examination of the report on the typhus epidemic in Upper Silesia. *Annals of Diagnostic Pathology*, **1**: 65–71.

Banwell, C., Lim, L., Seubsman, S.-A., Bain, C., Dixon, J. and Sleigh, A. (2009). BMI and health-related behaviors in a national cohort of 87,134 Thai open university students. *Journal of Epidemiology and Community Health*, **63**: 366–372.

Buck, C., Llopis, A., Najera, E. and Terris, M. (1988). *The Challenge of Epidemiology. Issues and Selected Readings*. New York: Pan American Health Organization.

Carmichael, G. (2008). Demographic disequilibrium in early twentieth century Thailand: falling mortality, rising fertility, or both? *Asian Population Studies*, **4**: 161–176.

Drotman, D. P. (1998). Emerging infectious diseases: a brief biographical heritage. *Emerging Infectious Diseases*, **4**: 372–373.

Franco, E. L. and Tota, J. (2010). Invited commentary: human papillomavirus infection and risk of cervical precancer – using the right methods to answer the right questions. *American Journal of Epidemiology*, **171**: 164–168.

Frankel, S., Gunnell, D. J., Peters, T. J., Maynard, M. and Davey Smith, G. (1998). Childhood energy intake and adult mortality from cancer: the Boyd Orr cohort study. *British Medical Journal*, **316**: 499–504.

Horgan, J. (1996). *The End of Science. Facing the Limits of Knowledge in the Twilight of the Scientific Age*. London: Abacus.

Janssen, I., Boyce, W. B., Simpson, K. and Pickett, P. (2006). Influence of individual- and area-level measures of socioeconomic status on obesity, unhealthy eating, and physical activity in Canadian adolescents. *American Journal of Clinical Nutrition*, **83**: 139–145.

Jordan, S., Lim, L., Vilainerun, D. *et al.* (2009). *Breast cancer in the Thai Cohort Study: an exploratory case-control analysis. The Breast*, **18**: 299–303.

Jordan, S. J., Whiteman, D. C., Purdie, D. M., Green, A. C. and Webb, P. M. (2006). Does smoking increase risk of ovarian cancer? A systematic review. *Gynecologic Oncology*, **103**: 1122–1129.

Kelly, M., Strazdins, L., Dellora, T., Khamman, S., Seubsman, S. and Sleigh, A. (2010). Thailand's work and health transition. *International Labour Review* (in press).

Kuh, D. and Ben-Shlomo, Y. (Eds) (2004). *A Life Course Approach to Chronic Disease Epidemiology*, 2nd edn. Oxford: Oxford University Press.

Kuller, L. H. (1999). Invited commentary: circular epidemiology. *American Journal of Epidemiology*, **150**: 897–903.

Lim, L., Kjellstrom, T., Sleigh, A. *et al.* (2009). Associations between urbanisation and components of the health-risk transition in Thailand. A descriptive study of 87,000 Thai adults. *Global Health Action*, epub, doi: **10**.3402/gha.v52i0.1914.

McMichael, A. J. (1999). Prisoners of the proximate: loosening the constraints on epidemiology in an age of change. *American Journal of Epidemiology*, **149**: 887–897.

Michels, K. B. (2001). A renaissance for measurement error. *International Journal of Epidemiology*, **30**: 421–422.

Pachanee, C.-A., Lim, L., Bain, C., Wibulpolprasert, S., Seubsman, S.-A. and Sleigh, A. (2010). Smoking behaviour among 84,315 open-university students in Thailand. *Asia Pacific Journal of Public Health ONlineFirst*, May 11, doi: **10**.1177/1010539509349148.

Peto, R., Doll, R., Buckley, J. D. and Sporn, M. B. (1981). Can dietary beta-carotene materially reduce human cancer rates? *Nature*, **290**: 201–208.

Rothman, K. J, Adami, H.-O. and Trichopoulos, D. (1998). Should the mission of epidemiology include the eradication of poverty? *Lancet*, **352**: 810–813.

Seubsman, S. and Sleigh, A. (2009). Height transition in Thai military recruits over three decades (1972–2006), *Journal of Epidemiology*, **19**: 196–201.

Sleigh, A. C., Suebsman, S., Bain C. and the Thai Cohort Study Team. (2008). Cohort profile: the Thai cohort of 87,134 open university students. *International Journal of Epidemiology*, **37**: 266–272.

Susser, M. (1998). Does risk factor epidemiology put epidemiology at risk? Peering into the future. *Journal of Epidemiology and Community Health*, **52**: 608–611.

Virchow, R. L. Report on the typhus epidemic in Upper Silesia. Translated in: Rather, L. J., Ed. (1985). *Rudolf Virchow: Collected Essays on Public Health and Epidemiology*, 2 vols. Canton, MA: Science History Publications.

Yiengprugsawan, V., Lim, L. L., Carmichael, G. A., Seubsman, S. and Sleigh, A. C. (2009). Tracking and decomposing health and disease inequality in Thailand. *Annals of Epidemiology*, **19**, 800–807.

Answers to questions

Chapter 2

1. (a) Cumulative incidence $= 15$ cases $\div 1,000$ women $= 1.5\%$ in 8 years.
   (b) Incidence rate $= 75$ strokes $\div 5,000$ person-years
   $$= 1.5/100 \text{ person-years } or$$
   $$15/1,000 \text{ person-years } or$$
   $$1,500/10^5 \text{ person-years}$$
   (c) Incidence rate $= 27$ cases $\div 50,000 = 54$ per 100,000 per year

2. (a) Prevalence at age $55 = 100 \div 2,000 = 0.05$ or 5%
   Prevalence at age $65 = 400 \div 2,000 = 0.20$ or 20%
   (b) Number of women 'at risk' $= 2,000 - 100$ (who already had high blood
   pressure)
   $$= 1,900$$
   (c) Cumulative incidence $= 300 \div 1,900 = 0.16$ or 16% in 10 years
   It is a measure of cumulative incidence because the same women have
   been followed for the 10-year period.
   (d) We could estimate the total number of person-years at risk by assuming that all 1,900 initially healthy women were followed for the whole 10 years, giving

   $$1,900 \times 10 = 19,000 \text{ py}$$

   but 300 of the women developed high blood pressure and so were not at risk for the whole period. If we assume that, *on average*, they developed it half way through the follow-up period, we can improve our estimate of the number of person-years to

   300 women who developed high blood pressure $\times 5$ years $= 1,500$
   $+ 1,600$ women with no high blood pressure $\times 10$ years $= 16,000$

   giving a total of 17,500 py.
   (e) Incidence rate $= 300 \div 17,500 = 17.1/1,000$ person-years or $1,710/10^5$ person-years (actually 1,714 but we have rounded this off to 1,710).

3. Answer = (a) community A has a younger population than community B.

   If a disease is more common in older people (true for most diseases, including IHD), then if the age-standardised rate is *higher* than the crude rate this tells us that the average age in the standard population is higher than that in the community. Conversely, if the age-standardised rate is *lower* than the crude rate, then the average age in the standard population is lower than in the community. The age-standardised rate was higher in community A but lower in community B so community A must have a younger population.

4. Table 2.10 shows that IHD is the most common cause of mortality causing 7.2 million deaths worldwide each year while diarrhoeal diseases are responsible for about 2.2 million deaths. But, if we consider the burden of each disease measured in DALYs, diarrhoeal diseases account for greater loss of healthy life (72.8 million DALYs) than IHD (62.6 million DALYs). This is because IHD is primarily a disease of older age while deaths from diarrhoeal disease are more common in children; as a result, more years of life are lost following the death of a child from diarrhoeal disease than following the death of an adult from IHD.

Chapter 4

1. This is not a straightforward task and there are no absolute right or wrong answers – it will always be partly a matter of judgement depending on the specific circumstances. A completed version of Table 4.1 on the next page shows the main issues and some specific exceptions are noted below.

Comments and exceptions

Ecological study: it may be possible to study rare diseases and exposures if the populations are large enough. If it uses routinely available data it may also be quick and cheap to run; however, if new data collection is required the converse may be true. The major drawbacks are that populations often differ in many ways other than the characteristic of interest and the results seen at the population level may not apply to the individual.

Cross-sectional study: relatively simple, cheap and quick to conduct. Not good for studying rare conditions and hard to establish temporality. The ethical issues are likely to be minor although for any study, collection of blood samples for genetic testing adds ethical complexity.

Case–control study: good for studying multiple causes of rare diseases. Ensuring that exposure occurred before the disease can be a challenge but is less

Table 4.1 Comparing the strengths and weaknesses of different study designs.

	Ecological	Cross sectional	Case–control	Cohort	Randomised controlled trial	Nested case–control
Investigation of rare disease or outcome	4	2	5	2	1	2
Investigation of a rare exposure	1	1	1	2–5	5	2
Testing multiple effects of an exposure	2–4	3	1	5	3	1
Study of multiple exposures	2–4	5	5	3	1	3
Establishing temporality[a]	N/A	1	1–3[a]	4	5	4
Give a direct measure of incidence	N/A	1	1	5	5	3
Explore exposures which change over time	1	1	2	5	1	5
Time required[b]	4	4	3	1	1	4
Costs[b]	1–3	4	3	1	1	4
Ethical problems[b]	N/A	4	4	4	1	4

[a] i.e. that the exposure came before the outcome. N.B., even in a case–control study, some exposures will clearly pre-date the development of disease; for example, gender, genetic characteristics, blood group.

[b] For these attributes, a score of 1 = poor indicates a lot of time required, high costs or major ethical problems; a score of 5 = excellent indicates least time required, lowest costs or no ethical problems.

of an issue for things that do not change over time (e.g. blood type, genetic markers, early life exposures). Not good for studying rare exposures. In a true population-based study it is possible to estimate disease incidence.

Cohort study: population-based cohort studies are not very good for studying rare exposures, but rare exposures can be studied if participants are selected to over-represent those who are 'exposed' to the factor of interest, for example an occupational cohort exposed to a specific chemical. Very large cohort studies (such as EPIC and the Million Women Study), with sufficient follow-up, can investigate rare outcomes. If information is collected at regular intervals it is possible to study effects of exposures that change over time. Establishing temporality can still be a problem for cases diagnosed very early in the follow-up period.

Randomised controlled trial: this shares many of the attributes of a cohort study except it is an excellent design to study rare exposures (because a large proportion of the population can be intentionally exposed) but is usually less good for studying multiple outcomes of one exposure as an RCT will usually be designed to focus on a small number of 'end-points'. However, the ethical implications and, because of the increased regulatory issues, sometimes the cost are much greater.

Nested case–control study: this combines many of the benefits of the cohort and case–control designs but can only be conducted in the context of an existing cohort study. The incremental costs are likely to be low.

2.

Nuremberg Code statement	Relevant moral principle
1. Requirement for voluntary consent	Respect for autonomy
2. The experiment should yield fruitful results	Beneficence
3. The experiment should be designed based on prior knowledge so the results justify performing the experiment	Beneficence and non-maleficence
4. Avoid unnecessary suffering	Non-maleficence
5. Experiments should not be conducted if death or disabling injury is a possibility	Non-maleficence
6. The degree of risk should not exceed the importance	Beneficence and non-maleficence
7. Proper precautions should be taken to avoid adverse events	Non-maleficence
8. Scientists should be properly qualified	Beneficence and non-maleficence
9. The subject should be able to withdraw at any time	Respect for autonomy
10. The scientist should discontinue the study if continuation is likely to risk in injury/death	Non-maleficence

Note that the principle of *Justice* is not explicitly covered by any of the statements, although it could be seen as implicit in some. This is because the primary focus is on protecting the individual, reflecting the circumstances from which the Nuremberg Code arose.

Chapter 5

1. (a) $$\text{Cumulative incidence} = \frac{\text{Number of people who get disease}}{\text{Number of people at risk at the start of the period}}$$

   So the cumulative incidence in

   (i) exposed workers $= 40 \div 2{,}500 = 1.6\%$ in 10 years
   (ii) unexposed workers $= 60 \div 7{,}500 = 0.8\%$ in 10 years
   (iii) all workers $= 100 \div 10{,}000 = 1.0\%$ in 10 years

   (b) The relative risk $= \dfrac{\text{Incidence in exposed group}}{\text{Incidence in unexposed group}}$

   $$= CI_e \div CI_o$$
   $$= 1.6 \div 0.8 = 2.0$$

   Workers exposed to pesticides were twice as likely to develop the disease as those not exposed.

(c) The attributable risk

Incidence in exposed group – Incidence in unexposed group

$CI_e - CI_o$

$1.6 - 0.8 = 0.8\%$ in 10 years

An additional 0.8 cases of disease will occur in every 100 men (or 8 in 1,000 men) exposed to pesticides for 10 years (over and above the background rate of disease in the unexposed group). This is the amount of disease that can be said to be *attributable to the pesticides* assuming that we believe that pesticide exposure is actually causing the disease.

Note: the attributable fraction would be $0.8 \div 1.6 = 50\%$

(d) The population attributable fraction $= (CI_T - CI_o) \div CI_T$

$$= (1.0 - 0.8) \div 1.0$$
$$= 0.2 \text{ or } 20\%$$

This tells us that *if pesticide exposure is a cause of the disease* then 20% of all cases occurring among the workers (regardless of whether they were exposed to pesticides) could be attributed to pesticide exposure.

Note: the population attributable risk would be $1.0 - 0.8 = 0.2\%$ in 10 years.

The difference between the *population attributable fraction* (PAF) and the *attributable fraction* (AF) depends on the prevalence of the exposure. An exposure with a high AF may have a low PAF if the exposure is very rare (very few of the cases in the whole population could be attributed to the exposure). Conversely, an exposure with a lower AF may have almost as high a PAF if the exposure is very common.

2. (a) Relative risk $= IR_e \div IR_o = 53 \div 6 = 8.8$

  (b) (i) RR for low-dose versus never used $= 39 \div 6 = 6.5$

      (ii) RR for high-dose versus never used $= 62 \div 6 = 10.3$

Results such as these are often presented as follows:

OC use	Incidence rate	Relative risk (versus never/past user)
Never/past user	6	1.0
Low-dose user	39	6.5
High-dose user	62	10.3

(*Note:* the relative risk in never/past users is set as 1.0 because this is the reference to which we are comparing the other groups; $IR_o \div IR_o = 1.0$.)

(c) The results suggest that, compared with women who have never used OCs, users of low-dose oestrogen OCs have a 6.5 times higher risk of thromboembolism and users of high-dose oestrogen OCs have a 10.3

times higher risk of thromboembolism. The risk of thromboembolism therefore increases with increasing level of oestrogen. This pattern is called a 'dose–response' relationship.

3. (a) A case–control study of smoking and lung cancer

	Cases	Controls	Total
Ever smokers	647	622	1269
Never smokers	2	27	29
Total	649	649	1298

(b) To answer this question you need to calculate the *odds ratio*:

$$\text{Odds ratio} = \frac{a \times d}{b \times c} = \frac{647 \times 27}{622 \times 2} = 14.0$$

(c) and (d) You need to calculate first the *attributable fraction* and then the *population attributable fraction*:

$$\text{Attributable Fraction} = \frac{(OR - 1)}{OR} = \frac{(14 - 1)}{14} \times 100 = 92.9\%$$

If smoking is a cause of lung cancer then 93% of lung cancers *among smokers* can be attributed to their smoking and, theoretically, would not have occurred if the men had never smoked.

$$\text{Population Attributable Fraction} = \frac{P_e(OR - 1)}{P_e(OR - 1) + 1}$$

$$= \frac{(0.958 \times 13)}{(0.958 \times 13) + 1} \times 100 = 92.6\%$$

where P_e = prevalence of exposure among controls = $622 \div 649 = 0.958$.

While the AF told us the proportion of lung cancers *among smokers* that could be attributed to smoking, the PAF tells us the proportion of *all* lung cancers attributable to smoking. In this particular example the prevalence of exposure is so high that the AF and PAF are almost identical.

4. (a) The incidence rates can be calculated as follows:

	Cases	Person-years (py)	Incidence rate (per 100,000 py)	Rate ratio
7–8 hours sleep	541	451,393	120	1.0
6 hours sleep	267	175,629	152	1.27
$\leq$ 5 hours sleep	67	30,115	222	1.85
All women	875	657,137	133	

(b) The rate of CHD increases as the length of time a woman sleeps decreases. A woman who sleeps for 6 hours is 27% more likely, and a woman who sleeps for 5 hours or less is 85% more likely, to develop CHD than a woman who sleeps for 7–8 hours.

(c) To answer this you need to calculate the *population attributable fraction*:

$$PAF = (CI_T - CI_o) \div CI_T$$
$$= (133 - 120) \div 133$$
$$= 0.098 \text{ or } 9.8\%$$

The PAF is quite low because most women, or at least most of the person-time is for women who sleep for 7–8 hours.

Chapter 6

1. The results from the first study suggest that alcohol is associated with an 80% increase in risk of the cancer. The confidence interval is quite narrow, suggesting that the study was fairly large and the estimate of the RR is quite precise. The results of the second study suggest that caffeine may also be associated with an 80% increase in risk of the cancer, but in this case the confidence interval is very wide, implying that it was a small study and hence that the estimate of the OR is very imprecise. It is possible that the association seen in the second study could simply represent the play of chance since the confidence interval includes the no-effect value of 1. Overall, the data suggest that there is a moderately strong association between alcohol and the cancer (although we would still like to see additional data to support this), but they tell us little about the risks of caffeine other than to flag a possible association that needs evaluating in a larger study.

2. The answer is (b). There will always be some random sampling error in a study even when study participants are selected at random and a 95% confidence interval will just give an indication of how much random sampling error is present. Exposure measurement is a completely different issue.

3. The answer is (c). The 'no-effect' value for a relative risk is 1.0 – this means that the risk is the same in the two groups being compared. Because the confidence interval does not include the value 1.0 (both the lower and upper bounds are below 1.0), this means that the result is statistically significant. Without having more information about the size of the relative risk we cannot say whether this is clinically significant.

4. If a result is statistically significant it means that it is unlikely to have arisen by chance while clinical significance describes whether or not a result is clinically or practically meaningful. In a large study even quite small differences can be

statistically significant, but if the difference is so small that it has no practical effect, e.g. a drug that reduces the duration of flu symptoms by only a couple of hours, then it may not be clinically significant. Conversely, a study may see a large difference that would be clinically meaningful but, if the study was quite small, this may not be statistically significant and it would be hard to be sure the difference had not arisen just by chance.

Chapter 7

1. Women who read health magazines obviously have an interest in health and so are probably more likely to be vegetarian than women who do not read such magazines. On top of this, the vegetarian readers may also be more likely to respond to the questionnaire. Both of these biases would mean that the percentage of vegetarians in the community would be overestimated. Note also that the study would provide information just about women and men might be very different.

2. (a) People with high alcohol intake are probably less likely to agree to take part.
   (b) Alcohol consumption in the control group is, therefore, likely to be lower than in the whole community.
   (c) Assuming that patients with liver disease tend to have a higher than average alcohol consumption, the difference between the cases and controls would be exaggerated because of the falsely low level of consumption among the controls. This would make the association between alcohol consumption and liver disease look stronger than it really was.

3. (a) The misclassification is *systematic* (because the measurement instrument *systematically* overestimated people's exposure) and *non-differential* (because it has occurred among both cases and controls).
   (b) In the presence of non-differential misclassification, the observed odds ratio is likely to underestimate the true odds ratio.
   (c) In this situation, (i) 15% or 15 of the 100 unexposed cases and (ii) 15% or 23 of the 150 unexposed controls would have been misclassified as exposed.
   (d) The best way to answer this is to draw up a 2 × 2 table showing the results that would have been obtained:

	Cases	Controls	Total
Exposed	300 + 15 = 315	250 + 23 = 273	588
Unexposed	100 − 15 = 85	150 − 23 = 127	212
Total	400	400	800

Therefore, in this situation, (i) 315 of the cases would be classified as exposed and 85 as unexposed, and (ii) 273 of the controls were exposed and 127 were unexposed.

(e) $OR = \dfrac{315 \times 127}{85 \times 273} = 1.7$

This compares to the 'true' value of 1.8. *Non-differential* misclassification will usually bias the results towards the null value regardless of whether it is random (as you saw in Table 7.5) or systematic, as in this example.

4. (a) The misclassification is *systematic*, because cases systematically under-estimated their exposure, and is *differential*, because it occurred only among cases, and not controls.

(b) There are 300 exposed cases so if misclassification affects 20% this means that 60 cases will be misclassified as unexposed. We can draw up a 2 × 2 table to show the results that would be obtained:

	Cases	Controls	Total
Exposed	300 − 60 = 240	250	490
Unexposed	100 + 60 = 160	150	310
Total	400	400	800

$OR = \dfrac{240 \times 150}{160 \times 250}$

$= 0.89$

The observed OR is therefore much lower than the true OR of 1.8 (in fact the bias is so great that the observed OR is less than 1.0 when the true OR is greater than 1.0).

(c) This contrasts with the situation in Table 7.7, where cases systematically *overestimated* their exposure to the same extent and the OR was biased *upwards* to 2.40.

5. (a) The misclassification is *systematic* because non-exposed people are mis-classified as exposed but the reverse is not occurring. It is *non-differential*, as would be expected in a cohort study, because it affects *all* exposed peo-ple regardless of whether or not they go on to develop disease.

(b) If exposed people, who have a higher incidence of disease, are misclassi-fied as unexposed then the incidence of disease in the unexposed group will increase, i.e. it will be greater than 1.0%. The incidence in the exposed group should not be affected.

(c) The effect of the misclassification will therefore be to make the two groups look more similar than they really are and the observed RR will be *lower* than the true RR. In this situation it is likely that it would be about 1.8 instead of 2.0.

Misclassification is just as much a problem in cohort studies as it is in case–control studies.

6. (a) In the situation where 20% of the controls are misclassified with regard to their exposure status, 50 of 250 exposed controls will be misclassified as unexposed and 30 of 150 unexposed controls will be misclassified as exposed:

	Cases	Controls	Total
Exposed	300	$250 - 50 + 30 = 230$	530
Unexposed	100	$150 - 30 + 50 = 170$	270
Total	400	400	800

$$OR = \frac{300 \times 170}{100 \times 230}$$
$$= 2.22$$

(b) This misclassification is *differential*; exposure measurement among the cases was perfect, and the misclassification only occurred among controls.

(c) Differential random misclassification can make an association look stronger or weaker than it really is. In this situation, we would observe a higher odds ratio (2.2 compared to the 'true' odds ratio of 2.0), making the association seem stronger than it really is.

(d) If we had misclassified cases instead of controls the bias would have gone the other way and we would have underestimated the 'true' odds ratio (an observed OR of 1.11), making the association seem weaker than it really is.

Chapter 8

1. Odds ratio $= \dfrac{a \times d}{b \times c} = \dfrac{20921 \times 94183}{64422 \times 7827} = 3.9$

2. (i) Moped drivers:

   Odds ratio $= \dfrac{17869 \times 86212}{51900 \times 7342} = 4.0$

   (ii) Moped passengers:

   Odds ratio $= \dfrac{3052 \times 7971}{12522 \times 485} = 4.0$

3. The crude and stratum-specific odds ratios are almost identical, suggesting that position on the moped does not confound the association between not wearing a helmet and head injury.

4. The crude association between rider position (drivers versus passengers) and head injury:

   Crude odds ratio $= \dfrac{25211 \times 20493}{138112 \times 3537} = 1.1$

(i) No helmet:

$$\text{Odds Ratio} = \frac{17869 \times 12522}{51900 \times 3052} = 1.4$$

(ii) Helmet:

$$\text{Odds Ratio} = \frac{7342 \times 7971}{86212 \times 485} = 1.4$$

The crude odds ratio suggests that rider position does not affect their risk of head injury (OR = 1.1) but when we stratify by helmet use we see that moped drivers have a 40% higher risk of head injury (OR = 1.4) than moped passengers regardless of whether or not they wear a helmet. The crude association was therefore confounded by helmet wearing.

5. For something to be a confounder it must be (i) a risk factor for disease among those who are not exposed to the factor of interest; (ii) be associated with the exposure of interest; and (iii) not lie on the causal pathway between exposure and outcome. Therefore, in the situation of drinking coffee and heart disease:

(a) Heart disease occurs more frequently in older people, and among males. It is possible that older people might drink less coffee than younger people, or that men might drink more (or less) coffee than women. If either of these conditions is true then the potential confounding effects of *age* and/or *sex* should be considered (certainly age and sex do not lie on the causal pathway between coffee drinking and heart disease).

(b) The confounding effects of *smoking* should definitely be considered. As you have seen in previous chapters, heart disease occurs more frequently in smokers, and those who drink coffee may be more likely to smoke. Also, while coffee drinking and smoking often go together, coffee drinking does not 'cause' someone to smoke.

(c) Heart disease occurs more frequently among those who do not exercise, and people who drink coffee may exercise less (for example, people who work in an office may drink more coffee and have less opportunity to exercise). Therefore the confounding effects of *physical activity* should also be considered.

(d) While consumption of fruit and vegetables may be protective against heart disease, it is also possible that people who drink a lot of coffee eat less of these foods so *fruit and vegetable intake* might confound the effects of coffee drinking on heart disease.

6. If either (i) half as many people participated in the study, or (ii) twice as many people participated in the study, the odds ratios will not change. Increasing or decreasing the size of a study will not make any difference to the amount of confounding (except in the context of a randomised controlled trial, when the bigger the study is, the less likely it is that there will be any confounding).

Results of the study shown in Table 8.8 assuming that the study had half as many people.

Energy intake	Total		High physical activity		Low physical activity	
	Heart disease	Controls	Heart disease	Controls	Heart disease	Controls
High	236	116	26	26	210	90
Low	605	398	5	8	600	390
OR	1.3		1.6		1.5	

Results of the study shown in Table 8.8 assuming that the study had twice as many people.

Energy intake	Total		High physical activity		Low physical activity	
	Heart disease	Controls	Heart disease	Controls	Heart disease	Controls
High	944	462	104	102	840	360
Low	2,420	1,590	20	30	2,400	1,560
OR	1.3		1.5		1.5	

Chapter 12

1. There are two clear clusters of cases, one starting in late December and the other about a month later. The girls in the first cluster must have been infected before the holiday and those in the second peak must have been infected when they returned to school. The occurrence of the second peak 4–8 weeks after the girls had returned to school on 7 January 1943 gives the clearest indication of the incubation period. Some girls infected early in the first cluster must have been exposed in November; i.e. the teacher must have been infectious then but became much more so when she developed the cold in mid December.

2. Overall this was an informative 'natural experiment', comparing children with different exposure categories for the *agent* (produced by the teacher), *environment* (the basement classroom) and *host* (different immune states, including that conferred by BCG vaccine). The March 1943 analysis was a *retrospective cohort study* of the 105 girls who were skin-test negative in December 1942. This enabled calculation of the cumulative incidence of infection (skin-test conversion) according to the four exposure categories (Table 12.2).

The 12-year follow-up was a *prospective cohort study* of the incidence of progressive post-primary pulmonary tuberculosis among 368 girls attending the school in March 1943. The exposures measured at the start were the initial immunological states (skin test, BCG) and evidence of recent infection (Table 12.3).

The incidence of infection (skin-test conversion) among those taught by the positive teacher was very high (86.6%). Environmental conditions in the basement were suitable for transmission (no ultraviolet light, probably high humidity and no ventilation) and the high infection rate among those entering the basement after the teacher was there (58.5%) supports this.

This study revealed the natural history of primary TB. A high proportion (20%) of the epidemic-infected girls developed post-primary TB over 12 years, nearly half within the first three years. The risk attenuated over time, but continued. Several features should be noted. The study involved adolescent girls; after infection, they are known to have higher rates of post-primary TB than boys. Also, the girls may have been malnourished due to wartime food shortages. This would boost post-infection disease rates even higher than usual.

The classification of skin-test positives is likely to have some inaccuracy; it is a difficult test to standardise and the old tuberculin test used then was more heterogeneous than the equivalent used today. Those negative in December 1942 included children whose parents had refused to have them vaccinated with BCG. These girls may have been socioeconomically distinct (poorer or richer) and this (via nutrition) could influence the course of events after infection – confounding the comparison of disease rates among skin-test positives in Table 12.3.

3. They are attack rates or measures of cumulative incidence (the proportion of girls who converted from negative to positive between December and March).
4. The numbers in groups C and D are small, but the percentage conversion rates in the other groups were very high (60%–85%), so we would have expected to see some converters if they really did have the same rates as groups A and B. (Note: formal statistical tests give the following results: C versus A, $p = 0.03$; D versus A, $p = 0.06$; and C + D versus A, $p = 0.002$, suggesting that the results are not likely to be due to chance.)
5. Preferences: (1) tuberculin negative (0% risk); (2) BCG-induced positive (2.2% risk); (3) 'naturally' positive (6.9% risk); (4) recent converters (20% risk).
6. Tuberculosis (TB) was transmitted in the basement classroom with highest risk to those actually taught by the infected teacher, next highest to those who occupied the room after she had used it that day (the air took time to clear after she had left the room), but not affecting those taught in the morning before she arrived (infected air settled overnight). This defines airborne transmission due to infectious droplet nuclei, respiratory droplets (10–100 micrometres in diameter) containing viable TB organisms from which water

molecules evaporated until they reach a size of 1–5 micrometres. Droplet nuclei are small enough to stay suspended in the air for many hours and are easily inhaled to reach the lung alveoli and cause TB infection. The fluctuating infectiousness of the teacher is not unusual with pulmonary tuberculosis.

Chapter 14

1. Relative measures (e.g. relative risk, RR; odds ratio, OR) evaluate the relative *strength of an association* between exposure and disease, and they are most useful for identifying the causes of a disease. Absolute or difference measures (e.g. attributable risk, AR; population attributable risk, PAR) are a better measure of the *burden of disease attributable to an exposure* and, therefore, potentially preventable by removal of that exposure. The attributable risk or attributable fraction tell us how much disease in an exposed group can be attributed to the exposure and the population attributable risk or population attributable fraction tell us how much disease in the whole population can be attributed to the exposure. Of all these measures, the PAR is most directly useful to assess the likely benefits of a prevention programme for the whole community.

Chapter 15

1. (a) The 2 × 2 table for repeat Pap smear:

| Pap smear | Colposcopy | | |
	Positive	Negative	Total
Positive	12	72	84
Negative	1	25	26
Total	13	97	110

 (b) Sensitivity and specificity for Pap smear:
 Sensitivity = 12 ÷ 13 = 0.923 or 92%
 Specificity = 25 ÷ 97 = 0.258 or 26%
 (c) Positive predictive value = 12 ÷ 84 = 14%
 (d) Probability of high-grade disease in women testing negative by Pap smear = 1 ÷ 26 = 0.038 or 4%
 (e) The repeat Pap smear had low specificity. In this population with a prevalence of 11.8% (pre-test probability), the positive predictive value is low, and all women testing positive would still have to go on to colposcopy. So,

although only 8% of higher-grade lesions would have been missed, this is not a very helpful extra step to add to the diagnostic process.

2. The first thing to do is complete a 2×2 table based on an artificial population of, say, 1,000 people. We know that 3% or 30 will be hepatitis B-positive and that the test will detect 82% or about 25 of them, leaving 5 false negatives. With a specificity of 93%, 902 of the 970 who are truly hepatitis B negative will correctly test negative, leaving 68 false positives:

	True status		
Hepatitis B test	Positive	Negative	Total
Positive	25	68	93
Negative	5	902	907
Total	30	970	1,000

   (a) The probability that an individual with a positive test result does not have hepatitis B is thus $68 \div 93 = 73\%$.

   (b) In a population free of hepatitis B, 7% ($68 \div 970$) of people would falsely test positive.

3. (a) The prevalence of prostate cancer in men over 60 years is 4% so 400 of a group of 10,000 men would be expected to have prostate cancer ($4\% \times 10,000$). The test has a sensitivity of 85% so 340 of the men with prostate cancer ($85\% \times 400$) would be expected to have a positive PSA test.

   (b) The remaining 9,600 men would not have prostate cancer and, as the test has a specificity of 80%, 7,680 of them ($80\% \times 9,600$) would be expected to have a negative PSA test and the remaining 1,920 would test positive.

   (c) The table below summarises the results.

Properties of the PSA screening test			
	Prostate cancer		
PSA test	Yes	No	Total
+	340	1,920	2,260
−	60	7,680	7,740
Total	400	9,600	10,000

The PPV is the proportion of all positive test results that are true positives $= 340 \div 2,260 = 15.0\%$.

   (d) The positive predictive value of 15% tells us that for every prostate cancer the PSA test identifies in this population ('true positives'), another 6 or 7 more men without cancer will also test positive and thus have to be investigated ('false positives'). The PPV is low because of the combination of relatively poor specificity and quite a low prevalence of disease (although 4% is higher than for many other cancers). Whether this means the programme should be abandoned depends on the amount of harm suffered by the false positives and the benefits of detecting the disease earlier in the minority who do have cancer. Widespread screening for e.g. breast and large bowel cancer is conducted with PPVs of this order; however, the public should be made more aware of the likelihood of false positive results when involving them in a decision of whether to screen or not.

On a more positive note, someone who has a negative test result is not too badly off. The negative predictive value of the test is very high (7,680 ÷ 7,740 = 99%), although you can see that the test would will still miss 60 cancers in every 10,000 men screened.

(e) If the prevalence of disease is higher, then the positive predictive value will also increase – in this case to 43% (1,275 ÷ 2,975). Now only about one in two PSA-positive men will be incorrectly labelled as having prostate cancer, a far more acceptable situation. However, as can be seen from the table below, we now miss more cases (225 instead of 60), and have a slightly reduced NPV of 97% (6,800 ÷ 7,025). And of course we have missed the opportunity for any early detection of prostate cancers in men in their 60s. Neither choice will please everyone!

Properties of the PSA screening test among men aged over 70 years

PSA test	Prostate cancer		Total
	Yes	No	
+	1,275	1,700	2,975
−	225	6,800	7,025
Total	1,500	8,500	10,000

(f) For a disease to be considered for a screening programme it should be a serious threat to health (and be perceived as such by the population); be reasonably common (but this can still mean very low prevalence in practical terms) and have a fairly well-understood natural history/clinical course. There must also be a good screening test for it and it should have been demonstrated, ideally in randomised trials, that outcomes are improved if treatment is initiated sooner.

Appendix 1: Direct standardisation

To use direct standardisation you need to know:

(1) the age-specific disease rates in your study population and

(2) the age distribution of the standard population

An example: standardising the IHD mortality rate for males in Germany to the world standard population

See Table 1. You first multiply each age-specific rate (Column D) by the number of people in that age group in the standard population (Column E) to calculate the number of events that you would expect to see in the standard population if it had the same rates as your study population (Column F).

You then divide the total number of events expected (the total of column F) by the total number of people in the standard population (the total of Column E) to calculate the standardised rate.

Crude mortality rate = Total deaths ÷ total population
= 211 per 100,000 per year

Standardised mortality rate = Expected deaths ÷ standard population
= 121 per 100,000 per year

Table 1 Standardising the IHD mortality rate for males in Germany to the world standard population.

A Age group (years)	B Number of IHD deaths (males) in Germany	C Number of males in Germany	D Mortality rate in Germany (per 100,000) (B ÷ C)	E World standard population	F Cases expected in standard population (D × E)
0–4	0	2,032,000	0.00	12,000	0.00
5–9	0	2,296,000	0.00	10,000	0.00
10–14	0	2,362,000	0.00	9,000	0.00
15–19	11	2,353,000	0.47	9,000	0.04
20–24	15	2,283,000	0.66	8,000	0.05
25–29	42	2,990,000	1.40	8,000	0.11
30–34	142	3,722,000	3.82	6,000	0.23
35–39	407	3,548,000	11.47	6,000	0.69
40–44	839	3,061,000	27.41	6,000	1.64
45–49	1,484	2,801,000	52.98	6,000	3.18
50–54	2,396	2,295,000	104.40	5,000	5.22
55–59	5,352	2,903,000	184.36	4,000	7.37
60–64	8,080	2,505,000	322.55	4,000	12.90
65–69	11,562	1,844,000	627.01	3,000	18.81
70–74	12,605	1,350,000	933.70	2,000	18.67
75–79	12,700	869,000	1461.45	1,000	14.61
80–84	12,727	403,000	3158.06	500	15.79
85+	16,213	376,000	4311.97	500	21.56
Total	84,575	39,993,000	211.47	100,000	120.89

(*Source for raw data:* Global Cardiovascular Infobase, www.cvdinfobase.ca, accessed 23 September 2003.)

Appendix 2: Standard populations

Table 2 Examples of some commonly used standard populations.

Age (years)	World standard[a]	African standard[a]	European standard[a]	New WHO world standard[b]
0–4	12,000	10,000	8,000	8,860
5–9	10,000	10,000	7,000	8,690
10–14	9,000	10,000	7,000	8,600
15–19	9,000	10,000	7,000	8,470
20–24	8,000	10,000	7,000	8,220
25–29	8,000	10,000	7,000	7,930
30–34	6,000	10,000	7,000	7,610
35–39	6,000	10,000	7,000	7,150
40–44	6,000	5,000	7,000	6,590
45–49	6,000	5,000	7,000	6,040
50–54	5,000	3,000	7,000	5,370
55–59	4,000	2,000	6,000	4,550
60–64	4,000	2,000	5,000	3,720
65–69	3,000	1,000	4,000	2,960
70–74	2,000	1,000	3,000	2,210
75–79	1,000	500	2,000	1,520
80–84	500	300	1,000	910
85+	500	200	1,000	635
Total	100,000	100,000	100,000	100,000[c]

[a] From Waterhouse *et al.* (1976); [b] From Ahmad *et al.* (2002); [c] The numbers do not sum to exactly 100,000 because of rounding.

REFERENCES

Ahmad, O., Boschi-Pinto, C., Lopez, A., Murray, C., Lozano, R. and Inoue, M. (2002). *Age Standardization of Rates: a New WHO Standard.* EIP/GPE/EBD World Health Organization. *Report No.: GPE Discussion Paper Series: No. 31.* Geneva: World Health Organization.

Waterhouse, J., Muir, C., Correa, P. and Powell, J. (Eds) (1976). *Cancer Incidence in Five Continents,* Vol. **III.** *IARC Scientific Publication No.* 15. Lyon: International Agency for Research on Cancer.

Appendix 3: Calculating cumulative incidence and lifetime risk from routine data

The 'quick and dirty' method

If a disease is rare, it is possible to make a rough estimate of the cumulative incidence by adding up the incidence rates for *each year* of life from 0 to 74. Since incidence rates are usually presented for 5-year age groups, e.g. 0–4 years, 5–9 years, etc., the rate at age 0 is the same as that at ages 1, 2, 3 and 4 years; similarly the rate at age 5 is the same as that at ages 6, 7, 8 and 9 years; and so on for each 5-year age-group. This means that, if the incidence in a 5-year band is 3/100,000, the chance a person develops disease during one of the 5 years is 3/100,000 and it is 15/100,000 for the whole 5-year period. One way to add up all the incidence rates to age 74 is therefore to multiply each of the age-specific rates by 5 (assuming that they are for 5-year age groups) and then to add them up. Or, to save time, you can do it the other way around and add up the 5-year rates and then multiply by 5 to obtain the same answer. This is then usually presented as a percentage:

$$\text{Cumulative incidence (CI)} \approx 5 \times (\text{sum of rates from 0 to 74}) \times 100 \qquad \text{(A3.1)}$$

As an example, consider the age-specific IHD mortality rates in Germany shown in Appendix 1. If we add up the rates from ages 0–4 up to 70–74, we find a total of 2,270/100,000 = 0.0227, so

$$\text{Cumulative incidence (CI)} \approx 5 \times 0.0227 \times 100 = 11.4\%$$

The proper method

Technically, the measure above is called the 'cumulative rate' because it is just the incidence rates summed or 'accumulated' for all ages from 0 to 74 years. To calculate a more accurate estimate of the cumulative incidence you have to use a slightly more complicated formula:

$$\text{Cumulative incidence (CI)} = 1 - \exp(-\text{cumulative rate}) \qquad \text{(A3.2)}$$

Where $\exp(x)$ means e^x, where $e = 2.7183$, the base for *natural* logarithms (as opposed to 10, which is the base for standard logarithms).

So, if the cumulative rate of IHD mortality is 11.4% (=0.114) then the cumulative incidence is

Cumulative incidence (CI) $= 1 - e^{(-0.114)} = 1 - 0.892 = 0.108$ or 10.8%

Note that this figure of 10.8% is slightly lower than the 'quick and dirty' value of 11.4% we calculated above. This difference arises because IHD is quite common. The rarer the disease and, therefore, the lower the cumulative incidence, the closer the answers from the two methods will be.

Lifetime risk

Lifetime risk can then be calculated by dividing 1 (or 100% if the cumulative incidence is expressed as a percentage) by the cumulative incidence:

Lifetime risk $= 1$ in $(1 \div$ cumulative incidence) (A3.3)

So the lifetime risk of IHD mortality in Germany is:

1 in $(1 \div 0.108) = 1$ in 9

It is important to note that, in this context, the cumulative incidence and lifetime risk are artificial measures. They assume that people do not die of any other causes along the way and they are also based on the current rates of disease without taking into account the fact that these may change over time. However, despite these limitations they can be a useful measure for comparing the burdens of various diseases within a population or for comparing the same disease across different populations.

Appendix 4: Indirect standardisation

To use indirect standardisation you need to know
(1) the age distribution of your study population and
(2) the age-specific disease rates in the standard population.

An example: calculating the SMR for IHD in males in Brazil compared with Germany

See Table 3. You first multiply each age-specific rate in the standard population (Column C) by the number of people in that age group in the study population (Column B) to calculate the number of events you would expect to see in the study population *if* it had the same rates as the standard population (Column D). You then divide the total number of events actually *observed* in the study population by the number of events *expected* (the total of column D) if the study population had had the same rates as the standard population. This gives you the *standardised mortality ratio* (SMR) or *standardised incidence ratio* (SIR) if you are using incidence rates.

Observed number of deaths in Brazil $= 39,437$
Expected number if Brazil had same mortality rates as Germany $= 70,978$
$\therefore$ Standardised mortality ratio (SMR) $= O \div E = 39,437 \div 70,978 = 0.56$

The *crude* mortality rate from IHD in Brazilian men was less than one-quarter of that in Germany (47 versus 211/100,000 per year) but the average age of the population is much lower in Brazil than in Germany. When we standardise for age, the SMR $= 0.56$ suggests that IHD mortality in Brazil is about half that in Germany.

Table 3 Calculating the SMR for IHD in males in Brazil compared with Germany.

A Age group (years)	B Male population in Brazil ($\times$1000)	C Mortality rate (males) in Germany (per 100,000)	D Expected deaths in Brazil ($C \times B$)
0–4	9,025	0.00	0.00
5–9	8,703	0.00	0.00
10–14	8,604	0.00	0.00
15–19	8,109	0.47	37.91
20–24	7,360	0.66	48.36
25–29	6,841	1.40	96.09
30–34	6,642	3.82	253.40
35–39	5,622	11.47	644.91
40–44	4,707	27.41	1290.16
45–49	3,745	52.98	1984.14
50–54	2,912	104.40	3040.15
55–59	2,454	184.36	4524.22
60–64	1,957	322.55	6312.40
65–69	1,583	627.01	9925.51
70–74	1,138	933.70	10625.55
75–79	721	1461.45	10537.05
80+	583	3715.02	21658.57
Total	80,706	211.47	70978.43

(*Source for raw data:* Global Cardiovascular Infobase, www.cvdinfobase.ca, accessed 23 September 2003.)

Appendix 5: Calculating life expectancy from a life table

Life expectancy is calculated based on what we expect to happen to a hypothetical cohort of 100,000 newborn infants if they experience the same mortality rates that currently operate within the population. (The cohort size is often denoted I_x where x is the age of interest, thus at the start age $= 0$ and $I_0 = 100,000$.) The table shows the first and last few rows of a standard life table for Australian males based on mortality rates from 2005–7.

If the probability of a male dying before his first birthday (q_0) is 0.00527 then we would expect 527 deaths in our cohort in the first year of life ($d_0 = I_0 \times q_0$) leaving 99,473 survivors at age $= 1$ (i.e. $I_1 = 99,473$). We can also estimate the numbers of years of life lived between the ages of 0 and 1. Because most infant deaths occur shortly after birth this is estimated as 99,535 years, but for older ages we assume that those who died did so, on average, halfway through the year and thus contribute 0.5 years of life. Thus, for example, at age $= 3$ the total years of life $L_3 = 99,409 - (19 \div 2) = 99,399$. If we repeat these calculations for each year of age up to 100 we end up with 1,412 men from our original cohort of 100,000 who survive to age 100, 445 of whom will die before their 101st birthday.

We then go on to calculate the total number of years lived by our cohort. Most life tables do not go beyond 100 years although there are still some survivors at this point. We therefore have to estimate the total amount of life they have left; in this case 3,429 years. We can then add on the total years of life lived at every other year of life, giving a total of 7,902,203 years for the entire cohort. By dividing the years of life remaining at any given age by the number of survivors at that age ($T_x \div I_x$), we can then calculate life expectancy at that age. For example, at age 3 the 99,409 survivors have a total of 7,603,796 years life remaining, giving a life expectancy at age 3 of 76.5 years.

Table 4 Life table for Australian males, 2005–7.

Age	Life table cohort I_x	Probability of dying q_x	Number of deaths $d_x = I_x \times q_x$	Years of live lived $L_x = I_x - (d_x \div 2)$	Cumulative years of life $T_x = T_{x+1} + L_x$	Life expectancy $e_x = T_x \div I_x$
0	100,000	0.00527	527	99,535	7,902,203	79.0
1	99,473	0.00040	40	99,452	7,802,668	78.4
2	99,434	0.00025	25	99,420	7,703,216	77.5
3	99,409	0.00019	19	99,399	7,603,796	76.5
...	...	...	...	...	...	...
97	3,879	0.27159	1,054	3,330	10,862	2.8
98	2,825	0.28593	808	2,403	7,532	2.7
99	2,018	0.30026	606	1,700	5,129	2.5
100	1,412	0.31460	445	3,429	3,429	2.4

Where: I_x = the proportion of persons surviving to that age

q_x = the proportion of persons dying between exact age x (I_x) and exact age x + 1 (I_{x+1})

d_x = the number of deaths occurring between exact age x and exact age x + 1

L_x = the years of life lived by the cohort between exact age x and exact age x + 1

(*Source for raw data:* Australian Bureau of Statistics. (2007). Life Tables Australia: 2005–2007. ABS Publication 3302.0.55.001. Accessed from http://www.abs.gov.au on 12 September 2009.)

Appendix 6: The Mantel-Haenszel method for calculating pooled odds ratios

When you do a stratified analysis to control for confounding you end up with a number of different odds ratios – one for each stratum. If these are all fairly similar, the next stage is to combine them into a single **adjusted odds ratio** that summarises the effect of the exposure *adjusted* for the confounder. Note that it is practical to do this only when you have a fairly small number of strata; once you need to adjust for more than one or two confounders it is better to use multivariable modelling techniques.

An adjusted odds ratio is essentially a *weighted average* of the stratum specific odds ratios. We calculate a weighted average rather than a straight average so that strata with more people (and therefore greater precision) have a bigger influence on the final result than small strata. To calculate a weighted average, each individual value is multiplied by its weight and these new values are then added up and divided by the sum of the weights. Various sets of weights can be used for pooling odds ratios, but those proposed by Mantel and Haenszel (1959) are commonly used.

Imagine a case–control study with a total of T people in each stratum (T may be different for each stratum) as follows:

	Cases	Controls
Exposed	a	b
Unexposed	c	d

$T = a + b + c + d$

The odds ratio in each stratum is

$$OR = \frac{a \times d}{b \times c}$$

The weight for each stratum is

$$w = \frac{b \times c}{T} \tag{A5.1}$$

So for each stratum we calculate:

$$\text{OR} \times w = \frac{a \times d}{b \times c} \times \frac{b \times c}{T} = \frac{a \times d}{T} \tag{A5.2}$$

We then add these values up for each stratum ($= \Sigma[(a \times d) \div T]$, where Σ (sigma) means summed over all strata, and divide by the sum of the weights $= \Sigma[(b \times c) \div T]$, so:

$$\text{Mantel–Haenszel pooled OR} = \frac{\Sigma[(a \times d) \div T]}{\Sigma[(b \times c) \div T]}$$

As an example, imagine a case–control study in which we are concerned about possible confounding by socioeconomic status (SES) because high SES is associated with a lower risk of disease but an increased risk of exposure:

Table 5 A hypothetical case–control study, stratified by SES.

	High SES		Low SES		Total	
	Cases	Controls	Cases	Controls	Cases	Controls
Exposed	460	490	90	45	550	535
Unexposed	60	150	70	95	130	245
Total	520	640	160	140	680	245
Odds ratio	2.35		2.71		1.94	

To calculate the Mantel-Haenszel adjusted odds ratio:
1. first calculate *for each stratum separately:* $(a \times d) \div T$ and add these up for all of the strata,
2. then calculate *for each stratum separately:* $(b \times c) \div T$ and add these up for all of the strata, and
3. then divide (1) by the result from (2).

Table 6 Calculation of the Mantel-Haenszel adjusted odds ratio.

	High SES	Low SES	Total
(1) $(a \times d) \div T$	$(460 \times 150) \div 1{,}160 = 59.48$	$(90 \times 95) \div 300 = 28.50$	$59.48 + 28.50 = 87.98$
(2) $(b \times c) \div T$	$(60 \times 490) \div 1{,}160 = 25.34$	$(70 \times 45) \div 300 = 10.50$	$25.34 + 10.50 = 35.84$
(3) $\dfrac{\Sigma[(a \times d) \div T]}{\Sigma[(b \times c) \div T]}$			$87.98 \div 35.84 = 2.45$

In this example the pooled or adjusted OR of 2.45 is higher than the crude OR of 1.94, confirming that there was some confounding by SES. The adjusted OR is much closer to the OR in the low SES group (2.35) than it is to the OR in the high SES group (2.71) because the low SES group is much larger.

Meta-analysis

Exactly the same method can also be used to pool odds ratios from different studies in a meta-analysis.

REFERENCE

Mantel, N. and Haenszel, W. (1959). Statistical aspects of the analysis of data from retrospective studies of disease. *Journal of the National Cancer Institute*, **22**: 719–748.

Appendix 7: Formulae for calculating confidence intervals for common epidemiological measures

Although statistical packages routinely calculate confidence intervals for you, it is helpful to understand where they come from and sometimes useful to be able to calculate them by hand. We show below the formulae for estimating confidence intervals for some of the most common measures. The general rule for a 95% confidence interval is that the lower bound is equal to the point estimate minus 1.96 × the standard error and the upper bound is equal to the estimate plus 1.96 × the standard error. For 90% intervals you simply substitute 1.645 for 1.96 (giving a narrower interval but less certainty that it contains the correct value) and for 99% intervals you use 2.575 (giving a wider interval and more certainty that it contains the correct value).[1]

i.e. 95% confidence limits = estimate ± 1.96 × standard error

It is important to remember though that some intervals have to be calculated on a log scale and then back-transformed to the original scale (see, for example, the formula for the odds ratio below).

So, assuming that your data are set out in a standard way as follows:

	Cases/ affected	Controls/ unaffected	Total people	Total person-years
Exposed	a	b	N_1	PY_1
Unexposed	c	d	N_0	PY_0

Then Table 7 below shows you how to calculate the standard error for some common epidemiological measures:

---

[1] These intervals are calculated on the assumption that the estimate comes from a 'normal' distribution or bell-shaped curve and this distribution can therefore be used to identify the multiplier for any width of CI although 90%, 95% and 99% are those most commonly used.

Table 7 Formulae for calculating the standard error for some common epidemiological measures.

Measure	Estimate	Standard error
Risk (in exposed)[a]	$\dfrac{a}{N_1}$	$\sqrt{\dfrac{a(N_1 - a)}{N_1}}$
Incidence rate (in exposed)	$\dfrac{a}{PY_1}$	$\sqrt{\dfrac{a}{PY_1^2}}$
Log odds ratio	$ln\left(\dfrac{a \times d}{b \times c}\right)$	$\sqrt{\dfrac{1}{a} + \dfrac{1}{b} + \dfrac{1}{c} + \dfrac{1}{d}}$
Log risk ratio	$ln\left(\dfrac{a}{N_1} \div \dfrac{c}{N_0}\right)$	$\sqrt{\dfrac{1}{a} - \dfrac{1}{N_1} + \dfrac{1}{c} - \dfrac{1}{N_0}}$
Log rate ratio	$ln\left(\dfrac{a}{PY_1} \div \dfrac{c}{PY_0}\right)$	$\sqrt{\dfrac{1}{a} + \dfrac{1}{c}}$

[a] Can be used for any proportion, e.g. cumulative incidence or prevalence.

So if a case–control study gives the following results:

Table 8 Hypothetical results from a case–control study.

	Cases	Controls	Total
Exposed	130	45	175
Unexposed	87	198	285

$$\text{Odds ratio} = \frac{130 \times 198}{87 \times 45} = 6.57$$

$$\text{Log odds ratio} = \ln(6.57) = 1.883$$

$$\text{Standard error of log odds ratio} = \sqrt{\frac{1}{130} + \frac{1}{45} + \frac{1}{87} + \frac{1}{198}} = 0.216$$

So to calculate the 95% confidence interval for the log odds ratio:

$$\text{Lower bound} = 1.883 - (1.96 \times 0.216) = 1.460$$

$$\text{Upper bound} = 1.883 + (1.96 \times 0.216) = 2.306$$

And the 95% confidence interval for the odds ratio itself is then obtained by exponentiating to move back from the (natural) log scale to the more familiar arithmetic scale:

Lower bound $= \exp^{1.460} = 4.3$

Upper bound $= \exp^{2.306} = 10.0$

The final result might thus be presented as OR $= 6.6$ (95% CI 4.3–10.0).

Glossary

Note: We have used italics to indicate other terms that are defined in this glossary.

Absolute risk reduction (ARR), Absolute risk increase (ARI) – clinical epidemiology terms for the *attributable risk*, used when then the risk in the exposed group is lower (ARR $= I_o - I_e$) or higher (ARI $= I_e - I_o$) than the risk in the control group.

Accuracy – this is achieved when the observed result is close to the true value. See also *precision*.

Adjustment – the process of correcting an estimate (e.g. odds ratio or relative risk) to reduce the *confounding* effects of some other factor; analogous to the process of *standardisation*.

Age-specific rate – incidence or mortality rate calculated for a specific age-group (usually a one, five or 10 year age band) to remove the *confounding* effects of age. See also *crude rate, age-standardised rate.*

Age-standardised rate – incidence or mortality rate that has been standardised for age by the process of *direct standardisation.* In practice an age-standardised rate is a weighted average of the *age-specific rates* where the weights are obtained from the age-distribution of a pre-defined standard population. See also *crude rate, standardised incidence (mortality) rate.*

Airborne transmission – transmission of an infectious agent via infectious droplet nuclei that can be inhaled. See also *direct transmission* and *indirect transmission.*

Ascertainment bias – see *selection bias.*

Attack rate – a measure of *cumulative incidence* often used for an *outbreak* that occurs over a relatively short time period. See also *secondary attack rate.*

Attributable fraction – the proportion of all disease occurring in an exposed group that can be attributed to their exposure; equal to the *attributable risk* $(I_e - I_o)$ divided by the incidence of disease in the exposed group (I_e).

Attributable risk – a measure of the excess amount of disease occurring in one group over and above that in a comparison or reference group $(I_e - I_o)$.

It can be calculated using *incidence rates* in which case it is also known as a *rate difference* or *cumulative incidence* in which case it is a *risk difference*.

Background rate or risk – the rate or risk of disease in an unexposed population; i.e. the amount of disease that will occur in the absence of the exposure or risk factor of interest.

Case-cohort study – a study conducted within the context of a *cohort study*, where cases are all those diagnosed with a particular disease and the comparison group is a random sample (sub-cohort) of the whole cohort population. The main difference from a *nested case-control study* is that the sub-cohort may include some people with the disease of interest; also, because it is selected to represent the whole cohort, the same sub-cohort can be used for studies of different outcomes.

Case-control study – a study where a group of people with disease (cases) are compared to a group without the disease (controls), selected to represent the population from which the cases came.

Case-crossover study – a study where each case acts as their own control thereby controlling for many known and unknown confounders. Exposure in a defined period prior to disease onset is compared with exposure in a defined 'control' period. Only suitable for studying transient exposures – for example studies of sexual activity and myocardial infarction.

Case-fatality ratio (CFR) – the proportion of people with a given disease or condition who die from it in a given period. It is a common measure of the short-term severity of an acute disease and allows a direct assessment of the effectiveness of an intervention.

Case-finding – opportunistic attempts at early detection of disease when someone comes into contact with the health system for another reason.

Cause – something (an event, condition, characteristic or combination of these) that plays an essential role in producing an effect (e.g. the occurrence of disease). See also *component cause, necessary cause, sufficient cause*.

Cluster – a group of cases of a rare (usually non-infectious) disease that occur in the same area or time period at a level greater than would be expected by chance.

Cohort study – a study where a sample of people (the cohort) are followed up over time to see who develops the disease of interest. The cohort may be a single population group who are then stratified on the basis of their exposure level, or it may be a group who have experienced a specific exposure (for example an occupational or military group) who are then compared with e.g. the general population.

Common-source epidemic – see *point-source epidemic*.

Community trial – a trial in which the intervention is implemented at the community level, usually because it would be impossible to offer (or evaluate) the intervention at the individual level; for example studies of water fluoridation and dental health.

Competing cause – a cause of death other than the disease of interest. For example, in a long-term cohort study some people will die from other causes before they develop the condition of interest and in this case the investigator will never know if they might have developed the condition if they had lived longer.

Component cause – something (an event, condition, characteristic or combination of these) that, in conjunction with other factors, plays a role in producing an effect (e.g. the occurrence of disease). However it is neither necessary to cause disease, nor sufficient to cause disease on its own. See also *necessary cause, sufficient cause.*

Confidence interval (CI) – the range placed around a *point estimate* in which the true result is likely to lie and a way of quantifying the amount of *random sampling error* in a study or, conversely, the *precision* of an estimate. Most common are 95% confidence intervals and these are often interpreted as the range that will include the true value 95% of the time. However what they really mean is that if we were to repeat a study many times with different samples of people, then 95% of the 95% confidence intervals we calculated would include the true value. Other percentages can also be used for example 99% intervals are wider but more likely to include the true value whereas 90% intervals are narrower but less likely to include the true value.

Confounding – a mixing or muddling of effects that can occur when the relationship we are interested in is confused by the effect of something else – the 'confounder'.

Confounding by indication – a type of confounding common in non-randomised studies looking at the effects of treatment. It occurs because, even among a group of people who all have the same medical condition, those who choose to take or who are prescribed a particular medication may well differ from those who do not take it or who are not prescribed it. For example, most drugs have one or more contra-indications and people with these conditions would not be prescribed that drug and so would all be in the non-exposed group.

Contagious epidemic – see *propagative epidemic.*

Control event rate (CER) – a term sometimes used in clinical trials to describe the *cumulative incidence* of the outcome of interest in the control or placebo group. See also *experimental event rate.*

Correlation study – see *ecological study.*

Critical point – the theoretical (and usually unknown) point during the development of disease after which the disease process is irreversible and treatment will confer little or no benefit. Depending on the disease, this may occur very early in the disease process or may not occur at all.

Crossover trial – a clinical trial where the same group of participants forms both the experimental and the control group. Participants are randomised such that they either receive the active treatment for the first time period and placebo for the second, or to receive placebo for the first study period and the active treatment for the second. This design can only be used for exposures that have a fairly transient effect such that the effect of treatment does not carryover from one time period to the next.

Cross-sectional study – a survey of a random sample or cross-section of the population where information about potential *exposures* and outcomes is collected at the same time. Distinct from *cohort studies* and most *case-control studies* because it does not just consider *incident* (new) *cases* but all those in the population at the time of the survey (*prevalent cases*).

Crude estimate – an unadjusted measure of disease occurrence or association that has been calculated without consideration of the potential *confounding* effects of other variables.

Crude rate – overall incidence or mortality rate calculated for a whole population (IR = number of events in one year ÷ total population or IR = number of events ÷ person-time at risk) with no *adjustment* for the potential *confounding* effects of other variables e.g. age. See also *age-specific rate, age-standardised rate, standardised incidence (mortality) rate*.

Cumulative incidence – the proportion of a defined population that develops the outcome of interest in a specified time period (CI = number of cases in a given time period ÷ number of people at risk during the same period).

Diagnostic test – a definitive test used to diagnose disease in those suspected of being affected. See also *screening test*.

Differential error or misclassification – measurement error or *misclassification* that occurs to a greater extent in one study group than another, for example it is more likely to occur in cases than controls (or *vice versa*) in a *case-control study*.

Direct standardisation – the process where the rate of disease (or mortality) in a population is calculated on the assumption that the population had a standard age-sex distribution. If this is done for several different study populations then the resulting *standardised incidence (mortality) rates* can be directly compared because any differences in age/sex between the populations have been removed. Direct standardisation is most commonly performed for age and sex but can be performed for other characteristics such as race, socioeconomic status. See also *indirect standardisation*.

Direct transmission – transmission of an infectious agent through close personal contact with an infected individual, for example by touching infectious secretions or excreta. See also *indirect transmission* and *airborne transmission*.

Disability-adjusted life year (DALY) – a measure of the burden of a disease or risk factor on a population that counts not only years of life lost completely due to premature death, but also years of health lost through disability where the extent of disability is weighted from zero (perfect health) to one (death). See also *quality-adjusted life year*.

Disability-free life expectancy – the number of years of life an individual of a given age is expected to live free of disability, based on current morbidity and mortality rates. See also *life expectancy* and *health adjusted life expectancy*.

Ecological fallacy – an error made when information about groups of people is used to make inferences about individuals. For example, if suicide rates are lower in areas with high unemployment it would be tempting to assume this means that the unemployed are less likely to commit suicide than the employed. However, we do not know who is actually committing suicide. It is possible that it is unemployed people committing suicide, but that they are more likely to do so if they live in an area where the overall unemployment rate is low.

Ecological study – a study comparing the levels of exposure and or disease across populations rather than individuals. For example a study relating average income to child mortality rates in different countries. Susceptible to *ecological fallacy*.

Effect modification – when the association between an *exposure* and outcome (the 'effect') differs across levels of a third variable – the 'effect modifier'.

Eligibility criteria – criteria used to define the target population and establish whether an individual is eligible to participate in a study. See also *exclusion criteria*.

Endemic disease – a disease that is constantly present in a given population.

Epidemic – the occurrence of disease at a level greater than would normally be expected.

Excess rate – see *rate difference*.

Excess risk – see *risk difference*.

Exclusion criteria – criteria on which potential participants who are eligible for a study are excluded, usually for practical reasons such as their level of health, ability to give informed consent, ability to complete the study requirements. See also *eligibility criteria*.

Expected years of life lost (EYLL) – the number of years of expected life lost due to a death at a given age; equal to the life expectancy at that age. See also *potential years of life lost*.

Experimental event rate (EER) – a term sometimes used in clinical trials to describe the *cumulative incidence* of the outcome of interest in the treatment or intervention group.

Exposure – a generic term used to describe the genetic, phenotypic, behavioural, lifestyle, environmental factors (or potential *causes*) being studied in relation to an outcome of interest.

Extended-source epidemic – see *point-source epidemic*.

External validity – the degree to which the results of a study can be reliably applied to a broader population than that included in the study. This depends on how representative the study population is of the target population (i.e. the response rate) and also how representative the target population is of other populations of interest. When applied to a causal association it is usually a decision based on judgement – for example can the results of a study of American men be applied to men (or women) in Russia?

False negative – a negative test result in a person who actually has the condition being tested for and thus should have tested positive.

False positive – a positive test result in a person who does not actually have the condition being tested for and thus should have tested negative.

Force of morbidity – a synonym for the *incidence rate*.

Generalisability – see *external validity*.

Health-adjusted life expectancy (HALE) – the equivalent number of years an individual can expect to live in full health based on current morbidity and mortality rates. Unlike *disability-free life expectancy* where years of life lived with disability are ignored, HALE includes this extra time but includes a weighting to allow for the fact that it is not lived in full health. See also *life expectancy*.

Health expectancy measures – measures that focus on what is being achieved such as *life-expectancy*. See also *health gap measures*.

Health gap measures – measures that focus on what is not being achieved such as *years of potential life lost*. They have the useful property that they can be calculated separately for different diseases or for different causes of disease. See also *health expectancy measures*.

Healthy worker effect – a problem that arises in occupational studies because workers are inherently healthier than the general population which includes all those too sick to work. As a result, employed groups will naturally tend to have lower morbidity/mortality rates than the overall population and it can be difficult to know whether this might mask an increase in risk due to a specific occupational *exposure*. Similar issues arise in comparisons of other healthy groups, such as the armed forces, to the general population.

Heterogeneity – when something varies across different groups it is heterogeneous.

Historical (or retrospective) cohort study – a *cohort study* where participants are identified in the present and historical records are used to measure their *exposure* in the past. This past measure of exposure can then be linked to the incidence of disease over the intervening years. This preserves the major benefit of a cohort study in that exposure is documented prior to the outcomes occurring, but avoids the lengthy time delay in that the outcomes have already occurred.

Homogeneity – when something is constant across different groups it is homogeneous.

Host – the human or animal to which an infectious agent acquires entry and in which it multiplies.

Hypothesis test – a statistical test to assess the probability that the observed result would have arisen if the true result was something different. Usually calculated to assess the probability that a result as great as or greater than that observed would have arisen if there is really no association (the *null hypothesis*).

Incidence – new cases of disease; somewhat confusingly the term is commonly used to describe the actual number of new cases and also as a synonym for both the *incidence rate* and *cumulative incidence*.

Incidence density – see *incidence rate*.

Incidence density sampling – a scheme for selecting controls for a *case-control study* (or *nested case-control study*) where controls are selected from all those in the population who are disease-free but at risk of developing the disease at the time when a case is diagnosed. In practice this means that someone can be recruited as a control for a study and then recruited again as a case if they go on to develop the disease of interest.

Incidence rate – the rate at which new cases of disease occur in a population. Can be calculated from population data as IR = number of new cases in a one-year period ÷ the number of people at risk during the same period. If it is not reasonable to assume that everyone has been at risk for the whole period, for example in a *cohort study* where people have been recruited to the study over a period of time, then it can be calculated as IR = number of new cases in a one-year period ÷ total *person time* at risk.

Incident case – a new case of disease that is diagnosed during a specified time period.

Incubation period – the time between initial infection (entry of an infectious agent into a susceptible host) and the onset of clinical disease (symptoms).

Indirect standardisation – the process where the observed number of events in a study population is compared to the number of events that would have been expected to occur if the study population had the same incidence/mortality rates as a reference population. Indirect standardisation is most commonly performed for age and sex but can be performed for other characteristics such as race, socioeconomic status. The results are usually presented as a *standardised incidence (mortality) ratio*. See also *direct standardisation*.

Indirect transmission – transmission of an infectious agent that involves a *vehicle* which may be inanimate, such as bedding, clothes or utensils (collectively called 'fomites'), food or water, or the soil; or alive in which case it is called a *vector*. See also *direct transmission* and *airborne transmission*.

Infection – the entry of a microbial agent into a higher-order host and its multiplication within the host.

Infectivity – the ability of an organism to invade and multiply in a host. It is the proportion of exposures that result in infection.

Infestation – when a lower organism lives on an external surface of another (usually higher) organism, for example, lice and scabies.

Intensity (of infection) – a measure of the number of organisms infecting an individual.

Intention to treat analysis – analysis of data from a randomised trial that compares the groups as they were originally randomised, regardless of whether people actually received the intervention or not. Usually the most appropriate way to analyse data from a randomised study because if only those who actually received the intervention are compared with the rest, the benefits of the randomisation in terms of controlling for confounding and avoidance of selection bias are lost.

Internal validity – the degree to which the results of a particular study are free from bias and confounding.

Interval case – a case of disease that is diagnosed clinically between routine visits for screening.

Interviewer (observer) bias – a bias that can arise in exposure (disease) measurement when an interviewer (or observer) is aware of the disease (exposure) status of an individual. For example: an interviewer may ask questions somewhat differently, and thus potentially get different answers, when they are talking to someone they know has disease; a clinician may be more likely to diagnose disease in someone they know has been exposed to a particular factor.

Latent period (of an infectious agent) – the time from entry of an infectious agent into a host until the onset of infectiousness; may be longer or shorter than the *incubation period*. If it is shorter then infected persons may pass on the infection before they become ill (as with influenza) and if it is longer they will be ill before they are very infectious (as with SARS).

Lead time – the period between the first detectable signs of disease (i.e. detection by screening is possible) and the overt symptoms that normally lead to diagnosis.

Lead time bias – bias introduced into screening studies when groups of screened and unscreened individuals are compared without consideration of *lead time* such that screened individuals appear to do better simply because their disease was detected earlier than among those who are not screened.

Length bias – the over-representation of slowly progressing disease, which is more likely to have a favourable outcome, among cases detected by *screening*.

Life expectancy – the average number of years that an individual of a given age is expected to live if current mortality rates continue; see also *health adjusted life expectancy*.

Life table – a table that shows, amongst other things, the probability that an individual of any given age will die before reaching their next birthday (or the next age-group if the table is not calculated for individual years of age), and their future life-expectancy. Also known as a mortality table or actuarial table.

Measurement error – any error in the measurement of either *exposure* or disease. Can lead to *misclassification* of exposure or disease status.

Meta-analysis – a technique for combining the results of multiple different studies into a single estimate, essentially a weighted average of the study-specific results where more reliance is placed on bigger studies with more precise estimates.

Migrant study – a comparison of disease incidence/mortality between groups who have migrated to a new country and those who stayed in their home country, for example Japanese people in Hawaii and Japanese in Japan. As both groups are likely to be genetically similar, differences between the groups suggest the condition under study is at least partly determined by environmental causes.

Misclassification – occurs when errors in measurement of exposure or outcome mean that people are classified into the wrong groups. For example someone with disease is wrongly classified as disease-free or *vice versa*, or someone who has been exposed to the factor of interest is wrongly classified as unexposed, or exposed at a lower level. See also *non-differential misclassification, differential misclassification*.

N-of-1 trial – a *crossover trial* involving a single patient who serves as their own control such that they are randomised to periods of active treatment and placebo and their outcomes during the different time periods are compared. This design can only be used for exposures that have a fairly transient effect such that the effect of treatment does not carryover from one time period to the next.

Necessary cause – a *component cause* that is necessary for an outcome to occur; for example infection with influenza virus is a necessary cause of influenza.

Negative predictive value (NPV) – a measure of the performance of a screening programme; the NPV of the test is the probability that someone who tests negative truly does not have the condition of interest. See also: *sensitivity, specificity, positive predictive value*.

Nested case-control study – a study conducted within the context of a *cohort study*, where cases are all those diagnosed with a particular disease and the comparison group is selected from those without disease at the time the cases were diagnosed. For this reason, the comparison group is specific to the particular case-group and cannot be used to study other outcomes as is possible in a *case-cohort study*.

Non-differential error or misclassification – measurement error or *misclassification* that occurs to the same extent in all study groups, for example in both cases and controls in a *case-control study*.

Null hypothesis – the hypothesis that there is no difference between the groups being studied or no association between an exposure and outcome.

Null value – the value that indicates no effect or association between two factors; equal to 0 for a difference measure (*absolute risk*) and 1.0 for a relative measure (*relative risk*).

Number needed to treat – the estimated number of people who would have to be given a new treatment in order to save one life (or prevent one adverse event if death is not the relevant outcome) in a specified time period, often one year. Calculated as $1 \div absolute\ risk\ reduction$.

Odds – the ratio of the number of people within a particular group who meet a specified condition divided by the number of people in the group who do not meet that condition. Identical to the odds commonly used in betting.

Odds ratio – the *odds* of disease in a group of people exposed to a potential risk factor divided by the odds of the same disease in a second or reference group who are unexposed. In practice this is equal to the odds that someone with disease (case) is exposed to a potential risk factor divided by the odds that someone without the disease is exposed to the same factor. In some circumstances (the outcome is rare or controls in a case-control study are selected via *incidence density sampling*) the odds ratio is equal to the *relative risk*.

Outbreak – the occurrence of cases of disease in a community or region where it would not normally be expected, or at a much greater level than expected. See also *epidemic*.

Pathogenicity – the power of an organism to produce overt illness among those infected. It is measured as the proportion of those exposed to infection that goes on to develop clinical or overt illness.

Period prevalence – the proportion of a population affected by the condition of interest at any point during a specified time interval; period prevalence = the *prevalence* at the start of the time interval + the *incidence* of new cases during the time interval. See also *point prevalence*.

Person-time or person-years – the total amount of time lived by a defined group of people. For example, if 100 people are followed for an average of 5.7 years this is a total 570 person-years (100×5.7) of follow-up.

Point estimate or effect estimate – the main measure of association calculated in a study, for example an *odds ratio* or *relative risk.*

Point prevalence – the proportion of a population affected by the condition of interest at a specific point in time.

Point-source epidemic – an epidemic that occurs when many people are suddenly exposed to the same source of infection, leading to a clear increase in incidence of disease. May also be called a common-source or extended-source epidemic, the latter implying that the exposure may be spread over a period.

Population attributable fraction – the proportion of disease occurring in a population that can be attributed to the exposure of interest. Equal to the *population attributable risk* ($I_T - I_o$) divided by the incidence of disease in the whole population (I_T). See also *population attributable risk, attributable fraction.*

Population attributable risk – the amount of disease (usually measured as *incidence rate* or *cumulative incidence*) occurring in a population that can be attributed to the exposure of interest ($I_T - I_o$). See also *population attributable fraction, attributable risk.*

Positive predictive value (PPV) – a measure of the performance of a screening programme; the PPV of the test is the probability that someone who tests positive actually has the condition of interest. See also: *sensitivity, specificity, negative predictive value.*

Post-test probability – a clinical epidemiology term for the probability that someone has disease based on the results of a specific test; a synonym for the *positive predictive value.*

Potential years of life lost (PYLL) – also known as years of potential life lost; the number of years of life lost because of deaths that occur prior to some pre-defined age.

Power – probability that the study will detect an association of a particular size if it truly exists in the general population.

Precision – little variation between the results; the converse of random error. A precise estimate will have a narrow *confidence interval*, conversely a wide confidence interval indicates a lack of precision.

Pre-test probability – a clinical epidemiology term for the probability that someone has disease based on the evidence available before a test is performed; often used synonymously with *prevalence.*

Prevalence – the proportion of a population affected by the condition of interest. See also *point prevalence, period prevalence.*

Prevalence ratio – the *prevalence* of disease in one group divided by the prevalence in a second or reference group.

Prevalent case – a case of disease that is already present in the population at a given point in time.

Primary prevention – all interventions that attempt to prevent disease from occurring, i.e., to reduce the incidence of disease.

Propagative epidemic – an epidemic that arises from the introduction of an infection into a susceptible population with subsequent transmission from person to person and a progressive increase in incidence. Also known as a contagious epidemic.

Proportional mortality ratio (PMR) – the proportion of deaths due to a specific cause in a group of interest divided by the proportion of deaths due to the same cause in a comparison group.

p-value (probability value) – the probability that we would have seen a difference as big as (or bigger than) we did if there were really no difference between the groups.

Quality-adjusted life year (QALY) – a measure of *life expectancy* that weights each year of life based on the quality of that life from one (perfect health) to zero (death). See also *disability-adjusted life year*.

Random error – or poor precision is the divergence, by chance alone, of a measurement from the true value.

Randomisation – the process of allocating study participants to different exposure groups (e.g. intervention and control) at random such that each person has an equal chance of being allocated to the intervention group. Not to be confused with *random selection*.

Randomised controlled trial – a study where people are allocated to the exposure and control groups at random; the best design to avoid *confounding*.

Random sampling error – the introduction of error into the results of a study because only a sample of the population was studied instead of the whole population, for example in a population-based case-control study where a sample of people without disease are recruited to represent the broader population. Random sampling error is unavoidable in most situations but can be minimised by taking as large a sample as possible. It can also be quantified by the use of *confidence intervals*.

Random selection – the selection of participants for a study on the basis of chance such that each person in the source population has the same chance of being included in the study. Note, this does not mean that exposure is assigned at random, see *randomisation*.

Rare disease assumption – when a disease (or any health condition) is relatively rare (e.g. <10%) then the *odds ratio*, *risk ratio* and incidence *rate ratio* will all be approximately equal and the odds ratio can be used as an estimate of the *relative risk* (the risk of disease in one group relative to a reference group).

Rate difference – the *incidence rate* of disease in one group minus the *incidence rate* in a second or reference group ($IR_e - IR_o$); also described as *attributable risk*.

Rate ratio – the *incidence rate* of disease in one group divided by the *incidence rate* in a second or reference group ($IR_e \div IR_o$); also described as *relative risk*.

Recall bias – a type of bias that occurs when one group in a study tends to recall or report information differently from the comparison group. Most likely in a *case-control study* (or *cross-sectional study*) when cases, who may have thought extensively about what caused their disease, may recall their past exposures differently from controls who do not have disease.

Relative risk – the term *relative risk* is synonymous with *risk ratio* but in practice it is also commonly used to describe a *rate ratio* and, in some circumstances, an *odds ratio* since all three measures compare the amount of disease in one group *relative* to that in another.

Relative risk reduction (RRR), Relative risk increase (RRI) – clinical epidemiology terms used to describe the reduction (or increase) in *relative risk* in a study group compared to the reference level of 1.0. For example, a RRI of 0.3 would mean that the relative risk in the study group was 1.3; a RRR of 0.3 would mean that the relative risk was 0.7.

Relative survival rate – the *survival rate* adjusted to allow for the fact that some people would have died anyway from other causes. A relative survival rate of 100% thus does not indicate that no-one has died, but that mortality did not differ from that experienced by the general population.

Reservoir – the natural habitat of an infectious agent; may be human, animal or environmental.

Residual confounding – in practice adjusting for a confounding variable is unlikely to remove its confounding effect completely. Any remaining confounding is known as residual confounding. The more a variable confounds an association (i.e., the bigger the change in an effect estimate when you adjust for the confounder), the more likely there is to be some remaining uncontrolled confounding.

Retrospective cohort study – see *historical cohort study*.

Risk difference – the *cumulative incidence* or risk of disease in one group minus the *cumulative incidence* or risk in a second or reference group ($CI_e - CI_o$); also described as *attributable risk*.

Risk factor – a factor (genetic, behavioural, environmental, societal) that is thought to increase risk of developing a particular health state. For example, smoking is a strong risk factor for lung cancer. The term was coined by investigators on the Framingham Heart Study.

Risk ratio – the *cumulative incidence* or risk of disease in one group divided by the *cumulative incidence* or risk in a second or reference group ($CI_e \div CI_o$); also described as *relative risk*.

Screening – the widespread use of a simple test for disease in an apparently healthy (asymptomatic) population.

Screening programme – an organised system using a *screening test* among asymptomatic people in the population to identify early cases of disease in order to improve outcomes.

Screening test – a test, usually relatively cheap and simple, used to test large numbers of apparently healthy people to identify individuals suspected of having early disease who will then go on to have further *diagnostic tests* to confirm the diagnosis. A screening test differs from a diagnostic test in that there is greater emphasis on cost and safety (as large numbers may be tested and most will not have disease) and less on definitive diagnosis.

Secondary attack rate – the number of cases of infection that develop among the susceptible contacts of an infected case as a proportion of the total number of exposed contacts; a measure of *infectivity*.

Secondary prevention – efforts to reduce the burden of disease by detecting it sooner (e.g., by *screening*) and thereby making treatment more effective and improving outcomes. Secondary prevention does not affect the incidence of disease, in fact it may actually lead to a transient increase in incidence as more cases are detected quickly. See also *primary prevention*.

Selection bias – the introduction of bias into the results of a study because those selected to be in the study differ from those not selected in some systematic way. For example, those who agree to participate in a study may be more health conscious (e.g. less overweight, lower levels of smoking and alcohol consumption, higher levels of physical activity) than those who refuse to participate. If this affects recruitment of controls (but not cases) for a *case-control study* then comparisons between cases and controls will be biased.

Sensitivity – usually a measure of the performance of a screening test; the sensitivity of the test is the probability that someone with the condition of interest will return a positive test result. See also: *specificity, positive predictive value, negative predictive value*.

Sensitivity analysis – the process of repeating the analysis of a study to see how the results are affected if different assumptions are made. If the results are similar regardless of the assumptions then we can be more confident in them; if they differ greatly then we would be less confident that we were seeing a real effect.

Simpson's paradox – where the crude association observed in a study is in the opposite direction to the true association due to *confounding*.

Source (of infectious agent) – the person, animal or object from which the host acquires the infection.

Specificity – usually a measure of the performance of a screening test; the sensitivity of the test is the probability that someone without the condition of interest will return a negative test result. See also *sensitivity, positive predictive value, negative predictive value*.

Standardisation – see *direct standardisation, indirect standardisation.*

Standardised incidence (morbidity) ratio (SIR, SMR) – the number of new cases of disease observed in a study population over a specified period of time compared with the number that would have been expected if the study population had had the same incidence rates as a standard or comparison population (often the general population). Calculated by the process of *indirect standardisation.* Note: confusingly, both standardised morbidity ratios and the *standardised mortality ratio* (see below) are sometimes abbreviated as SMR.

Standardised incidence (mortality) rate – an incidence or mortality rate that has been *adjusted* by the process of *direct standardisation* to remove the potential *confounding* effects of another variable, usually age. In practice, the standardised rate is the rate that would have been seen in a population with a pre-defined distribution of the factor of concern (e.g. age). See also *age-standardised rate.*

Standardised mortality ratio (SMR) – the number of deaths observed in a study population over a specified period of time compared with the number that would have been expected if the study population had had the same mortality rates as a standard or comparison population (often the general population).

Stationary population – a population that does not change in size over time i.e. the number of people entering the population (e.g. by birth or immigration) approximately equals the number of people leaving the population (death or emigration).

Stratification – a process in which we divide or stratify the study participants into two or more separate groups or strata and calculate measures of association separately in each group. Used to assess whether an association (or effect) varies among different subgroups of the population, i.e. there is *effect modification.* For example, if an association differs between smokers and non-smokers (stratification by smoking status).

Sufficient cause – a *component* cause or group of causes that will inevitably lead an outcome to occur.

Survival rate – proportion of patients in a group who are still alive a specified period after diagnosis.

Systematic error – occurs when observations in a study differ from the truth in a non-random way. For example, if those who agree to take part in a study are less likely to be smokers than those who do not agree to take part; or if cases are more likely to over-estimate their past exposure to second-hand smoke than non-cases.

Target population – the population that we want to study.

True negative – a negative test result in a person who is truly free of the condition being tested for.

True positive – a positive test result in a person who truly has the condition being tested for

Type I error – the error that occurs when the results of a study suggest there is a relationship between exposure and outcome but the truth is that there is none (also called alpha error).

Type II error – the error that occurs when the results of a study suggest there is no association between exposure and outcome when, in truth, there is an association (also known as beta error).

Validity – see *external validity, internal validity.*

Vector – a living organism that transmits an infectious agent, for example mosquitoes that transmit malaria and dengue, ticks.

Vehicle – something that transmits an infectious agent from one host to another. It may be inanimate (e.g. food, water, the soil) or it may be alive in which case it is called a *vector.*

Virulence – the ability of an organism to produce serious disease; measured by the proportion of those who are infected (determined by immunoassay) who develop severe overt disease.

Volunteer bias or volunteerism – bias introduced because people who volunteer for a study or attend for screening are likely to be different from those who do not volunteer.

Years of potential life lost (YPLL) – see *potential years of life lost.*

Index